Global Mental Health
and Neuroethics

Global Mental Health and Neuroethics

Edited by

Dan J. Stein

Ilina Singh

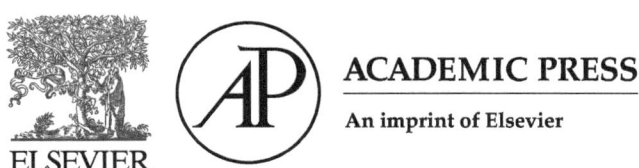

ACADEMIC PRESS

An imprint of Elsevier

ELSEVIER

Academic Press is an imprint of Elsevier
125 London Wall, London EC2Y 5AS, United Kingdom
525 B Street, Suite 1650, San Diego, CA 92101, United States
50 Hampshire Street, 5th Floor, Cambridge, MA 02139, United States
The Boulevard, Langford Lane, Kidlington, Oxford OX5 1GB, United Kingdom

Notices
Knowledge and best practice in this field are constantly changing. As new research and experience
broaden our understanding, changes in research methods, professional practices, or medical treatment
may become necessary.

Practitioners and researchers must always rely on their own experience and knowledge in evaluating
and using any information, methods, compounds, or experiments described herein. In using such
information or methods they should be mindful of their own safety and the safety of others, including
parties for whom they have a professional responsibility.

To the fullest extent of the law, neither the Publisher nor the authors, contributors, or editors, assume
any liability for any injury and/or damage to persons or property as a matter of products liability,
negligence or otherwise, or from any use or operation of any methods, products, instructions, or ideas
contained in the material herein.

Library of Congress Cataloging-in-Publication Data
A catalog record for this book is available from the Library of Congress

British Library Cataloguing-in-Publication Data
A catalogue record for this book is available from the British Library

ISBN 978-0-12-815063-4

For information on all Academic Press publications
visit our website at https://www.elsevier.com/

Publisher: Nikki Levy
Acquisition Editor: Nikki Levy
Editorial Project Manager: Megan Ashdown
Production Project Manager: Anitha Sivaraj
Cover Designer: Mark Rogers

Typeset by SPi Global, India

Transferred to Digital Printing in 2019

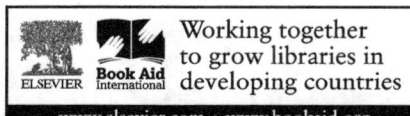

Contents

Contributors

Ronald Anguzu Public and Community Health Program, Institute for Health and Equity, Medical College of Wisconsin, Milwaukee, WI, United States

Anthony Barnett School of Psychological Sciences and Turner Institute for Brain and Mental Health, Monash University, Melbourne, VIC, Australia

Gillian Bartlett Department of Family Medicine, McGill University, Montréal, QC, Canada

Adrian Carter School of Psychological Sciences and Turner Institute for Brain and Mental Health, Monash University, Melbourne, VIC; University of Queensland Centre of Clinical Research, University of Queensland, Brisbane, QLD, Australia

Veljko Dubljević Science Technology and Society Program, Department of Philosophy and Religious Studies, North Carolina State University, Raleigh, NC, United States

Jantina de Vries Department of Medicine, University of Cape Town, Cape Town, South Africa

K.W.M. Bill Fulford Collaborating Centre for Values-based Practice, St Catherine's College, and Member of the Philosophy Faculty, University of Oxford, Oxford, United Kingdom

Wayne Hall Centre for Youth Substance Abuse Research, The University of Queensland, Brisbane, QLD, Australia; National Addiction Centre, Institute of Psychiatry, Psychology and Neuroscience, Kings College London, London, United Kingdom

Karen Herrera-Ferrá Asociación Mexicana de Neuroética, Atizapán, Mexico

Xanthe Hunt Institute for Life Course Health Research, Faculty of Medicine and Health Sciences, Stellenbosch University, Stellenbosch, South Africa

Judy Illes Neuroethics Canada, Department of Neurology, University of British Columbia, Vancouver, BC, Canada

Fabrice Jotterand Center for Bioethics and Medical Humanities, Institute for Health and Equity, Medical College of Wisconsin, Milwaukee, WI, United States; Institute for Biomedical Ethics, University of Basel, Basel, Switzerland

Cristina Longo Department of Family Medicine, McGill University, Montréal, QC, Canada

Alicja Malinowska Department of Psychiatry, University of Cambridge, School of Clinical Medicine and the Behavioural and Clinical Neuroscience Institute, Cambridge, United Kingdom

Doug McConnell Oxford Uehiro Centre for Practical Ethics, University of Oxford, Oxford, United Kingdom

Andrea C. Palk Department of Psychiatry, University of Cape Town, Cape Town, South Africa

Vasiliki Rahimzadeh Postdoctoral Fellow, Stanford Center for Biomedical Ethics, Stanford University, Stanford, CA, United States

Barbara J. Sahakian Department of Psychiatry, University of Cambridge, School of Clinical Medicine and the Behavioural and Clinical Neuroscience Institute, Cambridge, United Kingdom

Julian Savulescu Oxford Uehiro Centre for Practical Ethics, University of Oxford, Oxford, United Kingdom

George Savulich Department of Psychiatry, University of Cambridge, School of Clinical Medicine and the Behavioural and Clinical Neuroscience Institute, Cambridge, United Kingdom

Ayla Selamoglu Department of Psychiatry, University of Cambridge, School of Clinical Medicine and the Behavioural and Clinical Neuroscience Institute, Cambridge, United Kingdom

Abdul R. Shour Public and Community Health Program, Institute for Health and Equity, Medical College of Wisconsin, Milwaukee, WI, United States

Ilina Singh Department of Psychiatry, University of Oxford, Oxford, United Kingdom

Walter Sinnott-Armstrong Philosophy Department and Kenan Institute for Ethics, Duke University, Durham, NC, United States

Sarah Skeen Institute for Life Course Health Research, Faculty of Medicine and Health Sciences, Stellenbosch University, Stellenbosch, South Africa

Joshua August Skorburg Philosophy Department and Kenan Institute for Ethics, Duke University, Durham, NC, United States

Werdie van Staden Philosophy Department and Kenan Institute for Ethics, Duke University, Durham, NC, United States

Dan J. Stein Department of Psychiatry, University of Cape Town, Cape Town, South Africa

Mark Tomlinson Institute for Life Course Health Research, Faculty of Medicine and Health Sciences, Stellenbosch University, Stellenbosch, South Africa; School of Nursing and Midwifery, Queens University, Belfast, United Kingdom

Kevin Chien-Chang Wu Graduate Institute of Medical Education and Bioethics, National Taiwan University College of Medicine; Department of Psychiatry, National Taiwan University Hospital, Taipei, Taiwan

Foreword

Serendipitous discoveries in psychopharmacology have been important in advancing psychiatric science, but have had only partial success in reducing the burden of disease associated with mental disorders. Current advances in neuroscience and neurogenetics hold great promise for improving our understanding of these conditions and for advancing treatment outcomes. However, with this promise comes important conceptual and practical issues, which this volumes addresses.

A first question concerns how we ensure that the benefits of clinical neuroscience have global impact? Global mental health has appropriately focused on addressing the treatment gap across the world; advances in implementation science will be key in ensuring this important goal is attained. There is also a need for diverse populations from around the world to be included in clinical neuroscience research, in order to ensure that the benefits of discovery science in fields such as neurogenetics reach all communities. Priority settings exercises in mental health have correctly emphasized the importance of both discovery and implementation science across the globe. These are big, hard issues, but it is essential that they be raised.

We also have to ask how we ensure that as clinical neuroscience is used for assessment and treatment in a range of different settings it is done so ethically. More specifically, how can the growing field of neuroethics shed light on global mental health, and its approach to clinical research? Global mental health has been informed primarily by a communitarian ethics of justice: there is a need to ensure that mental health services are accessible to all. In contrast, neuroethics has been informed primarily by individualistic ethical concerns, including the importance of autonomy and privacy. These perspectives seem complementary, and both need to be addressed.

Stein and Singh's volume tackles these key issues at this intersection of global mental health and neuroethics. Contributors from a range of different disciplines and geographic regions address three important sets of questions. First, they discuss conceptual questions about the nature of mental disorder, and of psychiatric research and practice. Contemporary developments in global mental health and neuroethics provide a fresh perspective on perennial questions at the heart of the philosophy of psychiatry. Second, the contributors address the ethics of new neurotechnologies in a global context, providing interesting new arguments and insights. Finally, they address questions relevant to specific illnesses and populations, building on intersections between global mental health and neuroethics to provide new resources to address a variety of problems.

Global mental health and neuroethics are two novel and valuable approaches that can significantly advance our approaches to mental disorders and mental health. This volume is the first to bring these key disciplines into dialog; by doing so it provides novel insights into a range of conceptual and practical questions that will be key to the future of psychiatry and clinical neuroscience.

Harold Kincaid

Introduction

1

Dan J. Stein[a], Ilina Singh[b]
[a]Department of Psychiatry, University of Cape Town, Cape Town, South Africa,
[b]Department of Psychiatry, University of Oxford, Oxford, United Kingdom

Global mental health and neuroethics are two relatively new and highly influential transdisciplinary fields that are based on a solid foundation of prior work, and that have built on this foundation in novel and creative ways. Global mental health has built on earlier work in psychiatric epidemiology, cross-cultural psychiatry, and human rights, in order to emphasize the importance of addressing mental illness and well-being throughout the world. In short shrift, it has become a key approach to rethinking mental health. Neuroethics has built on moral philosophy, philosophy of science, and bioethics, developing key intersections between neuroscience and ethics, including both the ethics of neuroscience and the neuroscience of ethics. Again, although a new discipline, by focusing on these intersections, neuroethics has asked a range of important questions, and provided resources for addressing them.

This volume aims to develop a dialog between global mental health and neuroethics. Any such dialog must again draw on a range of earlier work that has been undertaken at the intersection of psychiatry, neuroscience, and ethics. Philosophy of psychiatry and psychology, psychiatric ethics, and philosophy of neuroscience have all made significant contributions to our understanding of the nature of mental disorder, our concepts of brain and mind, and our appreciation of the values entailed by psychiatric research and practice. With the advent of new ways of conceptualizing and approaching mental health and well-being around the world, and with advances in thinking through the relationships between neuroscience and ethics, it is now timely to bring global mental health and neuroethics into closer juxtaposition.

Global mental health and neuroethics are both exciting and productive transdisciplinary areas of investigation, that are asking and answering a range of overlapping questions. A dialog between them therefore has the potential to make substantial contributions to a number of long-standing debates as well as more recently emerging controversies about the nature of mental disorders and the mechanisms that underlie these conditions, and about the ethics of mental health research and intervention, particularly when considered in a global context. In this volume, three different sets of questions are addressed by a number of leading clinicians, public health practitioners and philosophers, who work in a range of different contexts around the world, and who bring a spectrum of disciplinary backgrounds to bear on the relevant debates and controversies.

A first set of questions are conceptual in nature. Psychiatry has long witnessed a debate between those who regard the field as a scientific endeavor that is making steady progress toward understanding and treating mental disorders, and those who

Global Mental Health and Neuroethics. https://doi.org/10.1016/B978-0-12-815063-4.00001-0

criticize the discipline as focused merely on constraining deviance and paternalisti-cally imposing one particular set of values. A first chapter by Stein and Palk addresses the intersection between global mental health and neuroethics from the contrasting perspectives of scientism and skepticism, arguing that each perspective has important insights which are useful for contributing to a more integrative and sophisticated posi-tion that conceptualizes psychiatry as both theory-bound and values-based.

In complementary vein, Fulford and van Staden, who have long emphasized the importance of both evidence-based and values-based practice, extend their conceptual framework to the arena of global mental health and neuroethics. They use tools from ordinary language philosophy to advocate for a Fact-plus-Value model to meet the challenges of global mental health and neuroethics. McConnell and Savulescu articu-late a critical view of contemporary psychiatry, and argue that a welfarist approach is useful in correcting these flaws and so provides a useful framework for global mental health. Finally, Tomlinson expands on the issue of the social determinants of health, exploring a range of social, economic, and environmental risks that global mental health and neuroethics will need to explore in the next two decades.

A second set of questions emerges from the juxtaposition of global mental health and neuroscience, addressing key questions about the nature of neuroscience research, and the ethics of various neurotechnologies, in a global context. Neurogenetics is a major focus of contemporary psychiatric research, and has raised a range of ethical issues. de Vries addresses the ethical issues that arise when such work is undertaken in under-resourced and diverse areas of the globe. Psychopharmacology is a major intervention in contemporary psychiatry, and has led to a neuroethics debate on the value of cosmetic psychopharmacology. Palk and Stein consider the ethics of cosmetic psychopharmacology in a global context, arguing for the value of a relational account, informed by an African moral framework, that in many ways complements a welfarist approach.

Deep brain stimulation is currently restricted to treatment of extremely refractory cases of mental disorder, but the potential use of such interventions raises a range of questions about whether and how this neurotechnology alters the self. In their contri-bution, Skorburg and Sinnott-Armstrong emphasize the importance of empirical work on changes in identity with deep brain stimulation, and highlight a range of ethical issues raised by such interventions, including cross-cultural considerations. Herrera-Ferrá proposes that it may be possible to draw on current knowledge and practices in neuroeducation, in order to facilitate efforts in global mental health to address the mental health treatment gap within a human rights framework. Finally, Jotterand and colleagues discuss some of the issues that arise in the context of civil unrest, political violence, and continuous exposure to stressors, addressing the question of how best to improve access to new neuroscientific knowledge and treatment options relevant to the impact of poverty and violence.

A third set of questions employs resources at the intersection of global mental health and neuroscience to address questions that are relevant to a number of specific ill-nesses and populations. Illes and colleagues discuss practical and theoretical strengths of role-playing games to understand health-related quality of life (HRQoL) in children with neurocognitive challenges; Sahakian and her colleagues discuss cannabis use and abuse in youth; Barnett, Hall, and Carter discuss addiction and substance use disorders in general; Dubljevic discusses dementia in the elderly; and Wu discusses focuses on individuals with disability. Taken together, these chapters therefore cover a number of important conditions, as well as various issues that are relevant to different stages of the human lifecycle.

Across each of the chapters in this third section of the volume there is an emphasis on advances in neurotechnologies (e.g., brain imaging), on the application of such technologies in a range of different contexts, and on the use of global mental health and neuroethics as resources that may be useful in addressing areas of controversy and debate. Thus, for example, in their chapter on childhood neurocognitive impairments, Illes and colleagues discuss the role of participant research, and the importance of children's rights. And, in their chapter on addiction, Barnett and colleagues explore the role of neuroethics in setting funding priorities and allocating scarce financial resources.

In a concluding chapter, Palk and Stein provide an overview of the broad intersection of global mental health and ethics, drawing on the work in this volume, and outlining a framework for ethical global mental health. Their discussion of key ethical issues in global mental health is organized in terms of ethical challenges associated with global collaboration in mental health, with global mental health research, and with global mental health care. They go on to support calls for a more appropriate bioethics paradigm for health on a global scale, justified by principles such as equity, inclusivity and rectification—which are central in global health. They conclude by arguing that the relational principle of solidarity is an appropriate guiding principle for global health in general, and for global mental health in particular.

Taken together, then, these chapters demonstrate the rich potential of discussions at the intersection of global mental health and neuroethics for addressing a range of long-standing psychiatric debates (e.g., about the nature and boundaries of mental illness), as well as new controversies raised by novel neurotechnologies (e.g., deep brain stimulation). While they undoubtedly do not provide the last word on these debates and controversies, the frameworks that they provide for addressing them, provide useful resources for global mental health, for neuroethics, and for work at the intersection of these two rapidly developing and impactful fields.

Section A

Conceptual issues

Moving beyond scientism and skepticism

Dan J. Stein, Andrea C. Palk
Department of Psychiatry, University of Cape Town, Cape Town, South Africa

Introduction

The philosophy of psychiatry has long been characterized by a debate between those who see psychiatry as an important branch of medicine, and those who regard psychiatry as simply a sociopolitical mechanism for addressing deviance. These contrasting positions, which we have previously termed "classical" and "critical" (Stein, 2012a), are in turn informed by various foundational oppositions in philosophy of science, philosophy of language, and moral philosophy. Furthermore, those who take classical and critical positions likely differ on a range of other issues, including their view of the nature of psychiatric diagnosis, causal mechanisms underlying psychiatric disorders, and the value of psychiatry research and treatment (Stein, 2008).

In this chapter we aim to apply this conceptual framework to addressing the intersection between global mental health and neuroethics, arguing for an integrative approach to debates in the philosophy of psychiatry and neuroscience that draws on valuable insights from both the classical and critical positions. We begin by outlining a number of characteristics shared by global mental health and neuroethics, which also help provide a foundation for an integrative position. We then go on to suggest that an integrative position in turn helps provide a useful conceptual foundation for global mental health, for neuroethics, and for their intersection.

Global mental health and neuroethics

Global mental health and neuroethics are relatively new multidisciplinary fields that have been widely influential, reshaping our approach to psychiatric disorders and to intersections between neuroscience and ethics. Importantly, although the two fields have disparate agendas and contents, they also share key features in their conceptual approach and focus (Stein & Giordano, 2015; Stein & Illes, 2015). In this section, we emphasize that both global mental health and neuroethics take a naturalistic and empirical approach, are concerned with both disease and wellness, and emphasize human rights and patient empowerment. A dialog between these fields may benefit from understanding their similarities, as well as their differences.

First, both global mental health and neuroethics have emphasized a naturalistic and empirical approach to investigating questions in their domains. Global mental health, for example, advocates for resources for mental health based on evidence about

Global Mental Health and Neuroethics. https://doi.org/10.1016/B978-0-12-815063-4.00002-2

the burden of mental disease, undertakes randomized clinical trials to assess whether interventions adapted for under-resourced contexts are feasible and effective, and advocates for more research in low and middle-income countries (Patel et al., 2018). Neuroethics, on the other hand, has emphasized that advances in neuroscience may shed light on philosophical questions, and has advocated for empirical approaches to addressing bioethical questions (Illes & Hossain, 2017).

Second, both global mental health and neuroethics are concerned not only with disease, but also with wellness. Global mental health has emphasized the spectrum ranging from distress and disease, through to health and well-being, and has argued that both ends of this spectrum need to be conceptualized and addressed using public health principles (Collins et al., 2011). It has also emphasized the importance of recovery, in a broad sense. Neuroethics, similarly, has focused not only on psychiatric and neurological disorders, but has also been concerned with normative questions regarding the enhancement of psychiatric and mental functioning (Sahakian et al., 2015). It has also emphasized the value of using neurotechnologies to maximize the potential of all.

Third, both global mental health and neuroethics have advocated for mental health as a human right and for patient empowerment. Global mental health has argued for the value of including patients and their families in discussions about mental health research, and has emphasized the value of shared decision-making and of social inclusion interventions in psychiatric practice (Kleinman, 2013). Similarly, neuroethics has emphasized the importance of the principle of autonomy in decision making around neurotechnologies, and has underscored the potential value of such neurotechnologies in empowering individuals and in strengthening societies around the globe (Shook & Giordano, 2014).

At the same time, it is important to recognize the different frameworks within which global mental health and neuroethics have emerged. Global mental health is closely allied with the larger field of public health, while neuroethics is much more closely aligned with clinical neuroscience. Global mental health has, for example, often focused on social determinants of mental disorders and on social and policy interventions, while neuroethics has often been concerned with individual's neurophysiology and neurogenetics and with pharmacological and other somatic interventions. Also, global mental health has emphasized collectivist considerations or welfarism, while neuroethics has emphasized individualist considerations such as autonomy and privacy. These differences also mean, however, that there is real potential for synergy between global mental health and neuroscience.

With these broad comments in mind, we now wish to consider a number of perennial debates in the philosophy of psychiatry, including related discussions about the best way of conceptualizing the diagnosis, pathogenesis, and treatment of mental disorders. For each of these issues we will outline a classical and a critical approach, before going on to delineate positions that have been put forward in the global mental health and in the neuroethics literature. We then suggest an integrative position, which we argue builds on the strengths of both the classical and critical views, and which is helpful for underpinning the dialog between global mental health and neuroethics.

What is psychiatric disorder?

Questions about the nature of disease and disorder lie at the heart of the philosophy of medicine and the philosophy of psychiatry (Stein, 2013; Stein et al., 2010). From a classical perspective, a disease can be conceptualized as an ideal or natural kind, and can be defined in terms of its necessary and sufficient features. Much as a square can be defined in terms of its equal sides and right angles, so any particular disease can be operationally defined. This perspective is informed by a positivist philosophy of science that emphasizes the importance of observing and measuring phenomena and developing operational definitions, and by a philosophy of language that associates meaning with empirical verifiability or falsifiability. The classical perspective has substantially influenced psychiatric classifications such as the Diagnostic and Statistical Manual of Mental Disorders.

From a critical perspective, a psychiatric disorder needs to be understood as merely a social convention. Much as the definition of a weed varies from time to time, and place to place, so any particular disease or disorder is bound to a particular geographical and historical context. This view is consistent with a more relativist philosophy of science which emphasizes the ongoing shifts from one scientific paradigm to another, and which argues that science provides only one of many alternative ways in which individuals and societies conceptualize the world. It is consistent with a philosophy of language and meaning that highlights the emergence of the latter from interpersonal relationships, emphasizing meaning as interpersonal validation. The critical perspective has provided support for a range of critiques of psychiatry.

An integrative perspective argues that disease constructs, like many other constructs in the human sciences, are both theory-bound and value-laden. Disease constructs are more likely of a practical kind than a natural kind (Kendler, Zachar, & Craver, 2011); although as we understand the mechanisms underlying diseases, and as we advance our discussion of relevant values, our classifications improve. This view is consistent with a philosophy of science that emphasizes that the world is comprised of real structures and mechanisms (that can be unraveled over time), however, it also acknowledges the importance of insights from the philosophy of language that emphasize empirical study of the use of words and metaphors (Bhaskar, 1978; Lakoff & Johnson, 1999). Cognizance of such insights is crucial because disease is generally conceptualized in highly metaphorical terms which have implications for how it is perceived and treated (Stein, 2008).

Our view is that this integrative approach draws on strengths of the classical approach (e.g., emphasis on empirical research) as well as the critical approach (e.g., emphasis on value clarification). At the same time, by acknowledging that science is a social activity it avoids the scientism of the classical position, and by emphasizing that science advances over time it avoids the skepticism of the critical approach. While a detailed defense of this position is beyond the scope of this chapter, we would note that it is consistent with the way in which science works; science is, for example, a social activity that advances by uncovering the structures and mechanisms of the world, and by providing increasingly powerful causal explanations of the phenomena that these underpin.

This debate about the nature of psychiatric disorders has played out in the arena of global mental health. Global mental health has, for example, drawn on the constructs of contemporary psychiatry, such as depression and anxiety disorders, and has argued that public health approaches are useful for addressing the burden of these conditions around the world. Such work has subsequently been criticized for relying on constructs that are highly constrained insofar as they are linked to particular (Western) cultures and so overemphasize individual vulnerabilities rather than social phenomena. The globalization of these constructs is also regarded, by some, as a form of neocolonialism whereby a limited and flawed perspective is exported around the world, to the benefit of the exporters, and to the detriment of its recipients (Summerfield, 2012).

In keeping with an integrative position, global mental health has, however, emphasized that sociocultural contexts certainly influence the experience and expression of mental disorders, and that there are key social determinants impacting on mental disorders that public health approaches which aim to decrease the burden of disease must address. Such ideas in global mental health are based on earlier work in cross-cultural psychiatry, where one influential position drew a contrast between objective biomedical constructs and the subjective experience of illness (Kleinman, 1991; Stein, 1993). Thus, although a critical perspective has argued that the global mental health agenda is approached from an overly narrow and localized perspective, there is a strong argument that this is not in fact the case.

Neuroethics has on occasion seen similar debates. For example, a distinction has been drawn between aspects of human functioning that require treatment, and aspects of human functioning that could be enhanced. Some have emphasized that human growth and development follows along "natural" or species-typical lines; treatment is necessary (and natural) when functioning grows awry, while enhancement of functioning may be problematic (and unnatural). These ideas are consistent with a line of argument in philosophy of psychiatry that diseases are physiological dysfunctions (Stein, 1998). However, defining the "natural" and the "dysfunctional" is far from straightforward; physiological alterations (for example, leading to phenotypes that differ markedly from the norm) are not necessarily harmful (e.g., Gilbert's syndrome).

In keeping with an integrative position, a clinical neuroscience perspective has, however, emphasized that symptoms fall on dimensions (Insel & Quirion, 2005). Clinical neuroscience has by and large focused on understanding the underlying mechanisms that contribute to such phenotypes rather than attempting to delineate the normal from the abnormal (Insel et al., 2010). Some researchers strongly influenced by evolutionary theory and neuroscientific perspectives have attempted to argue that this boundary is best explained by understanding evolved functions, and how these can go awry (Cosmides & Tooby, 1999; Wakefield, 1992). However, the lines between normal and abnormal are necessarily fuzzy; phenotypes that differ from markedly from the normal may be advantageous under particular contexts (e.g., gene variants that increase risk for sickle call anemia, may confer protection against malaria).

In summary, we would argue that concepts of disease are theory-laden (reflecting our understandings of underlying mechanisms) and value-bound (reflecting an appreciation of associated harms). The boundaries between normal and abnormal are necessarily fuzzy, but with advances in our understanding of the relevant mechanisms and values, our nosological constructs do improve over time. This view is based on an integrative position in philosophy of psychiatry, and is consistent with the focus of both global mental health and neuroethics on dimensional approaches to understanding disease and well-being, as well as with the appreciation that global mental health has for the impact of context on boundaries of illness. In turn, this view provides conceptual support for these fields.

What causes mental illness?

From a classical perspective, rigorous observations of phenomena allow scientists to put forward covering laws, which systematize the relationships between different phenomena. Physics is often favored by the classical position as an exemplary science; Newton developed laws that covered a range of physical phenomena, Einstein advanced this work by producing even more sophisticated equations that covered an even broader range of physical phenomena. According to a classical perspective, other sciences, including the medical sciences, should aspire to this approach, carefully observing the world around them, and developing laws which rigorously describe the relationships between these phenomena (Stein, 1991).

From a critical perspective, physics and psychiatry are entirely different fields of endeavor, and require entirely different methods. Whereas the natural sciences may yield to "erklaren" (explanation), the human sciences require "verstehen" (understanding). In approaching psychiatric symptoms, we need first and foremost to appreciate their meaning, within a particular sociocultural context. This is best done by immersing oneself into that context, as the meaning of symptoms change from place to place and from time to time. The humanities provide a useful exemplar for clinicians; the narrative structures of fiction, for example, are useful in understanding the stories behind patients' symptoms (Stein, 1991).

An integrative position holds that science makes discoveries about the structures and mechanisms of the world. At the same time, science is a social activity, and the study of human beings, in particular, necessarily involves appreciation of meanings and reasons. Psychiatry relies on both erklaren (in order to know and modify the relevant psychobiological mechanisms) and verstehen (in order to appreciate and influence the relevant interpersonal context). Biology is the science to which clinicians should aspire; the structures and mechanisms that are relevant to human disease also play out in other species, and they range from the neuroanatomical and neurochemical (e.g., brain changes may play a key role) all the way through to the social (e.g., affiliation mechanisms may play a key role) (Stein, 1991).

To some extent this debate about the nature of pathogenesis has played out the in area of global mental health. On the one hand, the focus of global mental health on DSM-5 and ICD-11 constructs like depression is consistent with a classical perspective. On the other hand, given its roots in cross-cultural psychiatry, global mental health has emphasized the importance of not reifying disease constructs, of appreciating the way in which idioms of distress are shaped by culture, and of understanding mental illness as a meaningful response to the social environment. It is notable that a good deal of research in global mental health relies on mixed methods; clinical trials, for example, often employ formative qualitative research to appreciate the local context, and then go on to quantitative work.

Global mental health has admittedly not always focused specifically on understanding causal mechanisms underlying disease, rather emphasizing the importance of implementation science; of taking what we know to scale, and figuring out problems that arise during this process. However, in keeping with an integrative position, global mental health has relied on both qualitative and quantitative methods to investigate a range of mechanisms that contribute to mental illness, including social determinants. It is also noteworthy that priority setting exercises in global mental health research have emphasized the need to understand both neurobiological and societal mechanisms underlying mental disorders (Collins et al., 2011).

Neuroethics, given its close alliance with clinical neuroscience, has implicitly if not explicitly accepted the importance of understanding brain structures and mechanisms. It has been interested, for example, not only in advances in the neuroscience of psychiatric and neurological disorders, but also in identifying the neural mechanisms that underpin ethical decision-making, the so-called neuroscience of ethics. From a neuroethics perspective, just as contemporary physics has led to better answers to age-old questions in metaphysics, so can modern biology and neuroscience provide novel insights into perennial questions about morality. At the same time, neuroethics has often emphasized the importance of avoiding neuroreductionism (e.g., explaining a complex phenomenon such as morality purely with reference to brain states) and investigating the full range of psychobiological mechanisms (Savulescu & Earp, 2014).

In keeping with an integrative position, clinical neuroscience has certainly focused on the importance of discovery science. The Research Domain Criteria (RDoC) framework put forward by the National Institute for Mental Health, for example, argues that by studying brain systems across species, we will be able to identify consistent neuroanatomical, neurochemical, and neurogenetic mechanisms that underlie phenomena such as reward processing, fear learning, and decision making as well as obtain insights into their abnormalities (Insel et al., 2010). The RDoC framework has been accused by some of being reductionist, but it is noteworthy that its authors have consistently emphasized the importance of both genetic and environmental mechanisms, and the value of using both clinician-rated and self-report measures to fully understand and investigate behavior and subjective experience.

In summary, we would argue that psychiatric science advances both by uncovering the psychobiological mechanisms that underpin mental disorders, and by appreciating the context in which these conditions manifest. The reliance of psychiatric science on both quantitative and qualitative measures, and its focus on both genetic and environmental mechanisms, is consistent not only with an integrative position, but also with positions taken by both global mental health and neuroethics. It also consistent with the growing focus on "convergence science" (Eyre et al., 2017). An integrative position, which emphasizes the real psychobiological structures and mechanisms of the world, and the need for both a focus on erklaren and verstehen in their investigation, in turn provides a conceptual resource for these two fields.

Interventions for mental disorders and well-being

From a classical perspective, clinical trials are key in determining whether any particular intervention is useful. The practice of medicine is focused on disease rather than on wellness, and most research therefore takes place on medical conditions. Nevertheless health practitioners have always had a valid interest in improving health; this is seen for example, in obstetric practice, in preventive medicine, and in public health. In medical practice, as well as in each of these arenas of practice, a process of trial and error, and rigorous observation of the effects of intervention, has led to ever-improving treatments, with universal benefits.

From a critical perspective, a focus on wellness, like a focus on disease, must be conceptualized as essentially socio-political. There is a vast medical-industry complex focused on happiness, and its claims should be taken with skepticism, given the enormous profits that are at stake. While a focus on disease may minimize an appreciation of patient resilience, the focus of positive psychology on altering individuals' perception of stressors, allows the power structures of societies to be maintained. It is important, therefore, to emphasize human rights and patient empowerment; this focus ensures that the paternalism of medical interventions is counter-acted. The goals of both health research and treatment need to be defined by patients and their advocates; these may differ markedly from those of professionals (Stein, Seedat, Iversen, & Wessely, 2007; Stein, Xin, Osser, Li, & Jobson, 2002).

From an integrative perspective, though the cut-points between disease and normality are fuzzy, the value of interventions to treat disease and to enhance well-being are open to empirical investigation and rational debate. For example, the introduction of statins meant that it was useful to assess cholesterol levels, and to intervene when justified. Introduction of generic statins altered relevant cost-benefit calculations, and thresholds for treatment were appropriately lowered. Similarly, in mental health, there is a significant cost-benefit for treating severe depression. However, there is less agreement about the parameters of well-being, and less data on cost-efficacy for milder or subthreshold symptoms. Understanding and addressing patient values is a key component of good clinical practice, and shared decision-making, aimed at recovery, is an important goal (Fulford, 2011; Slade, 2017).

Once again, these debates have played out in global mental health. A good deal of the global mental health literature has focused on severe mental disorders, and on the underdiagnosis and undertreatment of these conditions. At the same time, consistent with an integrative position, global mental health practitioners have emphasized that disease and wellness fall on a spectrum, and have strongly advocated for mental health and well-being as a human right and for patient empowerment. In addition, stepped care approaches have been delineated, suggesting the treatment of milder illness at a primary care level, and the treatment of more severe illness in better-resourced settings. Global mental health practitioners have emphasized that clinical goal setting involves shared decision-making, with recovery as the goal.

As noted earlier, neuroethics is aligned with clinical neuroscience, which is focused on understanding the mechanisms underlying disease in order to develop new clinical targets. At the same time, consistent with an integrative position, neuroethics has had a strong interest in the potential use of neurotechnologies for enhancement purposes, and the field has been a strong advocate for patient participation in research, and for consumer empowerment. While some might suggest that the increased use of neurotechnologies represents further advances in corporate capitalism, with the medicalization and commercialization of everyday emotions and their control, others have argued that the democratization of neurotechnologies provides an opportunity for consumers to increase their own control over their own lives.

In summary, we would argue that it is important for psychiatric science to focus not only on disease, but also on well-being. Nevertheless, the profession and the public may often have a shared view of treatment goals and their benefit when addressing serious mental illness, while the parameters of well-being may often be more contentious and the benefits of well-being interventions less clear (Stein, 2012b). In either case, interventions need to be studied rigorously, patient input is needed in order to help determine the goals of intervention, and protection of human rights and facilitation of patient empowerment is key in psychiatric research and practice. This view is consistent with an integrative philosophy of science, as well as with much work in both global mental health and neuroscience, and in turn supports these endeavors. It is also consistent with the growing interest in personalized public health interventions (Desmond-Hellmann, 2016).

Conclusion

This chapter has emphasized several perennial debates in psychiatry, where a classical and critical position have been taken on a range of matters, including psychiatric diagnosis, pathogenesis of mental disorders, and optimal intervention for mental conditions and well-being. It has been argued that it is possible to transcend the scientism of the classical position, and the skepticism of the critical position by taking a position that integrates the strengths of each. This integrative position is consistent with, and supportive of, work being done by global mental health and neuroethics on diagnosis, pathogenesis, and intervention. It is also consistent with exciting work being done on convergence science, on personalized public health, and on the integration of global mental health with clinical neuroscience (Stein et al., 2015). Our hope is that such an integrative position helps foster a productive relationship between these two fields.

References

Bhaskar, R. (1978). *A realist theory of science* (2nd ed.). Sussex: Harvester Press.
Collins, P. Y., Patel, V., Joestl, S. S., March, D., Insel, T. R., Daar, A. S., et al. (2011). Grand challenges in global mental health. *Nature, 475*(7354), 27–30.
Cosmides, L., & Tooby, J. (1999). Toward an evolutionary taxonomy of treatable conditions. *Journal of Abnormal Psychology, 108*(3), 453–464.
Desmond-Hellmann, S. (2016). Progress lies in precision. *Science, 353*(6301), 731.

Eyre, H. A., Lavretsky, H., Forbes, M., Raji, C., Small, G., McGorry, P., et al. (2017). Convergence science arrives: How does it relate to psychiatry? *Academic Psychiatry: The Journal of the American Association of Directors of Psychiatric Residency Training and the Association for Academic Psychiatry, 41*(1), 91–99.

Fulford, K. W. (2011). The value of evidence and evidence of values: Bringing together values-based and evidence-based practice in policy and service development in mental health. *Journal of Evaluation in Clinical Practice, 17*(5), 976–987.

Illes, J., & Hossain, S. (2017). *Neuroethics: Anticipating the future* (1st ed.). Oxford; New York: Oxford University Press [xxxiii, 643 pages, 4 unnumbered pages of plates p.].

Insel, T., Cuthbert, B., Garvey, M., Heinssen, R., Pine, D. S., Quinn, K., et al. (2010). Research domain criteria (RDoC): Toward a new classification framework for research on mental disorders. *The American Journal of Psychiatry, 167*(7), 748–751.

Insel, T. R., & Quirion, R. (2005). Psychiatry as a clinical neuroscience discipline. *JAMA: The Journal of the American Medical Association, 294*(17), 2221–2224.

Kendler, K. S., Zachar, P., & Craver, C. (2011). What kinds of things are psychiatric disorders? *Psychological Medicine, 41*(6), 1143–1150.

Kleinman, A. (1991). *Rethinking psychiatry: From cultural category to personal experience.* Free Press.

Kleinman, A. (2013). Implementing global mental health. *Depression and Anxiety, 30*(6), 503–505.

Lakoff, G., & Johnson, M. (1999). *Philosophy in the flesh: The embodied mind and its challenge to Western thought.* New York: Basic Books.

Patel, V., Saxena, S., Lund, C., Thornicroft, G., Baingana, F., Bolton, P., et al. (2018). The Lancet commission on global mental health and sustainable development. *Lancet, 392*(10157), 1553–1598.

Sahakian, B. J., Bruhl, A. B., Cook, J., Killikelly, C., Savulich, G., Piercy, T., et al. (2015). The impact of neuroscience on society: Cognitive enhancement in neuropsychiatric disorders and in healthy people. *Philosophical Transactions of the Royal Society of London Series B, Biological Sciences, 370*(1677), 20140214.

Savulescu, J., & Earp, B. D. (2014). Neuroreductionism about sex and love. *Thinking, 13*(38), 7–12.

Shook, J. R., & Giordano, J. (2014). A principled and cosmopolitan neuroethics: Considerations for international relevance. *Philosophy, Ethics, and Humanities in Medicine: PEHM, 9*, 1.

Slade, M. (2017). Implementing shared decision making in routine mental health care. *World Psychiatry: Official Journal of the World Psychiatric Association, 16*(2), 146–153.

Stein, D. J. (1991). Philosophy and the DSM-III. *Comprehensive Psychiatry, 32*(5), 404–415.

Stein, D. J. (1993). Cross-cultural psychiatry and the DSM-IV. *Comprehensive Psychiatry, 34*(5), 322–329.

Stein, D. J. (1998). Philosophy of psychopharmacology. *Perspectives in Biology and Medicine, 41*(2), 200–211.

Stein, D. J. (2008). *Philosophy of psychopharmacology.* Cambridge University Press.

Stein, D. J. (2012a). Psychopharmacological enhancement: A conceptual framework. *Philosophy, Ethics, and Humanities in Medicine: PEHM, 7*, 5.

Stein, D. J. (2012b). Positive mental health: A note of caution. *World Psychiatry: Official Journal of the World Psychiatric Association, 11*(2), 107–109.

Stein, D. J. (2013). What is a mental disorder? A perspective from cognitive-affective science. *Canadian Journal of Psychiatry. Revue Canadienne de Psychiatrie, 58*(12), 656–662.

Stein, D. J., & Giordano, J. (2015). Global mental health and neuroethics. *BMC Medicine, 13*(1), 274.

Stein, D. J., He, Y., Phillips, A., Sahakian, B. J., Williams, J., & Patel, V. (2015). Global mental health and neuroscience: Potential synergies. *Lancet Psychiatry*, *2*, 178–185.

Stein, D. J., & Illes, J. (2015). Beyond scientism and skepticism: An integrative approach to global mental health. *Frontiers in Psychiatry*, *6*, 166.

Stein, D. J., Phillips, K. A., Bolton, D., Fulford, K. W., Sadler, J. Z., & Kendler, K. S. (2010). What is a mental/psychiatric disorder? From DSM-IV to DSM-V. *Psychological Medicine*, *40*(11), 1759–1765.

Stein, D. J., Seedat, S., Iversen, A., & Wessely, S. (2007). Post-traumatic stress disorder: Medicine and politics. *Lancet*, *369*(9556), 139–144.

Stein, D. J., Xin, Y., Osser, D., Li, X., & Jobson, K. (2002). Clinical psychopharmacology guidelines: Different strokes for different folks. *The World Journal of Biological Psychiatry: The Official Journal of the World Federation of Societies of Biological Psychiatry*, *3*(2), 64–67.

Summerfield, D. (2012). Afterword: Against "global mental health". *Transcultural Psychiatry*, *49*(3–4), 519–530.

Wakefield, J. C. (1992). Disorder as harmful dysfunction: A conceptual critique of DSM-III-R's definition of mental disorder. *Psychological Review*, *99*(2), 232–247.

Finding a word for it: An ordinary language philosophical perspective on the role of values-based practice as a partner to evidence-based practice

K.W.M. Bill Fulford[a], Werdie van Staden[b]
[a]Collaborating Centre for Values-based Practice, St Catherine's College, and Member of the Philosophy Faculty, University of Oxford, Oxford, United Kingdom, [b]Philosophy Department and Kenan Institute for Ethics, Duke University, Durham, NC, United States

This chapter describes a new approach to working with values in healthcare called values-based practice (VBP) and explores through the lens of ordinary language philosophy its role as a partner to evidence-based practice in responding to the challenges of global mental health and neuroethics. VBP holds accordingly conceptual resources for: reconciling the psychobiological mechanisms of Western psychiatry with services that are culturally appropriate; balancing neuroscience and its technological advances with skepticism; drawing the line between disease and wellness, and between medicalization and over-medicalization. It also holds practical resources for challenges of social inclusion and empowerment; challenges arising from the social determinants of disease; and the neuroethical challenges of enhancement.

"Values-based practice and ordinary language philosophy" section gives an overview of values-based practice indicating how it builds on ordinary language philosophy. "Values-based practice in bodily health" section explores the development of values-based practice in bodily medicine. "Values-based practice in mental health" section examines the more complex values challenges presented by mental health. "Fact-plus-value: A conceptual framework for global mental health and neuroethics" section indicates how the model underpinning values-based practice meets the conceptual challenges presented by global mental health and neuroethics. "Values-based practice: A practical resource for global mental health and neuroethics" section illustrates the reciprocal relationship between values-based practice and the practical challenges of global mental health and neuroethics.

Values-based practice and ordinary language philosophy

Where evidence-based practice provides a process that supports clinical decision-making when complex evidence is in play, values-based practice provides complementary processes that support clinical decision-making when complex values are in play.

Global Mental Health and Neuroethics. https://doi.org/10.1016/B978-0-12-815063-4.00003-4

The processes are different. Evidence-based practice employs computer-assisted search engines to explore large volumes of high-quality published research in electronic databases. Values-based practice employs learnable clinical skills exercised within a particular model of service delivery.

A forced choice exercise

Values-based practice is better understood through "doing rather than saying." Hence you may like to try the following exercise for yourself. The exercise involves making a choice:

Imagine you have developed early symptoms of a potentially fatal disease. Best evidence suggests two possible treatments

- TREATMENT A gives you a guaranteed period of full remission but no cure
- TREATMENT B gives you a 50:50 chance of "kill or complete cure"

So you have to decide: how long a period of remission would you want from Treatment A to choose that treatment rather than go for the 50:50 "kill or cure" from Treatment B?

You may find this difficult. But avoid thinking about what "other people" or "people in general" would choose, or what the "right" answer would be. Ask yourself, "given *me* as *I am now*, at *my* age and in *my* life circumstances, what would *I* choose?"

Please write down your answer before turning to Fig. 1 to see how other people responded.

The headline message from Fig. 1 is the diversity of responses. In training programs guided discussion of this diversity has three learning outcomes important for values-based practice:

(1) *Values vary widely from one person to the next*
People come up with very different figures for their minimum period of remission essentially because what they value—what matters or is important to them—varies widely.

Choosing treatment A over B ...

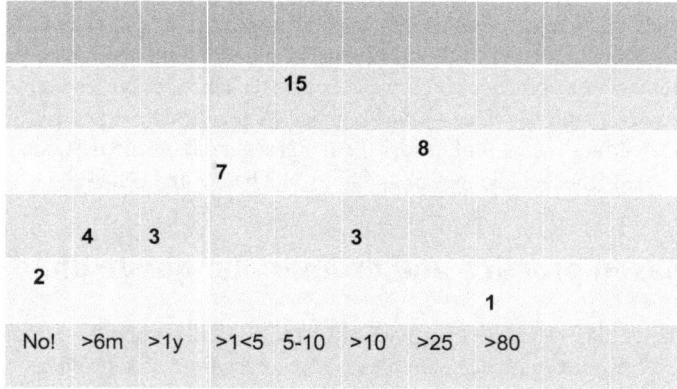

Fig. 1 Range of responses to the Forced Choice Exercise.

One person chooses, say, 20 years because they have young children and want to see them safely grown up. Another person may choose only a year because they need time to finish a research project. Yet another may choose the 50-50 Treatment B because what matters to them is to avoid having a (literal) deadline approaching however far away it might be.

It is natural in clinical contexts to equate values with ethics. This exercise allows participants to discover for themselves that while values include ethical values, they include much else besides. The question "what are values?" remains a matter of philosophical puzzlement. But for clinical purposes we can take "values" to mean anything that *matters or is important* from the perspective of the person concerned.

(2) *We cannot securely "second guess" each other's values*

Participants in the Forced Choice exercise are often surprised at the responses given by colleagues they thought they knew well.

A trainee surgeon described her "light bulb" moment when her partner of 6 years (also a trainee surgeon) responded very differently from how she expected (Handa et al., 2016). She chose 20 years minimum and had expected her partner to do the same. But he chose 6 months. This was a particular surprise to her because, she explained, they were due to get married in 6 months! They quickly came to understand each other's reasons: she had focused on having a family; he had focused on finishing his PhD. But as she wrote later: "If I could misjudge the values of the man I share my life with so profoundly, just how wrong might I be in assuming that I know what is important to my patients?"

This experience of surprise is important for values-based practice. We tend to assume we know what matters to other people. This is perhaps especially true of clinicians. Discovering for ourselves that we really do need to find out what is important to our patients is a key step toward training in values-based practice.

Being a surprise at the level of individuals, one may imagine how easily assumptions may be mistaken on what matters to communities and cultures, particularly relevant in the pursuit of global mental health and what would matter in the neuroethical choices afforded by neuroscientific technologies.

(3) *The diversity of people's responses has nothing to do with the evidence base being insecure*

In healthcare contexts the importance of evidence in clinical decision-making leads naturally to the idea that values come into play only where the relevant evidence-base is limited or unsatisfactory. But in the above exercise the evidence-base is exactly the same for everyone. The very different choices people make thus reflects very different values applied to the same evidence.

This third learning outcome is then readily summed up in the equation *"same evidence plus different values equals a different decision."* As we describe below, accounting for this equation is crucial in global health decisions and neuroethics.

An overview of values-based practice

The way values-based practice works is summarized in the flow diagram in Fig. 2. Its constituent elements are defined briefly in the accompanying Table 1. Full details are available from the sources given in the Further Reading at the end of the chapter.

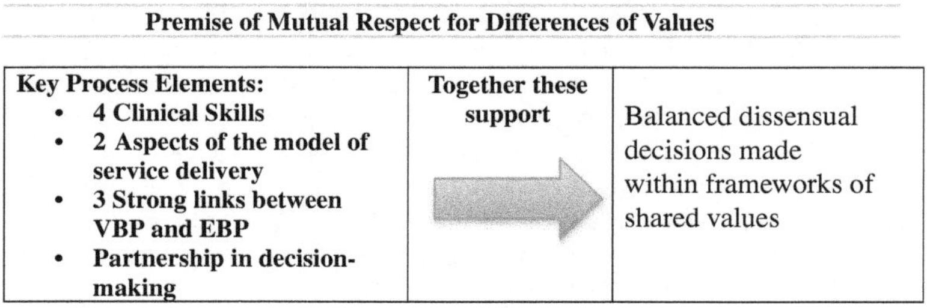

Premise of Mutual Respect for Differences of Values		
Key Process Elements: • **4 Clinical Skills** • **2 Aspects of the model of service delivery** • **3 Strong links between VBP and EBP** • **Partnership in decision-making**	**Together these support**	Balanced dissensual decisions made within frameworks of shared values

Fig. 2 A flow diagram of values-based practice.

Table 1   Brief definitions of the elements of values-based practice

Values-based practice	Brief definition
Premise of mutual respect	Mutual respect for differences of values
Skills—awareness	Awareness of values and of differences of values
Skills—knowledge	Knowledge retrieval and its limitations
Skills—reasoning	Used to explore the values in play rather than to provide answers
Skills—communication	Especially for eliciting values and conflict resolution
Patient-values-centered care	Care centered on the actual rather than assumed values of the patient
Extended MDT	MDT role extended to include a range of value perspectives as well as of knowledge and skills for interagency working
Two feet principle	All decisions are based on the two feet of values and evidence
Squeaky wheel principle	We notice values when they cause difficulties (like the squeaky wheel) but (like the wheel that doesn't squeak) they are always there and operative
Science-driven principle	Advances in medical science drive the need for VBP (as well as EBP) because they open up choices and with choices go values
Partnership	Decisions in VBP (although informed by clinical guidelines and other sources) are made by those directly concerned working together in partnership
Frameworks of shared values	Values shared by those in a given decision making context and within which balanced decisions can be made on individual cases
Balanced dissensual decision-making	Decisions in which the values in question remain in play to be balanced sometimes one way and sometimes in other ways according to the circumstances of a given case

The process of values-based practice includes ten elements: four areas of clinical skills, an appropriate service model (one that is person-centered and multidisciplinary), three principles linking values with evidence, and partnership in decision-making. Building on a premise of mutual respect, these elements together support balanced decision-making within frameworks of shared values.

We illustrate how values-based practice works out clinically with the case histories introducing the next two sections. First, though, in anticipation of our discussion of the relationship between values-based practice and global mental health and neuroethics, we will indicate briefly how values-based practice builds on its origins in ordinary language philosophy.

Roots of values-based practice in ordinary language philosophy

The roots of values-based practice lie in ordinary language philosophy (Fulford & Van Staden, 2013). Developed in the middle decades of the 20th century, by J.L. Austin and others of the "Oxford School," ordinary language philosophy explores the meanings of concepts by examining the ways they are *used* in everyday, or ordinary, contexts (Warnock, 1989, chap. 1). Austin suggested a number of sources for this philosophical "field work" as he called it (Austin, 1956–57, p. 25), including in particular case histories (Austin, 1956–57, p. 42).

Philosophical field work is one of a number of links between ordinary language philosophy and clinical practice (Fulford, 1990). Of particular significance in the context of global mental health and neuroethics is that focussing on language use leads to a more complete view of what another Oxford philosopher, Gilbert Ryle, called the "logical geography" (Ryle, 1963, p. 10).

Note Ryle's claim is that focussing on language use provides a "more complete" not a "complete," still less a "final," view. That a more complete view may nonetheless be helpful is indicated by the outcomes of the Forced Choice exercise. The exercise is in effect an exercise in ordinary language philosophy in that instead of reflecting on clinical decision-making it requires participants to actually make a choice. Correspondingly, then, its three learning outcomes add up to a more complete view of clinical decision-making: (1) that the operative values include anything that matters or is important to the person concerned; (2) that we cannot securely second guess another's values; and (3) that values are always important in clinical decision-making however well established the evidence-base may be.

Ordinary language philosophy, however, is as Austin put it, only a way of "making a start ..." (cited in Warnock, 1989, p. 5). It has always to be developed and built on collaboratively through teamwork and mixed methods approaches developed with disciplines appropriate to the problem in question. We will see later that there may be mutual benefit from teamwork of this ordinary language kind in the relationship of values-based practice with global mental health and neuroethics.

Values-based practice in bodily health

The case histories with which we start this section and the next are based on the stories of real people with biographical and other details changed to ensure confidentiality.

Case histories have a relatively low status in the "evidence hierarchy" of evidence-based medicine. In values-based practice by contrast, reflecting its origins in ordinary language philosophy, case histories have a central place.

Mrs. Jones' Knee

Mrs. Jones, a woman with painful arthritis in her left knee, consulted an orthopedic surgeon, Mr. Smith, for knee replacement. Mr. Smith explained that while all operations carried a degree of risk, knee replacement was now routine and had excellent outcomes, and he was happy to offer it in her case.

Mrs. Jones got up to leave looking pleased. As she reached the door she turned back saying "Thank you doctor, I'm so pleased I will be able to get back to my gardening." Hearing this Mr. Smith invited Mrs. Jones to sit down again and tell him more. She explained that although her knee was painful, what really mattered to her was that she could not bend well enough for gardening. We have a problem, then, Mr. Smith responded, because with the artificial joints currently available Mrs. Jones was likely to end up no more mobile than before, and possibly less so.

So they agreed on conservative management using anti-inflammatory medication and physiotherapy. This worked. Eighteen months later Mrs. Jones still had a painful knee but her mobility was sufficiently restored that she was happily gardening again.

This may perhaps seem an unlikely case study for a chapter on values-based practice. Mrs. Jones' values, it will be acknowledged, the issues that mattered or were important to her, were central to the decision not to operate. But where, it may be asked, are the values *issues*? Where correspondingly is the need for values-based practice? Surely, it may be said, this is "just good practice."

Values-based practice is indeed about good practice. In this instance good practice meant shared decision-making based on evidence and values. Mr. Smith was an expert in the evidence on options for treating arthritis of the knee. For most people with this condition, what matters or is important to them (what they value) is pain relief. But Mrs. Jones had *different* values from most people. What mattered to Mrs. Jones was gardening. This is why for Mrs. Jones, mobility trumped pain relief. This in turn is why bringing together Mr. Smith's expert knowledge of the evidence with Mrs. Jones' values (what really mattered to her) led to their shared decision to proceed conservatively.

As in the Forced Choice exercise, therefor, the importance of values in Mrs. Jones' story had nothing to do with the evidence-base being inadequate. To the contrary, consistently with the Science Driven Principle ("Values-based practice and ordinary language philosophy" section, Table 1), it was the evidence that gave Mrs. Jones options and thus brought her values into play. Consistent with this strong link between evidence and values, is the fact that the lead discipline in Oxford's Collaborating Centre for Values-based Practice is the science-led discipline of surgery (see valuesbasedpractice.org; also Handa et al., 2016).

The result of shared decision-making in Mrs. Jones' story was a "win" for everyone. Mrs. Jones avoided a major operation from which she would have emerged (by her values) worse off. The local health service saved the costs of this counter-productive intervention. Mr. Smith and his team had extra operating time for other patients. Small wonder then that shared decision-making based on evidence and values has been widely adopted as good practice in both ethical guidance (General Medical Council, 2008) and legal standards (Herring, Fulford, Dunn, & Handa, 2017; Montgomery v Lanarkshire Health Board, 2015). Applying these standards in the more complex values environment of (global) mental health and neuroscience is however more challenging. It is to this that we turn in the next sections.

Values-based practice in mental health

As you read through the following story you may find it helpful to compare it with the story of Mrs. Jones Knee. In what ways are the two stories similar? In what ways different?

Simon the seer

Simon was a 40-year old, black, American lawyer from a middle-class, Baptist family. Although not a religious man he had occasional relatively minor psychic experiences that had led him to seek the guidance of a professional "seer."

Then, out of the blue, he found himself the subject of a malpractice legal action from a group of colleagues. Although he believed himself innocent, he knew that defending himself would be expensive and potentially dangerous. He responded to this crisis by sitting up all night praying in front of an impromptu altar on which he had placed an open bible between two candles. The next morning he found that wax from the candles had run down onto the bible marking out various words and phrases. He described his experiences thus: "I got up and I saw the seal that was in my father's bible (he called the wax marks 'seals' or 'suns') and I called my friend John and I said, you know, 'something remarkable is going on over here.' I think the beauty of it was the specificity by which the sun burned through. It was ... in my mind, a clever play on words."

Simon continued to receive "revelations" through the images left in melted candle wax. They meant nothing to anyone else including his Baptist friends and family. But for Simon they represented biblical symbols (the bull, the 24 elders, the arc of the covenant, etc.) signifying that "I am the living son of David ... (and) captain of the guard of Israel." When confronted with skepticism, he said simply "I don't get upset, because I know within myself, what I know."

A first point of similarity between Simon's story and Mrs. Jones' knee is that both are drawn from everyday practice. Mrs. Jones' story is about treatment in everyday surgical practice. Simon's story is about diagnosis in everyday psychiatric practice. Exhibiting as Simon does "delusional perception" (Wing, Cooper, & Sartorius, 1974, symptom 82, pp. 172–173), his story opens up the range of both mental and bodily conditions (including temporal lobe brain tumor) in the differential diagnosis of schizophrenia.

When it comes to values, though, there is a *prima facie* difference between the two stories. Mrs. Jones' story raised explicit value considerations, which are at face level about treatment options but at deeper also a matter of diagnostic understanding of what is *bad* for Mrs. Jones. But there are no such explicit value considerations in Simon's story. The differential diagnosis of schizophrenia, it would seem to many, is based on the facts: descriptively defined symptoms combined with a "physical" examination and investigations.

Values in Simon's story

This fact-only view of diagnosis is standard in psychiatry. It is reflected for example in the World Health Organization's ICD (International Classification of Diseases; World Health Organization, 1992). This in turn reflects the standard view in medicine that while values come into treatment choice, diagnosis is a matter for value-free science. Looking, however, at how Simon's story turned out, will suggest that this standard fact-only view is (in the terms of ordinary language philosophy) an incomplete view.

The messages Simon received from his "seals" guided him in defending his case. The guidance was very specific: for example leading him to key precedent cases. The result was that he won (the action was shown to be a racially motivated attempt to undermine his growing practice), his reputation as a lawyer was thus further enhanced, and he went on to make a great deal of money. When last heard of he had set up a research trust to support work not on schizophrenia but on religious experience.

This outcome is open to different interpretations. Many psychiatrists, holding to the standard fact-only view, might argue that Simon was fortunate in that his schizophrenia turned out to be unusually "benign." Others would reject disease labels outright arguing that far from an illness, Simon's experiences should be understood rather (as Simon himself understood them) in positive terms as being spiritual or religious in nature.

Note therefor that in framing these different ways of understanding Simon's story we fall naturally into the language of values ("fortunate," "benign," "positive terms"). Similar evaluative language is evident too in the language of the principal alternative classification to the ICD, the American Psychiatric Association's DSM (Diagnostic and Statistical Manual of Mental Disorders). The DSM-5 differs from ICD-10 in adding to its symptom-based diagnostic criteria, "criteria of clinical significance" based on functioning. For schizophrenia the relevant Criterion B (as it is called) reads as follows:

For a significant portion of the time since the onset of the disturbance, level of functioning in one or more major areas, such as work, interpersonal relations, or self-care, is markedly below the level achieved prior to the onset (or when the onset is in childhood or adolescence, there is failure to achieve expected levels of interpersonal, academic, or occupational functioning) (American Psychiatric Association, 2013, p. 99).

Simon therefor (to the extent at least of his occupational functioning) fails to satisfy DSM's Criterion B thus allowing for the possibility of understanding his story in terms of spiritual experience rather than pathology. But this possibility turns on how Simon's functioning is *evaluated*. Criterion B requires *impaired functioning*. This means that for a pathological understanding of his story Simon's functioning ("in one or more major areas, such as work, interpersonal relations, or self-care") has to have been not only changed (a matter of fact) but changed *for the worse* (a matter of *value*)—it must have been "*below* the level" previously achieved, or, if he were a child or adolescent, there must have been "*failure* to achieve" expected levels.

This is not as such to say that Simon's experiences were or were not spiritual or indeed pathological in nature. Certainly, his occupational functioning was enhanced rather than impaired. But the larger question of the status of his experiences is a question for, say, theology, epistemology or metaphysics. The point (the ordinary language philosophical point) is that the language of the DSM itself shows that any attempt to answer the larger question must start from a more complete view than that offered by the standard fact-only medical view of diagnosis. The language of DSM itself, that is to say, suggests a more complete view of diagnosis, a view that while indeed it includes the facts of the standard view, *includes values as well*. This more complete fact-plus-value view is further suggested by the many other instances of evaluative language occurring explicitly throughout DSM (Sadler, 2005) and implicitly in ICD (Fulford, 1994).

Values in psychiatric diagnosis

Just how the importance of values in psychiatric diagnosis should be understood is an open question that has figured prominently in the long-running debate about the concept of mental illness. Thomas Szasz, for example, regarded psychiatric diagnostic values as evidence that mental illnesses were different in principle from bodily illnesses (he called them "myths"; Szasz, 1960). Robert Kendell, opposing Szasz, argued that these same values were a reflection of the primitive state of psychiatric science (Kendell, 1975).

There is much to be said for both these positions and the debate in various forms continues. The issues turn on deeper issues in the even longer running is-ought debate in moral philosophy. One version of the latter debate is skeptical of its very terms of engagement, arguing that there is no essential separation between description and evaluation (Putnam, 2002).

Rather, though, than pursuing these debates we will turn instead to a third and quite different way of understanding the appearance of values in psychiatric diagnosis. This third interpretation, different from the interpretations equally of Szasz and of Kendell, will be worth considering in a little more detail. Derived as it is from ordinary language philosophy, it provides a more complete view of the medical model of diagnosis that, as we will see in later sections, is helpful in addressing the challenges of global mental health and neuroethics.

Third interpretation: Visible values = diverse values

The third interpretation of values in psychiatric diagnosis—to give the conclusion of this section first—is that *visible values indicate the presence of diverse values*.

This interpretation is based on the work of another Oxford philosopher, R.M. Hare. In the is-ought debate Hare argued in favor of an essential separation of description from evaluation (see e.g., Hare, 1963). The is-ought debate as already noted continues. But in pursuing the debate Hare and others made a number of novel observations about the language of values that, applied in turn to the language of medicine (Fulford, 1989; Fulford & Van Staden, 2013), led ultimately to values-based practice.

The relevant observation here is that while values are everywhere we tend to notice them only when they are diverse and hence come to our attention through disagreements. You may recognize this idea in the Squeaky Wheel Principle of values-based practice (Table 1, "Values-based practice and ordinary language philosophy" section).

The wheels on a car come to our attention only when they cause trouble (only when they squeak). Applying this observation to the debate about mental illness thus suggests that the appearance of values in psychiatric diagnosis (as in Criterion B) reflects the fact that psychiatry is concerned with areas of experience and behavior where our values are relatively diverse.

This is shown diagrammatically in Fig. 3. Adapting one of Hare's examples, Fig. 3 shows how from a values point of view, concepts of bodily disorder are like strawberries

Shared values = Implicit Values	Diverse Values = Explicit Values
Strawberries and Bodily Illness	**Pictures and Mental Illness**
• 'Good' in 'good strawberry' is a value term • But people have **shared** ideas about what kinds of strawberry are good (red, sweet, etc) • Hence 'good' in 'good strawberry' has factual associations ('red, sweet, tasty, etc strawberry') with its evaluative meaning becoming **implicit**	• 'Good' in 'good picture' is a value term • But people have **different** ideas about what kinds of picture are good • Hence 'good' in 'good picture' has no consistent factual associations and its evaluative meaning remains **explicit**
• Bodily illness is in this respect like strawberries • It involves areas of human experience and behavior (such as pain) where our values are largely **shared** • Hence the meaning of bodily illness has factual associations and its evaluative meaning becoming **implicit**	• Mental illness is in this respect like pictures • It involves areas of human experience and behavior (such as emotion, desire, beliefs, etc) where our values are highly **diverse** • Hence the meaning of mental illness has no consistent factual meaning and its evaluative meaning remains **explicit**

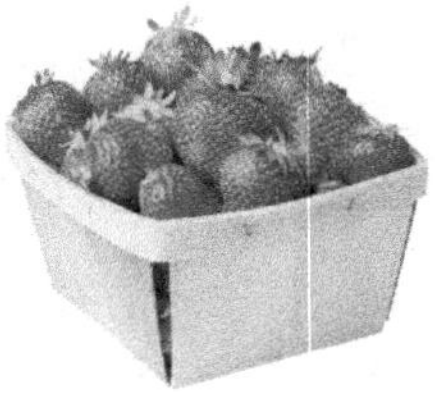

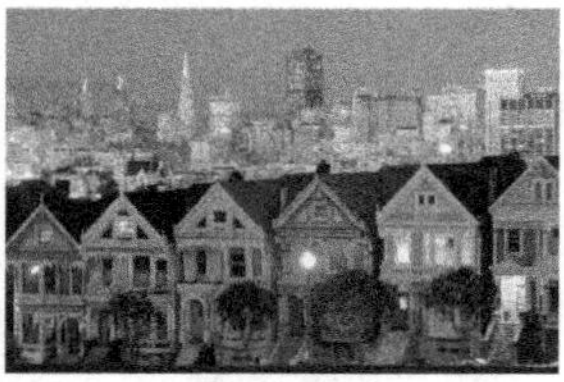

Fig. 3 Bodily disorders are like strawberries; mental disorders are like pictures.

(people have similar values) whereas concepts of mental disorder are like pictures (people have diverse values). Values are thus visible in the diagnostic terms of mental health not because (as Szasz argued) psychiatry is beyond the pale of scientific medicine, nor (as Kendell argued) because psychiatry is scientifically underdeveloped, but because psychiatry is concerned with areas of experience and behavior where our values are relatively diverse. Thus, bodily medicine deals with experiences like pain where our values are largely shared (pain is for most people a bad experience); psychiatry by contrast deals with emotion, desire, volition, belief, sexuality, responsibility and so forth, areas in which our values are widely diverse, notwithstanding that we may at times share a value in psychiatry too, for example, that someone's functioning has changed for the *worse*.

We have spelled out this third way of understanding the visibility of values in the diagnostic concepts of psychiatry in some detail because it provides what amounts to a depth dimension of ordinary language theory that is required for values-based practice to be applied successfully in the more complex values environment of mental health. In the next two sections we explore the importance of this depth dimension as the basis, respectively, of a conceptual model and of a practical resource for meeting the challenges of global mental health and neuroethics.

Fact-plus-value: A conceptual framework for global mental health and neuroethics

One major group challenges for global mental health and neuroethics is concerned with conceptual problems at the interface between Western science and diverse cultures. We can divide these conceptual problems into two main kinds, challenges of reconciliation and challenges of demarcation. Challenges of reconciliation include how to reconcile on the one hand the psychobiological mechanisms of Western psychiatry with, on the other hand, services that are culturally appropriate; and how to balance neuroscience and mental health sciences with skepticism. Challenges of demarcation in global mental health and exercising neuroethical choices include such problems as where to draw the line between disease and wellness; and between medicalization and over-medicalization.

These are multi-facetted challenges to which correspondingly multi-facetted answers are offered by the range of contributors to this volume. Ordinary language philosophy, as indicated earlier, lends itself to teamwork in exploring complex problems and is thus hospitable to the requirement for what is called in Chapter 1 "convergent methodologies." At the heart of this whole group of challenges, however, is the problem of how the very concept of mental disorder should be understood. It is with this problem in particular that ordinary language philosophy may be helpful in (as Austin put it) "making a start."

A fact-plus-value medical model

Making a start in understanding the concept of mental illness underpins the work described in earlier sections of this chapter culminating in the Fact-plus-Value medical model set out in "Values-based practice in mental health" section (Fig. 3). This model

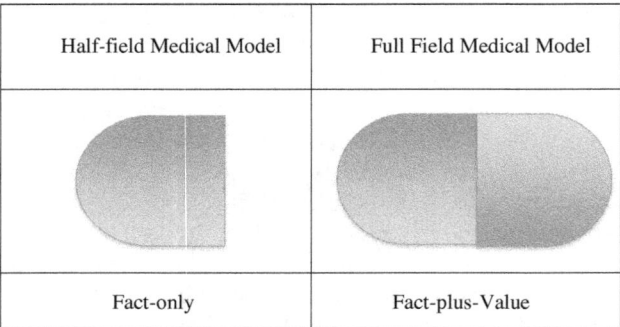

Fig. 4 Diagram comparing the Fact-only standard medical model with the more complete Fact-plus-Value medical model derived from ordinary language philosophy.

is compared diagrammatically with the standard Fact-only medical model in Fig. 4. Extending Ryle's metaphor of ordinary language philosophy as generating a more complete view, Fig. 4 represents the standard (Fact-only) medical model as a half-field or hemianopic view compared with the full-field (Fact-plus-Value) medical model derived from ordinary language philosophy.

Before looking at the implications of this Fact-plus-Value model, it will be worth reviewing briefly how the model builds on and reflects points made in earlier sections. First, the Fact-plus-Value model is as just noted a "more complete" but not final model. It has nothing to say for example about "disability." Second, its authority comes not from an external perspective on mental health but from the language of mental health itself (as represented in "Values-based practice in mental health" section by Simon's story and the language of DSM). Third, as a more complete view, it is inclusive not exclusive. That is to say, in making visible the values that are already there, it adds values to, rather than subtracting facts from, the standard view.

This is why both models shown in Fig. 4 are called "medical models." There is a tendency to equate the term "medical model" with a Fact-only (or at any rate Facts-central) model of medicine. This tendency goes with others: the tendency noted in "Values-based practice and ordinary language philosophy" section to think that values-based practice is required only where the evidence-base is inadequate; or to view values-based practice as a moderator of evidence-based practice; and a wider tendency to oppose the "science" and "art" of medicine. But fact and value, and with them evidence-based practice and values-based practice, are in the Fact-plus-Value model shown in Fig. 3 *equal* partners.

The "adds to not subtracts from" Fact-plus-Value medical model applies equally to bodily disorders as to mental disorders. There is a difference of degree, of course, as we saw in "Values-based practice in mental health" section, a difference in the degree of values agreement. This difference of degree also pertains among the various bodily disorders (compare for example the diagnostic value-ladenness of alcohol withdrawal versus metastatic cancer) and among the various mental disorders (compare for example the diagnostic value-ladenness of anti-social personality disorder and advanced Alzheimer's dementia). This difference of degree of values agreement will turn out in "Values-based practice: A practical resource for global mental health and neuro-ethics" section to be important for understanding the role of values-based practice in responding to the practical challenges of global mental health and neuroethics. First, though, in the remainder of this section, we will look at how a Fact-plus-Value medical model provides a powerful framework for responding to the two groups of conceptual challenges for global mental health and neuroethics outlined above, challenges of reconciliation, and challenges of demarcation.

Challenges of reconciliation

With a Fact-plus-Value medical model the problems of reconciliation simply do not arise. In a Fact-only model the challenge is how to incorporate values (including cultural values). In a Fact-plus-Value model the values are there already. So there are no dilemmas of as we put it in the introduction to this section, "on the one hand … and on the other hand." Both "hands," as it were, are there already. With the left hand (of facts) we hold on to the psychobiological mechanisms of contemporary psychiatry. With the right hand, we hold on to culturally appropriate services (to the extent that this means services that respect differences of cultural values).

As to mental health, neuroscience and skepticism, the model, again, offers a clear position, though in this instance one of exclusion rather than inclusion. Extending the above metaphor, in neither "hand" of the Fact-plus-Value medical model is there room for skepticism about science as such. If models are advanced that are skeptical of psychobiological mechanisms, for example global mental health models in which spirits are operative causal factors, then these models should be measured against the observational standards of science. This of course begs deep epistemological and, per-haps, political questions. These questions could indeed be pursued by way of further development of a Fact-plus-Value medical model. But they fall outside the "making a start" ordinary language status of the model as it stands. The model thus firmly excludes any form of cultural relativism in which "all world views are equal" (Van Staden & Fulford, 2015).

Challenges of demarcation

The Fact-plus-Value medical model is similarly uncompromising on the challenges of demarcation, though in this instance less hospitably to Western science.

First, as to the line between disease and wellness, this is to be drawn not with the fact-side but with the values-side of the model. Kendell, you will recall from "Values-based practice in mental health" section, attributed the values in psychiatric diagnosis to what he took to be the primitive state of psychiatric science. This is reasonable within a Fact-only or Facts-central medical model. A contemporary counterpart po-sition would be that with a sufficiently developed neuroscience, the differential di-agnosis in a case like Simon's would come down to a brain scan or other objective test obviating the need for any Criterion B. But the "visible values = diverse values" account shows this to be mistaken. According to this account the visibility of values in psychiatric diagnosis reflects the diversity of human values in the areas with which psychiatry is concerned. Short therefor of abolishing the diversity of human values, any future psychiatric science must encompass, rather than displace, the values in psychiatric diagnosis.

One corollary of this argument is that problems of over-medicalization may arise similarly from the values—rather than the fact-side of the model. This possibility is supported by the findings from an ordinary language study of abusive uses of psychiatry in the former Soviet Union (Fulford, Smirnov, & Snow, 1993). Western psychiatry at the time assumed that these abuses arose from Soviet diagnostic concepts being a product of inadequate Soviet psychiatric science. By looking at contemporary Soviet scientific publications (two of the study's authors were Russian speakers) the study showed to the contrary that Soviet diagnostic concepts were in fact closely equivalent to their Western counterparts. The conclusion therefor was that in this instance at least the vulnerability of psychiatry to abuse arose not from poor science but from a failure to attend to the evaluative aspects of psychiatric diagnosis (specifically, the unacknowledged influence of Soviet political values).

The importance of "visible values = diverse values" in psychiatric diagnosis has implications also for Western psychiatry and clinical neuroscience. It could be important in research, for example in the failure of translation of contemporary neuroscience to which both critics and supporters of DSM alike have recently drawn attention (see respectively, Kupfer, First, & Regier, 2002; Insel, 2013). It could be important too in clinical care. It is to the practical implications of the model that we turn next.

Values-based practice: A practical resource for global mental health and neuroethics

A second major group of challenges for global mental health and neuroethics is concerned not with concept but practice. This is where values-based practice, as the practical counterpart of a Fact-plus-Value medical model, comes into play. We consider the role of values-based practice here in relation to three main kinds of practical challenge: challenges of social inclusion and empowerment; challenges arising from the social determinants of disease; and challenges of enhancement.

Challenges of social inclusion and empowerment

With its premise of mutual respect, values-based practice is a ready resource for more effective shared decision-making between professionals and patients. In this respect psychiatry is once again no different in principle from bodily medicine. But it is more challenging in practice owing to its inherent values diversity. This is important for example in Western psychiatry in the need for what has become known as recovery practice.

"Recovery" in this context means recovering a good quality of life as judged by the values of (by what is important to) the person concerned. Mrs. Jones in "Values-based practice in bodily health" section "recovered" in this values-based sense. But in psychiatry patients have for too long expressed concern that they are treated (particularly with medications) without regard to what is important to them (Campbell, 1996). Values-based practice in engaging directly with what is important to the person concerned is thus inherently recovery-oriented. Resources for values-based recovery services extend to diagnosis (Fulford, Duhig, Hankin, Hicks, & Keeble, 2015) and, more surprisingly perhaps, to involuntary treatment (Fulford, Dewey, & King, 2015).

Here though we hit one of the limits of values-based practice as it has been developed thus far. For as the service user and mental health advocate, David Crepaz-Keay, has pointed out (Crepaz-Keay, Fulford, & Van Staden, 2015), while values-based practice is certainly helpful in supporting the move in recovery from dependence to independence, it lacks the conceptual resources to support the further move from independence to inter-dependence. This is an important limitation because moving on from individual independence to social interdependence is for most people essential to achieving a good quality of life.

We return below to how this limitation of values-based practice might be addressed. First we set the limitation itself in the context of a wider range of challenges arising from the social determinants of disease.

Challenges arising from the social determinants of disease

The limitation of values-based practice in recovery practice is an aspect of its wider limitations in focussing on the individual at the expense of the collective. This limitation was first pointed out by Sridha Venkatapuram, a philosopher working on the implications for global health equity (Venkatapuram, 2014) of the growing evidence, from Marmot (2006) and others, for the importance of social and political (as against individual and biological) determinants of disease. Venkatapuram argued in light of this evidence for a widening of the scope of values-based practice. Crepaz-Keay's point in relation to recovery is similarly motivated.

The individual focus of values-based practice reflects its origins in English and other languages reflecting the strongly individualist orientation of Western healthcare. But ordinary language philosophy means more than just ordinary English-language philosophy. As the philosopher Rom Harré first pointed out, concepts occur in other languages for which there are no English equivalents (Harré, 1983, pp. 85–92). Harré had in mind Inuit and Maori languages. In the case of values-based practice a particularly rich resource is offered by African languages.

African cultures are sometimes represented as being organized around the collective rather than the individual. But this is an over-simplification premised on non-African ways of thinking (Van Staden, 2011). African cultures are neither necessarily collective nor individualist but something different that incorporates both in a context responsive way. "Ubuntu" is one of a number of words expressing this idea in sub-Saharan African languages (Metz, 2011; Ramose, 2003; Schutte, 1993). Combined with practices such as the indaba (an isiZulu term for a particular kind of meeting involving a substantive communicative process, Van Staden, 2010, 2011), Ubuntu is the backdrop orientation of a social interconnectedness and communal responsibility to both individuals and society within which their respective values are balanced through communicative processes appropriate to a given situation. Embedded within the orientation of Ubuntu, the Sesotho term Batho Pele lends itself to a distinctive African form of values-based practice (Van Staden & Fulford, 2015).

VBP and its African form espouse the context dependence of values. In VBP, the context matters whether the values between individuals are shared or legitimately different. In its African form, the context matters in the relationship between (and practical processing of) individual and societal values. The context dependence of individual and societal values is an important pointer for global mental health—a pointer that may avert the mistaken attribution or assumption of a value as if pertaining globally or being (equally) important globally. By this pointer, the context matters, for instance, whether deploying lay health care workers, often advocated in global mental health (Wainberg et al., 2017), would be ethically sound.

Extending the "field work" of ordinary language philosophy from English to African languages thus builds on and enhances values-based practice. As such it provides additional resources for meeting the challenges arising from the social determinants of disease in the context not only of global mental health but of Western healthcare too.

Challenges of neuroethics exemplified in individual and global enhancement

Building on a Fact-plus-Value medical model, values-based practice offers a rich resource for meeting the challenges arising from the use of novel neuroscientific technologies for personal and/or collective enhancement, which are often considered by the neuroethics literature (for examples see Roco & Bainbridge's Converging Technologies Report, 2003).

The Science Driven Principle of values-based practice (Table 1, "Values-based practice and ordinary language philosophy" section) recognizes that new scientific technologies will generate more value-laden choices. This is nowhere more evident than where these technologies are used for enhancement. The very term "enhancement" (meaning *better*ment) is after all a value term. Values are thus squarely on the agenda from the beginning across the range of enhancements, physical, intellectual, cognitive, personality, or cosmetic. Even values themselves are included in the purview of potential enhancement, called moral enhancement (Canton, 2003; Persson & Savulescu, 2012) (chapter by Savulescu).

Values-based practice provides explicit processes to recognize, reason about and account for the diversity of values in play with issues of enhancement. As with other practical problems, this diversity should be addressed not only between individuals but between groups. For example, Canton (2003, p.78) anticipates that in the future, cultures will define enhancement based on their social and political values. One indication of the significance of social and political values in this context is the history of eugenics in the Second Reich where it was pursued as a form of enhancement in the name of medical science (Glover, 1999). In current times, decreasing the global mental health treatment gap may be seen as a global enhancement objective, pursued for example in the World Health Organization's Mental Health Gap Action Programme Intervention Guide (mhGAP-IG). This guide recognizes values diversity in its section "general principles of care" and by encouraging that the guide should be adapted to national and local needs (World Health Organization, 2016).

We thus come back to the importance of extending values-based practice from its current focus on the individual to encompass social and political values; or, as we might now put it, drawing on African concepts, extending values-based practice to a form of Batho Pele fit for purpose in meeting the challenges of global mental health and neuroethics.

Conclusions

This chapter has explored the relationship of values-based practice with global mental health and neuroethics. "Values-based practice and ordinary language philosophy" section used an interactive exercise (the Forced Choice exercise) to introduce values-based practice and to indicate its origins in ordinary language philosophy. "Values-based practice in bodily health" section described through the story of Mrs. Jones' Knee contemporary developments in values-based practice in bodily medicine. "Values-based practice in mental health" section drew out through Simon's story the sharper values challenges arising in mental health. Meeting these challenges required a depth dimension of theory derived from ordinary language philosophy of values. "Fact-plus-value: A conceptual framework for global mental health and neuroethics" section then showed how this depth dimension led to a Fact-plus-Value medical model that proved helpful in meeting some of the conceptual challenges presented by global mental health and neuroethics. "Values-based practice: A practical resource for global mental health and neuroethics" section turned from concept to practice, exploring the relationship between values-based practice, as the practical counterpart of a Fact-plus-Value medical model, and global mental health and neuroethics. The relationship proved to be reciprocal: each benefitted from but also offered resources for the other. African philosophy in particular—with its concepts of ubuntu and indaba—provided key resources for the further development of values-based practice.

Running through the chapter as a whole—as a golden thread if you will—has been the importance of words. We opened with the origins of values-based practice in ordinary language philosophy, these origins underpinned the successes of values-based practice as a partner to evidence-based practice in both bodily medicine and mental health, and it was with the potential of non-Western (particularly African) languages for the further development of values-based practice that we concluded "Values-based practice: A practical resource for global mental health and neuroethics" section.

Austin, the founding figure of ordinary language philosophy, would not have been surprised by this golden thread. "Words," he said, "are our tools" (Austin, 1956–57, p. 24). Extending Austin's metaphor, then, the conclusion to be drawn from this chapter is that global mental health and neuroethics provide a more extensive toolbox of words than the merely local (mainly Western) toolbox from which values-based practice has to date been developed. There are resources in the global toolbox that we have not had space here to consider: work on well-being (Fulford & Galvin, 2018); on the range of healing traditions represented by the rich variety of the world's religions (Atwell & Fulford, 2006); and on the diversity of cultural values to be found even within European traditions (Fulford, 2018; Fulford & Stoyanov, 2015). But the resources of African languages, illustrated here by "ubuntu" and "indaba," provide proof of product of this resource. The Western-derived toolbox of values-based practice has, as we have indicated, much to offer in a global context. The examples of ubuntu and indaba suggest, however, that where we find a tool missing from the toolbox of values-based practice, it is in the wider context of global mental health and neuroethics that we will find a word for it.

Acknowledgment

Fig. 1 is taken from a training template for Values-based Practice available on the website of the Collaborating Centre for Values-based Practice in Health and Social Care at St Catherine's College, Oxford (valuesbasedpractice.org) and is reproduced here by permission of the center.

References

American Psychiatric Association. (2013). *Diagnostic and Statistical Manual of Mental Disorders* (5th ed.). Arlington, VA: American Psychiatric Association. p. 99.

Atwell, R., & Fulford, K. W. M. (2006). The Christian tradition of spiritual direction as a sketch for a strong theology of diversity. In J. Cox, A. V. Campbell, & K. W. M. Fulford (Eds.), *Medicine of the person: Faith, science and values in health care provision* (pp. 83–95). London: Jessica. [chapter 6].

Austin, J. L. (1956–57). A plea for excuses. *Proceedings of the Aristotelian Society, 57*, 1–30. [Reprinted in A. R. White (ed.) (1968). The philosophy of action. Oxford: Oxford University Press, pp. 19–42].

Campbell, P. (1996). What we want from crisis services. In J. Read & J. Reynolds (Eds.), *Speaking our minds: An anthology* (pp. 180–183). Basingstoke: The Macmillan Press Ltd for The Open University.

Canton, J. (2003). The impact of convergent technologies and the future of business and the economy. In M. C. Roco & W. S. Bainbridge (Eds.), *Converging technologies for improving human performance: Nanotechnology, biotechnology, information technology and cognitive science* (pp. 71–78). Dordrecht: Kluwer Academic Publishers.

Crepaz-Keay, D., Fulford, K. W. M., & Van Staden, C. W. (2015). Putting both a person and people first: Interdependence, values-based practice and African Batho Pele as resources for co-production in mental health. In J. Z. Sadler, C. W. Van Staden, & K. W. M. Fulford (Eds.), *The Oxford handbook of psychiatric ethics*. Oxford: Oxford University Press. [chapter 4].

Fulford, K. W. M. (1989). *Moral theory and medical practice*. [Reprinted 1995 and 1999]Cambridge: Cambridge University Press.

Fulford, K. W. M. (1990). Philosophy and medicine: The Oxford connection. *British Journal of Psychiatry, 157*, 111–115.

Fulford, K. W. M. (1994). Closet logics: Hidden conceptual elements in the DSM and ICD classifications of mental disorders. In J. Z. Sadler, O. P. Wiggins, & M. A. Schwartz (Eds.), *Philosophical perspectives on psychiatric diagnostic classification* (pp. 211–232). Baltimore: Johns Hopkins University. [chapter 9].

Fulford, K. W. M. (2018). Cultural values and mental health: A manifesto for international values-based practice. *Eidos: A Journal for Philosophy and Culture, 2*(4), 136–147. https://doi.org/10.26319/4722.

Fulford, K. W. M., Dewey, S., & King, M. (2015). Values-based involuntary seclusion and treatment: Value pluralism and the UK's Mental Health Act 2007. In J. Z. Sadler, C. W. Van

Staden, & K. W. M. Fulford (Eds.), *The Oxford handbook of psychiatric ethics*. Oxford: Oxford University Press. [chapter 60].

Fulford, K. W. M., Duhig, L., Hankin, J., Hicks, J., & Keeble, J. (2015). Values-based assessment in mental health: The 3 keys to a shared approach between service users and service providers. In J. Z. Sadler, C. W. Van Staden, & K. W. M. Fulford (Eds.), *The Oxford handbook of psychiatric ethics*. Oxford: Oxford University Press. [chapter 73].

Fulford, K. W. M., & Galvin, K. T. (2018). Values-based practice: At home with our values. In K. T. Galvin (Ed.), *Routledge handbook of well-being* (pp. 230–240). London: Routledge. [chapter 23].

Fulford, K. W. M., Smirnov, A. Y. U., & Snow, E. (1993). Concepts of disease and the abuse of psychiatry in the USSR. *British Journal of Psychiatry, 162*, 801–810.

Fulford, K. W. M., & Stoyanov, D. (2015). Living at the edge of compromise: Balkan pluralism as a resource for new philosophy of mental health. In D. St. Stoyanov (Ed.), *Towards a new philosophy of mental health* (pp. 2–26). Newcastle upon Tyne: Cambridge Scholars Publishing. [chapter 1].

Fulford, K. W. M., & Van Staden, C. W. (2013). Values-based practice: Topsy-turvy take home messages from ordinary language philosophy (and a few next steps). In K. W. M. Fulford, M. Davies, R. Gipps, G. Graham, J. Sadler, G. Stanghellini, & T. Thornton (Eds.), *The Oxford handbook of philosophy and psychiatry* (pp. 385–412). Oxford: Oxford University Press. [chapter 26].

General Medical Council. (2008). *Consent: Patients and doctors making decisions together*. London: General Medical Council.

Glover, J. (1999). *Humanity: A moral history of the twentieth century*. London, London: Pimlico, Jonathan Cape.

Handa, I. A., Fulford-Smith, L., Barber, Z. E., Dobbs, T. D., Fulford, K. W. M., & Peile, E. (2016). The importance of seeing things from someone else's point of view. *BMJ*. http://careers.bmj.com/careers/advice/The_importance_of_seeing_things_from_someone_else's_point_of_view.

Hare, R. M. (1963). Descriptivism. *Proceedings of the British Academy, 49*, 115–134. [Reprinted in Hare, R. M. (1972) Essays on the moral concepts. London: The Macmillan Press Ltd].

Harré, R. (1983). *Personal being*. Oxford: Basil Blackwell.

Herring, J., Fulford, K. W. M., Dunn, M., & Handa, A. (2017). Elbow room for best practice? Montgomery, patients' values, and balanced decision-making in person-centered clinical care. *Medical Law Review, 25*(4), 582–603. https://doi.org/10.1093/medlaw/fwx029. https://academic.oup.com/medlaw/advance-articles.

Insel, T. R. (2013). *Transforming diagnosis*. http://www.nimh.nih.gov/about/director/2013/transforming-diagnosis.shtml.

Kendell, R. E. (1975). The concept of disease and its implications for psychiatry. *British Journal of Psychiatry, 127*, 305–315.

Kupfer, D. J., First, M. B., & Regier, D. E. (Eds.), (2002). *A research agenda for DSM-V*. Washington: American Psychiatric Association.

Marmot, M. (2006). Health in an unequal world: Social circumstances, biology and disease. *Clinical Medicine, 6*, 559–572.

Metz, T. (2011). Ubuntu as a moral theory and human rights in South Africa. *African Human Rights Law Journal, 11*, 532–559.

Montgomery v Lanarkshire Health Board. (2015). https://www.supremecourt.uk/cases/uksc-2013-0136.html.

Persson, I., & Savulescu, J. (2012). Unfit for the future: The need for moral enhancement. *Uehiro series in practical ethics*. Oxford: Oxford University Press.

Putnam, H. (2002). *The collapse of the fact/value dichotomy and other essays*. Cambridge, MA: Harvard University Press.

Ramose, M. B. (2003). The philosophy of ubuntu and ubuntu as a philosophy. In P. H. Coetzee & A. P. J. Roux (Eds.), *The African philosophy reader*. (2nd ed., pp. 230–238). New York/London: Routledge.

Roco, M. C. & Bainbridge, S. (Eds.), (2003). *Converging technologies for improving human performance: Nanotechnology, biotechnology, information technology and cognitive science*. Dordrecht: Kluwer Academic Publishers.

Ryle, G. (1963). *The concept of mind*. London and New York: Penguin Books Ltd. [1949; Penguin books].

Sadler, J. Z. (2005). *Values and psychiatric diagnosis*. Oxford: Oxford University Press.

Schutte, A. (1993). *Philosophy for Africa*. Rondebosch: UCT Press.

Szasz, T. S. (1960). The myth of mental illness. *American Psychologist, 15*, 113–118.

Van Staden, C. W. (2010). Stuck in the past or heading for flourishing people in diversity. *South African Journal of Psychiatry, 16*, 4–6.

Van Staden, C. W. (2011). African approaches to an enriched ethics of person-centred health practice. *International Journal of Person Centered Medicine, 1*, 11–17.

Van Staden, C. W., & Fulford, K. W. M. (2015). The indaba in African values-based practice: Respecting diversity of values without ethical relativism or individual liberalism. In J. Z. Sadler, C. W. Van Staden, & K. W. M. Fulford (Eds.), *The Oxford handbook of psychiatric ethics*. Oxford: Oxford University Press. [chapter 28].

Venkatapuram, S. (2014). Values-based practice and global health. In M. Loughlin (Ed.), *Debates in values-based practice: Arguments for and against*. Cambridge: Cambridge University Press. [chapter 11].

Wainberg, M. L., Scorza, P., Shultz, J. M., Helpman, L., Mootz, J. J., Johnson, K. A., et al. (2017). Challenges and opportunities in global mental health: A research-to-practice perspective. *Current Psychiatry Reports, 19*(5), 28.

Warnock, G. J. (1989). *J. L. Austin*. London: Routledge.

Wing, J. K., Cooper, J. E., & Sartorius, N. (1974). *Measurement and classification of psychiatric symptoms*. Cambridge: Cambridge University Press.

World Health Organization. (1992). *The ICD-10 classification of mental and behavioural disorders: Clinical descriptions and diagnostic guidelines*. Geneva: World Health Organization.

World Health Organization. (2016). *mhGAP intervention guide for mental, neurological and substance use disorders in nonspecialized health settings version 2.0*. Geneva: World Health Organization.

Further reading

For further details of values-based practice please see the website for the *Collaborating Centre for Values-based Practice in Health and Social Care* at St Catherine's College, Oxford University: valuesbasedparctice.org

The website includes a detailed Reading Guide covering the theory and practice of values-based practice and a number of down-loadable learning resources (see valuesbasedpractice.org and follow the links to 'More about VBP'/'Reading Guide' and 'More about VBP'/'Full text Downloads').

Fulford, Peile and Carroll's (2012) *Essential Values-based Practice: Clinical Stories Linking Science with People* (Cambridge: Cambridge University Press) illustrates through a series of extended case histories the applications of values-based practice across a number of clinical conditions in both primary and secondary care.

Welfarist psychiatry goes global

4

Doug McConnell, Julian Savulescu
Oxford Uehiro Centre for Practical Ethics, University of Oxford,
Oxford, United Kingdom

Introduction

Mental health problems represent a significant proportion of the global burden of disease (~10% disability-adjusted life years) yet receive a disproportionately low level of funding (less than 1% of most countries' healthcare budget) (Patel et al., 2016; Whiteford, Ferrari, Degenhardt, Feigin, & Vos, 2015). The situation is especially fraught in low- and middle-income countries (LMICs). Between 76% and 85% of people with severe mental disorders receive no treatment for their mental health problem in LMICs and untreated mental health problems account for 25.3% and 33.5% of all years lived with a disability in LMICs, respectively (World Health Organization, 2011). Governments from LMICs spend the lowest percentages of their health budgets on mental health worldwide and receive very little support from international aid and NGOs for mental health (Kakuma et al., 2011; Razzouk et al., 2010; Saxena, Thornicroft, Knapp, & Whiteford, 2007). Clinical trials are rarely conducted in low-income countries so the effectiveness of treatments in culturally diverse, low-income settings is largely unknown (Becker & Kleinman, 2013). Furthermore, a lack of appropriately trained health professionals in LMICs undermines the feasibility of a range of therapeutic approaches developed in the Western context (Becker & Kleinman, 2013; Saxena et al., 2007).

This situation has motivated a concerted effort to address global mental health by the WHO, the US National Institute of Mental Health, and the Global Alliance for Chronic Diseases, among others (Collins et al., 2011; World Health Organization, 2013). We argue that a welfarist approach to psychiatry will support this effort better than the dominant Western approach to psychiatry because it provides better tools to negotiate a variety of challenges. These challenges include the risk of entrenching flawed aspects of Western psychiatry in new populations, the neocolonial imposition of Western mental health norms, reducing stigma toward mental illness, and preventing the use of psychiatry for immoral or political ends. Welfarist psychiatry corrects these significant flaws in the Western psychiatric model, avoids neocolonialism by indexing aspects of patient welfare to the local sociocultural context, reduces stigma by abandoning the concept of "normal" mental health, and provides grounds to restrict the misuse of psychiatry by appealing to objective aspects of personal and social well-being.

We begin by describing welfarist psychiatry before outlining the relevant challenges to improving global mental health and explaining how welfarist psychiatry meets those challenges.

Global Mental Health and Neuroethics. https://doi.org/10.1016/B978-0-12-815063-4.00004-6

Welfarist psychiatry

Welfarist psychiatry (Roache & Savulescu, 2018) is a theoretical framework for psychiatry intended to replace the current dominant paradigm based on the concept of mental disorder.[a] The American Psychiatric Association's Diagnostic and Statistical Manual (DSM-5) defines a mental disorder as:

> A syndrome characterized by clinically significant disturbance in an individual's cognition, emotion regulation, or behavior that reflects a dysfunction in the psychological, biological, or developmental processes underlying mental functioning. Mental disorders are usually associated with significant distress or disability in social, occupational, or other important activities. An expectable or culturally approved response to a common stressor or loss, such as the death of a loved one, is not a mental disorder. Socially deviant behavior (e.g., political, religious, or sexual) and conflicts that are primarily between the individual and society are not mental disorders unless the deviance or conflict results from a dysfunction in the individual, as described above
>
> (American Psychiatric Association, 2013, p. 20)

In welfarist psychiatry, the concept of mental disorder is replaced with the much broader concept of psychological disadvantage (PD). A PD is a stable psychological trait that tends to worsen well-being given the social and environmental context. In contrast to mental disorders, PDs do not necessarily form part of a syndrome, involve no threshold between health and dysfunction, may include socially deviant behavior, and are not wholly attributable to the individual's "underlying mental functioning" because they involve a mismatch with the environment. In what follows, we elaborate on the attributes and implications of the concept of PD.

PDs are always a matter of degree and involve no distinction between mental disorder and mental health. This entails that each of us has a variety of PDs, i.e., a range of psychological traits that, if enhanced or improved, would increase our well-being. For example, one might be nervous about public speaking, or overly risk averse, impulsive, stubborn, and so on. Most PDs don't undermine our well-being too seriously but, nevertheless, we could all benefit from enhancing our PDs up to the point that further adjustment no longer provided any improvement in well-being. For legal purposes, it may sometimes be necessary to draw sharp dividing lines: between the ill and the healthy, the guilty and the not guilty, those who must be punished by imprisonment and those not, and so on. However, adopting welfarism would help discourage the belief that such lines correspond to ethically or medically significant divisions. By abandoning a conception of "normal" health, welfarist psychiatry doesn't distinguish between therapies (that aim to raise sub-normal health to normal health) and enhancements (that raise someone's well-being above normal levels). All effective psychiatric treatment of PDs can be considered enhancement in that all interventions aim to

---

[a] The welfarist account of psychiatry is an extension of the welfarist account of disability (Kahane & Savulescu, 2009; Savulescu & Kahane, 2011).

enhance well-being whatever the starting point. If we pair welfarist psychiatry with an egalitarian view of distributive justice (as is typical in healthcare), then we have reason to prioritize the treatment of more severe PDs that have a more serious impact on people's well-being. Therefore, psychiatric resources would still be weighted in favor of treating more severe PDs (including those that we currently recognize as "mental disorders") but, where cost-effective, resources would still be channeled toward milder PDs that we may not presently count as disorders proper.

PDs are context dependent. For example, the tendency to experience unusually high levels of social anxiety is a relatively severe PD for someone—like a politician—whose lifestyle involves many stressful social encounters but not for someone easily able to avoid such encounters, such as a forest worker.[b] Likewise, in some cases, having a diminished mental capacity can enhance well-being, for example, a decline in the specific recall of traumatic memories of someone with posttraumatic stress disorder may improve their wellbeing (Earp, Sandberg, Kahane, & Savulescu, 2014). For such a person a greater capacity for recall would count as a PD. PDs arise from mismatches between mental traits and the environment; they lack the essentialism of mental disorders that are assumed to be problems of "underlying mental functioning."[c] From the welfarist perspective, the debate over whether mental illnesses have organic pathologies or are just "problems in living" is irrelevant. If PDs happen to lack organic bases, the practice of psychiatry remains unthreatened as long as psychiatric methods (whether biological or interpersonal) prove effective in treating PDs.

Which traits are considered PDs and the relative and absolute severity of PDs depends on the conception of well-being the welfarist adopts. It is beyond the scope of the present work to defend a conception of well-being, but any feasible account of well-being must accommodate both subjective and objective perspectives. There is a subjective aspect to well-being because each person has a degree of first-person authority when they describe their subjective state as, say, distressed or content, and in establishing their own goals and values. There is an objective aspect to well-being because people can wrongly identify their subjective states, their best-interests, and the factors that influence attainment of those interests. Objective goods might include social relationships and personal development. For example, a dyspraxic stay at home mother may mistakenly believe that her dyspraxia reduces her capacity to care for the home, thus over-estimating the negative impact of dyspraxia on her well-being. It may be that her dyspraxia actually has no negative impact on her capacity to care for the home. In this case, she would be wrong to see her dyspraxia as a PD (assuming it didn't

---

[b] Even traits associated with (statistically) normal species functioning may qualify as PDs in certain conditions. For example, an IQ of 100 may constitute a PD in a culture where the only available jobs are either so boring that they leave all but the least intelligent people frustrated, or so difficult that they are unavailable to all but the most intelligent. Therefore, welfarist psychiatry is quite different to naturalist conceptions of mental illness which take mental illness to be an unnatural impediment to normal species functioning that are, inter alia, undesirable for their bearers (e.g., see Boorse, 1975).

[c] The welfarist can still distinguish between PDs that are predominantly caused by mental traits and those that are predominantly caused by the environment. Where a mental trait would result in a PD in a wide variety of the environments a person might realistically inhabit, it makes sense to say the PD is predominantly caused by the mental trait and vice versa.

undermine her well-being in other ways). More seriously, the value this woman places on caring for the home might be an "adaptive preference" (the phenomenon where people adjust their expectations to their circumstances). She might take herself to have relatively high well-being because she values caring for the home but, had she the option to pursue a profession, she might have enjoyed even greater well-being. Assuming that it is bad for people to live in deprived or disadvantageous circumstances, this indicates that well-being involves more than people's subjective assessments. Another reason not to rely solely on subjective considerations when assessing well-being is that subjective assessments of well-being tend not to be permanently affected either by catastrophe or good fortune. For example, people who become paraplegic suffer an initial decrease in happiness, but after a period of adaptation they report themselves to be about as happy as they were before becoming paraplegic (Kahneman & Varey, 1991); and winning the lottery only temporarily increases winners' happiness (Brickman, Coates, & Janoff-Bulman, 1978). Losing a loved one causes grief, but most people adapt. We want to allow for the possibility that becoming paraplegic or winning the lottery can have a long-term effect on well-being. This requires factoring objective elements into our conception of well-being; for example, allowing that loss of independence, loss of mobility, and increased financial security can affect a person's well-being in a way that does not depend entirely on how an individual responds emotionally to these things, or how happy that individual is. This conception fits with some plausible moral intuitions. For example, there are few who would not strongly condemn a surgeon who, in the absence of reasons making it very difficult or impossible to do so, failed to perform a procedure that could reverse a patient's paraplegia following an accident, and who defended this decision by observing that the patient will, in time, adapt to paraplegia. On the welfarist account, then, judgment as to whether someone has a PD depends on the patient's first-hand reports of their experience and their conception of a good life but also on an objective assessment of the patient's best interests. Clearly, subjective and objective elements of well-being can conflict. What a person most values and their happiness may conflict with their social relationships, or the capacity to develop their talents. It is beyond the scope of this chapter to try to address these fundamental value conflicts. For an evaluation of how different theories manage conflicts between subjective and objective components of well-being see Sarch (2012).

Considerations of well-being determine what counts as a PD, but they do not determine whether a PD should receive psychiatric treatment. The usual conditions of autonomous patient consent and consistency with distributive justice must also be met. Treatment cannot be forced on a patient even if it will increase his or her well-being and the patient might autonomously request treatments that will not address a PD or that risk undermining his well-being. We believe that doctors should accede to autonomous requests for such treatments (where they are legal) because supporting competent patients' autonomy over their bodies and psychologies is more important than increasing their welfare (Savulescu, 2007). However, those who believe that autonomy should sometimes be overridden in the name of welfare could still pursue a recognizable form of welfarist psychiatry. Similarly, different views of distributive justice will also yield variations in which PDs the welfarist should treat.

In addition to these familiar conditions on psychiatric treatment, however, there is a further condition that does not arise for the treatment of mental disorders. Whereas being diagnosed with a mental disorder entails that some form of psychiatric response is appropriate (given patient consent and distributive justice), having a PD underdetermines which institution is best suited to intervene. Somatic medicine, education, politics, and law are all motivated (at least in theory) by the general aim of improving people's lives, part of which involves preventing, mitigating, and treating PDs. Welfarist psychiatry is distinguished from these other fields, not by its aims, but its employment of psychiatric knowledge, techniques, and tools to achieve its aims.[d] So the category of PD is sufficiently broad that psychiatric treatment is not necessarily an appropriate response or the only appropriate response. This is especially clear when a PD is the result of prejudice. In a homophobic society, for example, being a homosexual is a PD because homosexuality reduces one's well-being in contrast to either being heterosexual in that society or being in a non-homophobic society.[e] Now, this PD could be resolved by changing people's sexuality with an as yet undiscovered psychiatric treatment (see Earp, Sandberg, & Savulescu, 2014) or by the elimination of prejudice, say through government-sponsored campaigns for gay rights. The welfarist can prioritize the governmental response over psychiatric responses on the grounds of justice; it is prejudiced society that is in the wrong, not the victims of that prejudice, and moral goodness is plausibly an element of objective well-being (Parfit, 1984). Furthermore, sometimes it is worth suffering with a PD because standing up for what is right is worth a cost to one's well-being. That said, the welfarist is more sanguine toward using psychiatry to help victims of prejudice than others might be. If there were poor prospects of alleviating a PD through non-psychiatric means (e.g., perhaps the government is complicit), there were psychiatric treatments that would improve well-being[f] and that were consistent with distributive justice, and the patient autonomously consented to treatment, then the welfarist position would recommend psychiatric treatment despite the PD being caused by prejudice (Earp, Sandberg, & Savulescu, 2014). To refuse to treat in these cases entails forcing a loss of well-being on victims of prejudice in order to fight prejudice.

To this point we have defined PDs as psychological traits that tend to undermine patient welfare. There is, however, another kind of PD—psychological traits that tend to undermine social welfare, e.g., impulsive and violent tendencies. Again, psychiatric treatment may not always be appropriate for such PDs or it may only form part of the response; the judicial system, for example, will often play a significant role. Two kinds of case where psychiatric resources are brought to bear are where a person displays pedophilic or psychopathic traits. In some cases, these PDs undermine the subject's well-being by causing distress but some pedophiles and most psychopaths are happy

---

[d] To avoid circularity here, we can understand "psychiatric knowledge, techniques, and tools" in the sort of sociological terms described in Cooper (2002).

[e] Kahane and Savulescu (2009) have argued that social prejudice should be excluded from the circumstances that are relevant to assessing disadvantageous states but here we follow Zohny (2016) in accepting that all circumstances are relevant.

[f] Given that such treatment involves an assault on self-concept it is only likely to improve well-being in inescapable contexts of relatively extreme prejudice.

with the way they are.[g] Whatever loss of personal welfare pedophiles and psychopaths suffer, clearly these conditions worry us most because of the potential for very serious losses of well-being for others. In fact, even if pedophiles and psychopaths suffered no loss in personal welfare we would still want to consider these PDs. By recognizing that social welfare contributes toward whether a condition counts as a PD, welfarism accommodates this intuition. The higher the risk of harm to others, the more severe the PD. When PDs pose sufficient risk to social welfare they can be treated for the benefit of others without patient consent and sometimes the patient may even be justifiably harmed. This concession doesn't necessarily pave the way for psychiatry to be used for morally dubious political ends. The limits of psychiatric power (like judicial power) can be set according to principles guiding the extent to which personal welfare can be overridden in the name of social welfare. Of course, there are disagreements over those principles and over how social welfare should be measured.[h] These issues are front and center when (below) we consider whether the West can justifiably limit the ways in which other cultures might want to use psychiatry.

Welfarist responses to global mental health challenges

Inadequacy of the Western psychiatric model

The Western psychiatric model based on the DSM-5 is the default conception of psychiatry that will be applied in the global context. This is because this model has become entrenched in the West and much of the funding and expertise for addressing global mental health will come from Western countries. However, the Western model is widely thought to have some serious flaws that undermine treatment and research which we should avoid passing on to other populations. One widespread concern is that many of the mental disorders described in the DSM-5 don't really exist.[i] The DSM-5 classifies and diagnoses mental disorders based on symptomatology which gives rise to two serious problems. First, we cannot be sure that we are correctly grouping symptoms together into different kinds of syndrome (Goldberg, 2010). Perhaps, for example, some of the instances of depressed thoughts, feelings, and behavior that we currently take to be part of the syndrome depression might actually be manifestations of different kinds of syndrome. A second problem is that the syndromes in the DSM have no connection to specific etiologies and so the DSM syndromes exhibit

---

[g] Accounts of well-being that include objective considerations such as "moral goodness" (Parfit, 1984) can say that there is a lack of well-being even in cases of happy pedophiles and psychopaths because neither are morally good (at least assuming they act on their harmful desires). If they resist acting on their impulses, then they would retain the objective quality of moral goodness but they would lose out on some well-being through having to struggle to control those impulses. A purely subjective account of well-being would be unable to say what is bad for the patient about being a happy pedophile or psychopath.

[h] In general, the Millian harm principle is a good place to start: that the sole ground for interference in liberty (and well-being) is significant harm to others (Mill, 2016).

[i] In what follows we focus on the DSM system but analogous arguments can be made against the World Health Organization's International Classification of Diseases system.

equifinality and multifinality. In equifinality, two cases with different etiologies present in similar ways. So when you classify disorders according to how they present, you end up with etiologically heterogeneous groups that are not helpfully treated in the same ways and that lead research astray (Uher & Rutter, 2012). In multifinality, the same underlying causes of mental disorder present in quite different ways depending on developmental context. When we group cases according to presentation, multifinality misleads us into dividing similar cases into different groups depowering research and misdirecting treatment. Equifinality and multifinality are problems for any nosology that first seeks valid classifications based on symptomatology and then moves to develop causal knowledge, e.g., Ghaemi (2012), Sinnott-Armstrong and Summers (2019), Banner (2013). The DSM system is also accused of facilitating the unjustified proliferation of new kinds of mental disorders and overdiagnosis because of the lack of a clear threshold between healthy and disordered states (McHugh & Treisman, 2007; Parker, 2005; Singh, Filipe, Bard, Bergey, & Baker, 2013).

The discovery of an underlying physiological pathology that characterized and caused each of the syndromes described by the DSM would go a long way toward resolving these problems. Such a pathology would validate the syndrome, create a clearer distinction between who had a disorder and who didn't, and specify an important part of syndrome etiology. It would also allow psychiatry to be easily applied in other contexts—if a population displayed the physiological pathology then they would have the syndrome (even if syndrome presentation varied somewhat by sociocultural context). Unfortunately, however, we have had little success in finding these biomarkers despite spending much time and effort searching for them. Nearly all the genetic risk factors we have found for schizophrenia for example, convey comparable risks for bipolar disorder, and for even other conditions such as depression, substance abuse and epilepsy (Insel et al., 2010). Despite this, many psychiatrists wishfully assume that physiological pathologies corresponding to each kind of mental disorder will be found. A growing body of research suggests that this assumption is likely to be false, e.g., Kendler and Gyngell (2019). The significant etiological influence of psychosocial factors is likely to entail that biological factors will be insufficient to explain which disorders develop and even whether a disorder develops (Levy, 2019). To continue to assume that the essential pathologies of each mental disorder are physiological over-emphasizes biological factors at the expense of psychosocial factors and encourages the view that psychiatric diagnosis is "an objective statement of fact" which is best treated by medication (British Psychological Society, 2013, pp. 2–3).[j]

So, to some extent, Western psychiatry is likely to be incorrectly pathologizing, misdiagnosing, overdiagnosing, and overtreating. Clearly, however, we cannot wait until we have developed a perfect form of psychiatry before we act to improve the treatment of mental illness in LMICs. Therefore, we will have to advance global psychiatry while simultaneously working to ameliorate the negative aspects

---

[j] It is often assumed that pharmacotherapy is the best way to treat physiological pathology but biological pathologies are not necessarily best treated by medication just because they are biological. For example, heart disease might be best treated by exercise and healthy diet.

of Western psychiatry. Welfarist psychiatry can help achieve this because it avoids a range of flaws in the Western psychiatric model.

Although welfarist psychiatry is symptom focussed, it does not make any assumptions regarding how PDs might be grouped into syndromes. Therefore, welfarist psychiatry just sidesteps the problem of correctly grouping symptoms into syndromes such as addiction, depression, bipolar disorder and so on. One might worry that this will mean that psychiatrists will often end up incompletely treating patients by only focussing on the most obvious symptoms of the patient's syndrome but this need not be the case. PDs will be statistically associated with one another so, based on the strength of those associations, the psychiatrist should look for any additional PDs associated with the presenting PD. In this way, the psychiatrist can treat the patient's particular constellation of symptoms without having to commit to labeling the patient with a particular syndrome that might be a poor fit. This leads to another concern that if welfarist psychiatry rejects the evidence-base developed to treat the DSM categories, then it will have to begin treatment design from scratch. Presumably, this would be grossly inefficient because there must be *some* truth in the research based on the DSM categories. The welfarist can, in fact, draw on the existing evidence-base but will do so with caution given multifinality and equifinality. Treatment guidelines developed for DSM syndromes are suggestive but must be taken with a grain of salt given that they have been tested on symptomatically heterogeneous groups of patients and those groups excluded people with similar symptoms but who failed to reach the DSM threshold. Therefore, the welfarist needn't abandon the existing evidence-base but would support further research to resolve the confusions built into that evidence by the DSM categories.

The dominant psychiatric paradigm is waiting on the discovery of essential etiology that will "validate" each kind of mental disorder and it is common to assume that the validating etiology will be an essential physiological pathology. PDs, in contrast, don't require such validation so the welfarist can get on with enhancing PDs without discovering their essential causes or if they are part of a wider syndrome. That said, the diagnosis of a PD underdetermines the etiology, the prognosis, and the most effective treatment so the welfarist is interested to discover these characteristics. However, the welfarist does not expect that the causes of PDs will be exclusively or even predominantly biological. The most significant causes may well be psychological and/or social especially since PDs are dependent on sociocultural context by definition.[k] Furthermore, it doesn't matter to the welfarist if the causes of a PD are essential to a *kind* of PD, it only matter what is causing *this* PD. This raises the objection that welfarist psychiatry will be inefficient, having to rediscover the causes of each kind of PD again and again. This isn't true, however. Although there is no assumption that PDs will fall into etiological kinds from the outset, if PDs happen to fall into etiological kinds, then the welfarist can take advantage of that by using similar treatments for each instance of the kind. A related concern is that the welfarist might end up

---

[k] As outlined above, even when we restrict ourselves to the narrower category of DSM defined disorders, the empirical evidence suggests that mental disorders are typically caused by a range of interacting factors across, biological, psychological and social levels.

inefficiently treating multiple symptoms that are downstream of a root cause rather than the root cause of the PDs. Again, although the welfarist has no preconception that different PDs will tend to arise together in a syndrome with a common cause, if such a syndromes exist, she can detect and address the common causes.

Moving away from the biology-focused disease model and considering instead the entire range of psychosocial factors that combine to reduce well-being, would reduce the current emphasis on medication as the primary means of treating PDs. A PD may be treated by addressing one or more of the biological, psychological, and/or sociocultural factors that contribute to a person's having a PD. The best form of treatment will be the one that best improves well-being. Someone whose high social anxiety qualifies as a PD, for example, could be helped by medication, talking therapy, or a career or other lifestyle change; none of which, in the absence of further information about the patient and his preferences, stands out as the best or most obvious option. That welfarism would widen the range of possible treatments for PDs would be a positive step for patient choice and autonomy. Welfarism discourages the view that a psychiatric diagnosis is always an objective statement of medical fact because well-being is partly subjective and dependent on local norms and social structures. The patient's own evaluation of how her well-being plays a key role in the diagnosis of a PD, and in the choice of treatment. On the welfarist approach, diagnosing a PD would simply not be possible without attending to the individual context of the patient. Doctors would be forced to look beyond the biological aspects of a psychological trait. The welfarist approach encourages doctors to get to know patients, which would be a step toward ensuring that those most in need of expert psychiatric assessment get the attention they require. This increased patient involvement should help address the marginalization of patients' views, experiences, and cultural context. To the extent that global mental health research already emphasizes psychosocial interventions and determinants of mental health it will fit more comfortably within the welfarist framework than the dominant psychiatric paradigm.

Another objection is that, even if welfarism doesn't prioritize pharmacotherapy, it may still worsen overtreatment and exaggerate the global mental health problem (Wakefield, 2007). This is because eliminating the distinction between serious mental disorders and less serious conditions removes one of the barriers to medicalization (Vilhelmsson, Svensson, & Meeuwisse, 2011, p. 213). Therefore, the welfarist sees opportunities to treat everywhere, including psychological traits above and beyond what we take to be normal healthy function. These concerns are misguided, however. The major concern with overtreatment is that people are receiving treatments (especially drugs) that are ineffective but welfarism only recommends treatment where it is expected to improve well-being. Welfarist psychiatry has the potential to target treatments to patients better than the DSM system because PDs are personalized while kinds of mental disorder are not. Additionally, considerations of distributive justice would ensure that resources were not disproportionately spent on milder PDs or PDs that would be more cost-effectively treated by other institutions, e.g., the judicial system. Welfarism won't exaggerate the scale of the global mental health problem because it aims to quantify the impact of PDs on well-being. The welfarist uses a continuum of severity so that milder PDs are counted for less and more severe PDs count for more.

Neo-colonialism

Even if Western psychiatry was perfectly calibrated to the Western context there would still be serious problems with the neocolonial imposition of Western conceptions of mental illness on non-Western contexts (Kopinak, 2015). The DSM diagnostic criteria are a distinctly American construction of mental illness, albeit one that has been largely adopted across the Western world. To the extent that mental illness is different in non-Western populations there will be a mismatch with the DSM system. There is good reason to think that mental illness will be different in non-Western populations because of the genetic and sociocultural variations between populations.[1] As already mentioned, there is a significant body of evidence indicating that the development of mental illness depends on the interaction between specific genetic and sociocultural factors, e.g., characteristics of peer groups and parents, cultural factors like gender-specific norms about smoking, and stressful life events (see for example, Bromet et al., 2011; Kendler & Gyngell, 2019; Tienari et al., 2004).

This data shows that the prevalence and severity of the DSM mental disorders vary by context but we should also expect to see different presentations of those disorders and even different *kinds* of disorder caused by interactions between unfamiliar genetic and sociocultural factors. There is evidence of culturally distinct forms of anorexia nervosa, PTSD, schizophrenia, depression, and social anxiety disorder (Kitanaka, 2012; Watters, 2010). In Japan, for example, taijin kyofusho appears to be a variant of social anxiety disorder where the sufferer has a fear of offending other people due to appearance or body odor. Perhaps this is created by a culture with a strong normative pressure to be sensitive to others' feelings.[m] Some syndromes may be sufficiently different from Western disorders to warrant separate diagnostic criteria, for example: "koro," found in Southeast Asia and Africa, involves a fear that one's sexual organs are disappearing or shrinking; "amok," found in Malaysia, where sufferers, typically males, withdraw and brood after a perceived slight and then erupt with a frenzy of violence; and "latah," found in Indonesia and Malaysia, where sufferers exhibit an exaggerated startle response while sometimes exclaiming normally inhibited sexually denotative words, but also often mimic others and readily obey others.[n]

A further consideration is that the local norms governing mentally healthy behavior vary somewhat independently of how psychological traits present. Certain behaviors

---

[1] Of course, this hasn't prevented studies based on DSM criteria from gathering results in non-Western populations. These studies appear to confirm the relevance of the DSM categories in non-Western populations but, in fact, they simply assume them; they lack the capacity to detect aspects of mental illness that don't conform to the DSM categories and so we cannot know the extent to which those categories distort reality. That said, there are certainly many common features to depression all around the world.

[m] There is also some evidence that the form of a disorder changes as the cultural context changes. The researcher Lee Sing contends that a form of anorexia existed in Hong Kong that wasn't characterized by unhappiness about being over-weight neither did it involve an unrealistic body image. In the mid-1990s this changed when the Western idea of anorexia was introduced by journalists and public health officials alarmed at the lack of preventative programs). Now most sufferers conform much more closely to the Western form of anorexia. (See Watters, 2010 for a summary of this research.)

[n] Despite clinical overlap with Tourette syndrome, it is now recognized as a distinct syndrome (Lanska, 2018).

may count as mentally unhealthy in one normative context, but are simply unusual in another, or are taken as a sign of being gifted in another. While there is a large literature on risk factors across regions, it is essential to bear in mind that what counts as a risk factor for mental illness depends on the correlation between that factor and behavior that breaks the local norms of mental health. If the norms of mental health are different between cultures, then so too are the factors that count as risk factors in that culture. Consequently, people who would never go on to be considered mentally ill by the local populace might be diagnosed as having a disorder or a risk factor by Western standards, while local variations in mental illness and associated risk factors might be awkwardly shoehorned into inappropriate DSM categories or left undiagnosed altogether (Bass, Bolton, & Murray, 2007).

Unfortunately, there are powerful political and economic motivations to impose Western psychiatric norms and categories globally (Singh et al., 2013). Pharmaceutical companies would prefer to sell the drugs they have developed for the Western market to the rest of the world because it is cheaper than investigating whether those drugs are effective in different contexts or developing new drugs (Jain & Jadhav, 2009). Similarly, governments and NGOs want to improve mental health as quickly and cheaply as possible so will be tempted to use the normative frameworks and treatments that are already available rather than spending the time and effort to calibrate them to the local populace. There is also pressure to quantify success in terms that make sense to Western donors and taxpayers. Furthermore, because Western psychiatry tends to assume the source of mental illness is at the level of the individual's biology; this directs focus away from the socio-political contexts that might significantly drive mental illness and makes it the individual's problem (Farmer, 2004; Summerfield, 2012). Therefore, repressive regimes and neocolonial interests may be eager to embrace this individualizing aspect of Western psychiatry for political gain and to the detriment of the local population's mental health. The welfarist approach can help resist these neocolonial political and economic forces and improve global mental health by rendering psychiatry sensitive to the local norms governing behavior and the local variations in the presentation of mental illness. Therefore, the welfarist approach should appeal to global mental health practitioners who are rightly concerned with addressing the social determinants of mental illness.

Welfarism is perfectly positioned to prevent neocolonial psychiatry because PDs are indexed to patient well-being and local patients' well-being is intimately connected with their particular sociocultural, environmental and genetic situation. Welfarist psychiatry is, therefore, open to the possibility that the kind of things undermining or promoting well-being in LMICs may be quite different from those in the West. The local variation in the factors that cause PDs presumably give rise to conditions such as koro, amok, and latah, as well as culturally specific variations on the conditions are familiar with in the West, e.g., taijin kyofusho. Where these conditions undermine well-being, they count as PDs. Clearly the symptoms of koro, amok, and latah undermine patient well-being and, in the case of amok, social welfare as well. The severity of these PDs depends on the extent to which it undermines personal and social well-being in the local context.

Welfarist psychiatry also accommodates the influence on PDs of the local norms governing behavior; the welfarist doesn't assume that the Western norms for behavior are universal. PDs typically develop when individuals consistently breach their society's norms, because individuals who fail to follow norms are exposed to distressing social opprobrium and threat of further sanction. Where these norms differ between cultures, so to do the range of behaviors that develop into PDs. For example, in cultures that expect long periods of mourning, long-running depressive symptoms that would be counted as PDs in the West will not cause much concern and so won't be PDs, or will count as less severe PDs. Indeed, to *not* exhibit depressive symptoms throughout the expected mourning period might count as a PD. Likewise, particular patterns of substance use might be PDs in one culture but not another depending on local norms governing intoxication and pleasure-seeking. Cultural differences in value entail that each culture will prioritize the treatment of PDs differently so that, from the perspective of outsiders, it will seem that relatively mild PDs are being treated while apparently more serious PDs are being neglected. These different prioritizations are justified as long as well-being is maximally enhanced in each normative context (within the limits of distributive justice).

Given this sensitivity to local variations in PDs and their causes, welfarist psychiatry highlights the risk of allowing pharmaceutical companies to sell existing drugs in new contexts without clinical testing. Of course, it may be better to allow distribution of drugs despite the risk rather than delay treatment and spend money on clinical trials. Nevertheless, the welfarist account makes this risk clear, whereas those who assume Western conceptions of mental disorders are universal are likely to cause harm through ignoring this risk. Furthermore, welfarist psychiatry is open to the potential efficacy of local treatments (pending clinical trials) given that they may well be more suited to the local conditions.

The welfarist's emphasis on the role of sociocultural context should also help avoid the detrimental power dynamic created when mental disorders are assumed to be inherent to individuals and so be an individual's problem rather than a social problem. Welfarist psychiatry like any form of psychiatry has limited political power. It is better placed to intervene at the level of the individual rather than the individual's sociocultural context. However, welfarist psychiatry doesn't make the bioreductive assumption that PDs develop exclusively at the individual level and so are problems only for, or related to, the individual. So, if certain political policies are causing PDs, welfarist psychiatry can highlight that publicly and can let individual patients know when their PDs are significantly caused by sociopolitical factors.

Avoiding prejudicial and harmful forms of psychiatry globally

Given the fundamental issues with Western psychiatry and the problems of neocolonialism, we might be tempted to simply adopt whatever conception of mental health and treatment is used locally. This, however, faces the problem that local norms of mental health are not necessarily right, and local treatments are not necessarily effective just because they are local. Such norms might create false mental illnesses out of prejudice or for political ends, e.g., homosexuality, or ignore real mental illness. After all, until

1973, the APA pathologized homosexuality which provided official support for humiliating and traumatic "conversion therapies." Even those Western psychiatrists who are suspicious of the DSM categories would feel certain that homosexuality is not a mental disorder. But what are the grounds for this certainty? Similarly, even where the presence of mental illness is not in dispute, the locally preferred means of treatment might, to Western eyes, appear ineffective or detrimental for patients, e.g., untested herbal remedies or spiritual interventions aimed at removing evil spirits. Are there objective grounds on which to exclude ineffective or harmful treatments? If well-being is at least partly objective, this would block objectively harmful treatments. For example, female infibulation might remove the capacity for sexual functioning, which is a part of the good life. Whether or not it is desired, it is harmful on an objective account of well-being, as we will argue in greater detail below.

A related concern is that many LMICs exhibit a strong stigma toward people with mental illness and a disinclination to care for them (Becker & Kleinman, 2013; Olugbile, Zachariah, Coker, Kuyinu, & Isichei, 2008; Razzouk et al., 2010; Shibre et al., 2001). Stigmatized individuals tend to adopt harmful coping mechanisms such as secrecy or withdrawal (Link, Cullen, Struening, Shrout, & Dohrenwend, 1989). Yet normative pressure and opprobrium, the close relatives of stigma, play an important social role. Sometimes normative pressure results in positive behavioral change and sometimes a society needs to exclude or marginalize dangerous or uncooperative people for social welfare. When individuals' behavior breaches social norms, what grounds are there to insist those people are mentally ill and require medical treatment when the local population sees them as dangerous, uncooperative and deserving of opprobrium and sanctions? Clearly, we need some objective standard to justify the imposition of norms and practices on other cultures. The welfarist account can provide a helpful solution as we describe below.

The welfarist's sensitivity to local norms raises the risk that the welfarist will accommodate *any* psychiatric practices and norms, even those that are clearly immoral, ineffective, or harmful. Welfarist psychiatry entails a default preference for treatments and norms favored by the local population because such treatments and norms will tend to be better received, and so result in greater personal and social welfare, than if one insists on disfavored treatments and norms. However, this default position can be overridden by consideration of objective aspects of well-being. The best treatments and norms are those that result in the greatest increases in well-being taking into consideration both subjective and objective aspects of well-being. So, the welfarist doesn't assume that patients and local populations are necessarily right in their assessments of well-being and what influences it.

To illustrate these points, reconsider the example where a culture is prejudiced against homosexuality and there is pressure to treat homosexuality with psychiatric interventions. As discussed above, homosexuality would count as a PD in this culture because the attitudes of others would clearly undermine the well-being of homosexual people. This wouldn't, however, necessarily justify psychiatric treatment primarily because treatment requires patient consent (and the patient would have several good reasons not to consent). But, as we have also seen, treatment without consent can be justified when a PD is a threat to social welfare. We can imagine a society where homosexuality is seen as such a threat to social welfare that the society believes the conditions are met to justify treatment without consent. The welfarist can reject this application of psychiatry, however, because this society is wrong that homosexuality risks social welfare.[o] Just as there are objective and subjective aspects to personal welfare there are objective and "subjective" aspects to social welfare. Social welfare would be undermined because of the distress felt by the prejudiced public based on their false beliefs about the threat of homosexuality but, objectively, homosexuality wouldn't undermine social welfare at all. In fact, social welfare would probably improve if homosexual people were treated as free and equal (and it would improve further if the prejudiced public accepted that).

Another kind of challenging case is where both the local public and the patient favor a form of ineffective, dubiously effective, or harmful treatment. For example, consider a homosexual man who agrees with his local culture's negative assessment of homosexuality and so would consent to conversion therapy if it were available. The objective evidence about these treatments is that they are ineffective in changing sexuality and cause serious harm (Beckstead & Morrow, 2004). In this case, the welfarist should restrict access to the treatment because it is highly likely that the objective harm to well-being will far outstrip the subjective benefit of receiving a favored treatment. Where favored treatments only risk a small amount of harm it might, on balance, be worth providing them for the subjective improvement in well-being. Where possible, welfare may be maximized by providing dubiously effective interventions that have a low risk of harm in parallel with treatments that are known to improve objective well-being. The promotion of treatments unpopular with the local culture will be justified to the extent that they are expected to raise objective aspects of well-being sufficiently that it will outweigh the subjective cost to well-being. But, of course, this would never justify forced treatment of autonomous patients.

One might object that the welfarist approach remains neocolonial because the supposedly objective assessment of well-being will be an inherently Western conception of well-being. In response, the welfarist can readily admit that epistemic humility requires the accommodation of reasonable disagreement over which factors influence well-being and how much they do so. Despite differences between reasonable assessments of well-being, there will be significant consensus especially over more serious mental illnesses (Stein, 2012). Nevertheless, some views of well-being will remain unreasonable. So, it is possible to accommodate different culture's views on well-being while still ruling out certain psychiatric practices and norms that would be bad for well-being on any reasonable view. Of course, this raises the issue of what counts as reasonable but we cannot do justice to that debate here.

Finally, welfarist psychiatry should help to reduce stigma against people with mental illness both in LMICs and the West. On the welfarist model, there would not be

---

[o] When working in such a society it might be tempting to appeal to the DSM position that homosexuality is not a disorder. Although this might be an expedient solution, it comes with the significant downside of reifying the authority of the DSM when there are serious concerns that it undermines good psychiatry. Of course, one might only appeal to the DSM when it happens to align with immediate goals and otherwise ignore it but such inconsistency undermines credibility.

a well-defined group of "mentally ill" people to stigmatize and there would be fewer accurate generalizations about what those diagnosed with PDs are like. This is because we all have psychological traits that, to a greater or lesser extent, make our lives worse given the environments we inhabit, and which limit the realization of our potential. These may be as debilitating as severe depression or as mild as a tendency to procrastinate. While this is unlikely to eliminate stigmatization and discrimination— these attitudes hardly require accurate generalizations about those at whom they are directed—emphasizing that PDs affect us all would be a step toward breaking down the perceived divide between the mentally ill and the normal. Treating people with stigma is not usually the result of careful reflection, however, it might be the case that certain populations would prefer to treat the mentally ill with stigma rather than psychiatric care. After all, many in the West continue to feel that addiction should be met with sanctions rather than healthcare. The welfarist can guide which PDs to treat with psychiatric care and when to use judicial sanctions or stigma based on the impact these interventions have on personal and social well-being. The promotion of psychiatric care for addiction and other PDs is justified where it improves personal and social well-being. For many kinds of PD, judicial sanction and stigma undermine well-being and when they do they would not be endorsed on a welfarist approach.

Conclusion

Welfarist psychiatry can be used to improve global mental health without passing on the problematic concept of "mental disorder," the contested DSM syndromes, and unhelpful bioreductionist assumptions; all of which haunt mainstream Western psychiatry. The welfarist also avoids the neocolonial imposition of Western norms and treatments on others by being sensitive to the relationship between the patient's psychological traits and his or her environmental context. This includes sensitivity to the local norms governing behavior and mental health. There is no assumption that the treatments and norms that have proven effective in the Western context will be effective in other contexts. But neither does the welfarist assume that the local population's preferences for mental health norms and treatments are ideal just because they have developed locally. By appealing to objective measures of personal and social well-being, welfarist psychiatry can prevent harmful applications of psychiatry without neocolonial imposition of the West's values. Finally, welfarist psychiatry contributes to reducing stigma by abandoning the strict distinction between "normal" mental health and "abnormal" mental illness.

Acknowledgments

The Wellcome Centre for Ethics and Humanities is supported by a Wellcome Centre Grant (203132/Z/16/Z). Julian Savulescu, through his involvement with the Murdoch Children's Research Institute, received funding through from the Victorian State Government through the Operational Infrastructure Support (OIS) Program.

References

American Psychiatric Association. (2013). *Diagnostic and statistical manual of mental disorders* (5th ed.). London: American Psychiatric Publishing.

Banner, N. F. (2013). Mental disorders are not brain disorders. *Journal of Evaluation in Clinical Practice, 19*(3), 509–513.

Bass, J. K., Bolton, P. A., & Murray, L. K. (2007). Do not forget culture when studying mental health. *Lancet (London, England), 370*(9591), 918–919.

Becker, A. E., & Kleinman, A. (2013). Mental health and the global agenda. *New England Journal of Medicine, 369*(1), 66–73.

Beckstead, A. L., & Morrow, S. L. (2004). Mormon clients' experiences of conversion therapy. *The Counseling Psychologist, 32*(5), 651–690.

Boorse, C. (1975). On the distinction between disease and illness. *Philosophy & Public Affairs, 5*, 49–68. Wiley.

Brickman, P., Coates, D., & Janoff-Bulman, R. (1978). Lottery winners and accident victims: Is happiness relative? *Journal of Personality and Social Psychology, 36*(8), 917–927.

British Psychological Society. (2013). *Classification of behaviour and experience in relation to functional psychiatric diagnoses: Time for a paradigm shift*. Leicester: British Psychological Society.

Bromet, E., Andrade, L. H., Hwang, I., Sampson, N. A., Alonso, J., de Girolamo, G., et al. (2011). Cross-national epidemiology of DSM-IV major depressive episode. *BMC Medicine, 9*(1), 90.

Collins, P. Y., Patel, V., Joestl, S. S., March, D., Insel, T. R., Daar, A. S., et al. (2011). Grand challenges in global mental health. *Nature, 475*(7354), 27–30.

Cooper, R. (2002). Disease. *Studies in History and Philosophy of Biological and Biomedical Sciences, 33*, 263–282.

Earp, B. D., Sandberg, A., Kahane, G., & Savulescu, J. (2014). When is diminishment a form of enhancement? Rethinking the enhancement debate in biomedical ethics. *Frontiers in Systems Neuroscience, 8*, 12.

Earp, B. D., Sandberg, A., & Savulescu, J. (2014). Brave new love: The threat of high-tech "conversion" therapy and the bio-oppression of sexual minorities. *AJOB Neuroscience, 5*(1), 4–12. https://doi.org/10.1080/21507740.2013.863242.

Farmer, P. (2004). An anthropology of structural violence. *Current Anthropology, 45*(3), 305–325.

Ghaemi, N. (2012). Taking disease seriously: Beyond "pragmatic" nosology. In K. S. Kendler & J. Parnas (Eds.), *Philosophical issues in psychiatry II: Nosology* (pp. 42–53). Oxford: Oxford University Press.

Goldberg, D. (2010). Should our major classifications of mental disorders be revised? *British Journal of Psychiatry, 196*(4), 255–256.

Insel, T., Cuthbert, B., Garvey, M., Heinssen, R., Pine, D. S., Quinn, K., et al. (2010). Research domain criteria (RDoC): Toward a new classification framework for research on mental disorders. *American Journal of Psychiatry, 167*(7), 748–751. https://doi.org/10.1176/appi.ajp.2010.09091379.

Jain, S., & Jadhav, S. (2009). Pills that swallow policy: Clinical ethnography of a community mental health program in northern India. *Transcultural Psychiatry, 46*(1), 60–85.

Kahane, G., & Savulescu, J. (2009). The welfarist account of disability. In K. Brownlee & A. Cureton (Eds.), *Disability and disadvantage* (pp. 15–53). Oxford: Oxford University Press.

Kahneman, D., & Varey, C. (1991). Notes on the psychology of utility. In J. Elster & J. E. Roemer (Eds.), *Interpersonal comparisons of well-being* (pp. 127–163). New York: Cambridge University Press.

Kakuma, R., Minas, H., Van Ginneken, N., Dal Poz, M. R., Desiraju, K., Morris, J. E., et al. (2011). Human resources for mental health care: Current situation and strategies for action. *The Lancet*, *378*(9803), 1654–1663.

Kendler, K. S., & Gyngell, C. (2019). Multi-level interactions and the dappled causal world of psychiatric disorders. In W. Davies, J. Savulescu, & R. Roache (Eds.), *Rethinking the biopsychosocial model*. Oxford: Oxford University Press.

Kitanaka, J. (2012). *Depression in Japan: Psychiatric cures for a society in distress*. Princeton: Princeton University Press.

Kopinak, J. K. (2015). Mental health in developing countries: Challenges and opportunities in introducing western mental health system in Uganda. *International Journal of MCH and AIDS*, *3*(1), 22–30.

Lanska, D. J. (2018). Jumping Frenchmen, Miryachit, and Latah: Culture-specific Hyperstartle-plus syndromes. *Frontiers of Neurology and Neuroscience*, *42*, 122–131.

Levy, N. (2019). The truth in social construction. In W. Davies, J. Savulescu, & R. Roache (Eds.), *Rethinking the biopsychosocial model*. Oxford: Oxford University Press.

Link, B. G., Cullen, F. T., Struening, E., Shrout, P. E., & Dohrenwend, B. P. (1989). A modified labeling theory approach to mental disorders: An empirical assessment. *American Sociological Review*, *54*(3), 400.

McHugh, P. R., & Treisman, G. (2007). PTSD: A problematic diagnostic category. *Journal of Anxiety Disorders*, *21*(2), 211–222.

Mill, J. S. (2016). *On liberty*. Los Angeles: Enhanced Media Publishing.

Olugbile, O., Zachariah, M. P., Coker, O., Kuyinu, O., & Isichei, B. (2008). Provision of mental health services in Nigeria. *International Psychiatry*, *5*(2), 32–34.

Parfit, D. (1984). *Reasons and persons*. Oxford: Clarendon Press.

Parker, G. (2005). Beyond major depression. *Psychological Medicine*, *35*(4), 467–474.

Patel, V., Chisholm, D., Parikh, R., Charlson, F. J., Degenhardt, L., Dua, T., et al. (2016). Addressing the burden of mental, neurological, and substance use disorders: Key messages from Disease Control Priorities, 3rd edition. *The Lancet*, *387*(10028), 1672–1685.

Razzouk, D., Sharan, P., Gallo, C., Gureje, O., Lamberte, E. E., de Jesus Mari, J., et al. (2010). Scarcity and inequity of mental health research resources in low-and-middle income countries: A global survey. *Health Policy*, *94*(3), 211–220.

Roache, R., & Savulescu, J. (2018). Psychological disadvantage and a welfarist approach to psychiatry: An alternative to the DSM paradigm. *Philosophy, Psychiatry, and Psychology*, *25*(4), 245–259.

Sarch, A. F. (2012). Multi-component theories of well-being and their structure. *Pacific Philosophical Quarterly*, *93*(4), 439–471. https://doi.org/10.1111/j.1468-0114.2012.01434.x.

Savulescu, J. (2007). Autonomy, the good life, and controversial choices. In R. Rhodes, L. P. Francis, & A. Silvers (Eds.), *The Blackwell guide to medical ethics*. Oxford: Blackwell.

Savulescu, J., & Kahane, G. (2011). Disability: A welfarist approach. *Clinical Ethics*, *6*(1), 45–51.

Saxena, S., Thornicroft, G., Knapp, M., & Whiteford, H. (2007). Resources for mental health: Scarcity, inequity, and inefficiency. *The Lancet*, *370*(9590), 878–889.

Shibre, T., Negash, A., Kullgren, G., Kebede, D., Alem, A., Fekadu, A., et al. (2001). Perception of stigma among family members of individuals with schizophrenia and major affective disorders in rural Ethiopia. *Social Psychiatry and Psychiatric Epidemiology*, *36*(6), 299–303.

Singh, I., Filipe, A. M., Bard, I., Bergey, M., & Baker, L. (2013). Globalization and cognitive enhancement: Emerging social and ethical challenges for ADHD clinicians. *Current Psychiatry Reports*, *15*(9), 385.

Sinnott-Armstrong, W., & Summers, J. (2019). Which biopsychosocial view of mental illness? In W. Davies, J. Savulescu, & R. Roache (Eds.), *Rethinking the biopsychosocial model*. Oxford: Oxford University Press.

Stein, D. J. (2012). Positive mental health: A note of caution. *World Psychiatry: Official Journal of the World Psychiatric Association (WPA)*, *11*(2), 107–109. Retrieved from: http://www.ncbi.nlm.nih.gov/pubmed/22654942.

Summerfield, D. (2012). Afterword: Against "global mental health". *Transcultural Psychiatry*, *49*(3–4), 519–530.

Tienari, P., Wynne, L. C., Sorri, A., Lahti, I., Läksy, K., Moring, J., et al. (2004). Genotype-environment interaction in schizophrenia-spectrum disorder. Long-term follow-up study of Finnish adoptees. *The British Journal of Psychiatry: the Journal of Mental Science*, *184*, 216–222.

Uher, R., & Rutter, M. (2012). Basing psychiatric classification on scientific foundation: Problems and prospects. *International Review of Psychiatry*, *24*(6), 591–605.

Vilhelmsson, A., Svensson, T., & Meeuwisse, A. (2011). Mental ill health, public health and medicalization. *Public Health Ethics*, *4*(3), 207–217.

Wakefield, J. C. (2007). The concept of mental disorder: Diagnostic implications of the harmful dysfunction analysis. *World Psychiatry: Official Journal of the World Psychiatric Association (WPA)*, *6*(3), 149–156.

Watters, E. (2010). *Crazy like us*. New York: Simon and Schuster.

Whiteford, H. A., Ferrari, A. J., Degenhardt, L., Feigin, V., & Vos, T. (2015). The global burden of mental, neurological and substance use disorders: An analysis from the global burden of disease study 2010. *PLoS ONE*, *10*(2), e0116820.

World Health Organization. (2011). *Global burden of mental disorders and the need for a comprehensive, coordinated response from health and social sectors at the country level*.

World Health Organization. (2013). *WHO comprehensive mental health action plan 2013–2020*.

Zohny, H. (2016). Enhancement, disability and the riddle of the relevant circumstances. *Journal of Medical Ethics*, *42*(9), 605–610.

The ethics of flourishing or failing: Social, economic and environmental determinants of global mental health in an uncertain future

Mark Tomlinson[a,b], Xanthe Hunt[a], Sarah Skeen[a]
[a]Institute for Life Course Health Research, Faculty of Medicine and Health Sciences, Stellenbosch University, Stellenbosch, South Africa, [b]School of Nursing and Midwifery, Queens University, Belfast, United Kingdom

Introduction

By most accounts, the last 60 years has been a period of increasing human flourishing. We have seen massive reductions in global poverty, improved communication and transportation infrastructure, overall reductions in levels of violence, and the establishment of a global political order overseen by the United Nations. In health, there have been remarkable declines in neonatal and child mortality, and a marked improvement in access to water and sanitation. This rosy picture however masks another bleaker view. In the area of human nutrition, a recent estimate is that there are approximately 800 million hungry people globally compared to 460 million in 1974 (Hickel, 2017). There are also currently more than 40 active conflicts across the world, coupled with a recent rise in populism and xenophobia. And all of this against a background of rapid technological and climatic change and a resulting set of potentially unprecedented threats to human well-being.

We are also experiencing global increases in mental ill health. The World Economic Forum estimates that between 2011 and 2030, mental health conditions will cost the global economy $16 trillion (Bloom et al., 2012), accrued primarily through lost labor and capital output (Jones et al., 2014). As a result of initiatives such as the World Health Organization's Commission on Social Determinants of Health (World Health Organization, 2008) and the work of Marmot and others (Marmot et al., 2008), we are beginning to better understand how poverty and adversity impact on mental health. However, significantly less is known about the social, economic and environmental factors that will underlie population mental health in the future, and how best to bolster potential protective factors and mitigate possible future threats. The Sustainable Development Goals (SDGs) provide a roadmap and indicators for improving human capital leading to 2030, and at the forefront of these goals is a recognition of systemic interactions between people and planet. It is an opportune time to consider these in relation to mental health.

Global Mental Health and Neuroethics. https://doi.org/10.1016/B978-0-12-815063-4.00005-8

These interactions will determine the types of questions neuroethicists will have to answer in the next decade and the challenges global mental health as a field will face. As we will show, the deep inequities across the world driven by developmental progress in some regions and within some countries, coupled with little or no progress in others, have created a host of economic, social and psychological factors that will drive human mental health in the future. Extreme inequality places some populations at increased risk, as others strive to ensure their own progress. The rise of nationalist populists is evidence for this shift away from the globalist vision that has dominated political and social worlds since the end of the Second World War. Balancing the imperative of development and the good it can do, with the unintentional harms and inequities that can result, will entail a contemplation of emergent risks.

A key aspect of neuroethics is a philosophical focus on what it means to be a human being, and not simply about understanding of the new technologies now being used in neuroscience and other disciplines (Levy, 2008). Climate breakdown, humanitarian crises and new emerging threats will undoubtedly pose complex questions about who we are as human beings and how we are to relate to one another in a global context of increasing fragility and conflict. This chapter will provide an overview of our current understanding of the social determinants of mental health, and provide a link to the future by way of an exploration of a selected group of social, economic and environmental risks that neuroethics needs to consider over the next two decades. We will conclude the chapter by suggesting a set of key actions to mitigate the effects of an uncertain future on global mental health.

Social determinants of mental health

Health status is strongly influenced by the social, economic and political forces that shape how people live (World Health Organization, 2008). Marmot's seminal work—the Whitehall Studies—showed that socio-economic position is a key determinant of health (Marmot et al., 1991). These studies showed how British civil servants at the "bottom" of the job ladder were in fact the ones suffering from poor health, rather than the so-called "stressed" leadership that conventional wisdom at the time dictated were the ones dying young from stress-induced heart failure and other health complaints. In fact, job insecurity and work characterized by low control and low satisfaction were the strongest predictors of poor health (Marmot et al., 1991). The mechanism that Marmot posited for this was the protective nature of "being in control of one's life" (Marmot, 2015). Subsequent research has unequivocally supported these findings and has been extended to mental health to show that people lower in socio-economic positions tend to have poorer mental health (Fryers, Jenkins, & Melzer, 2004; Fryers, Melzer, & Jenkins, 2003; Fryers, Melzer, Jenkins, & Brugha, 2005; Lund et al., 2010; Rubin, Evans, & Wilkinson, 2016; Rubin & Kelly, 2015; Rubin & Stuart, 2018). Depression for instance shows a clear poverty gradient with a wealth of evidence that shows higher rates of depression among poorer groups in high income countries (HIC) (Fisher et al., 2012), as well as higher rates in low and middle income countries (LMIC) compared to HIC (Cooper et al., 1999).

People living in poverty are vulnerable to a range of risk factors affecting their health, including poor education, food insecurity and malnutrition, poor household living conditions, environmental toxins, and lack of access to clean water and sanitation (Braveman & Gruskin, 2003; Marmot et al., 2008). For many, the costs of seeking healthcare may be unaffordable or even catastrophic (Saksena, Hsu, & Evans, 2014). Many protective behaviors, such as exclusive breast-feeding, school attendance, and sustained employment, which themselves depend on a good level of health, are under threat when living in poverty (Lu, Black, & Richter, 2016; Rollins et al., 2016). Prospective longitudinal studies have consistently shown that poor people are at increased risk of developing health problems, and this is also true for mental health specifically.

Poverty has been described as poison to the young human brain (Krugman, 2008; Lende, 2012), and it is well established that children living in poverty experience poorer development than peers not living in poverty. Yet, the mechanisms underlying this association have only more recently come into focus. The current model for conceptualizing the deleterious impacts of poverty on the developing brain, take into consideration a host of proximate and distal factors associated with impoverishment (Lende, 2012). Poverty associated with a host of household-level factors (violence exposure, insecure housing, food insecurity), directly impacts on the child's neurobiological and hormonal systems, through biological embedding (Miller & Chen, 2013). The mechanism by which poverty impacts on brain development is now understood to be the result of chronic stress (Garner, Shonkoff, Committee on Psychosocial Aspects of Child and Family Health, Committee on Early Childhood, Adoption, & Dependent Care and Section on Developmental and Behavioral Pediatrics, 2012; Shonkoff, Garner, Committee on Psychosocial Aspects of Child and Family Health, Committee on Early Childhood, Adoption, & Dependent Care and Section on Developmental and Behavioral Pediatrics, 2012).

Dohrenwend et al. (1992) were among the first to note the relationship between social causes and mental health, described an inverse relations between psychiatric disorders and socioeconomic status, and explored two competing causal pathways responsible for this phenomenon. More recently, researchers have shown how poverty and mental illness interact in a negative cycle (Patel & Kleinman, 2003). Lund and colleagues have expanded upon Dohrenwend et al.'s (1992) original pathways, postulating that these operate bi-directionally—the social drift/social selection pathway and the social causation pathway (Lund et al., 2011, 2018)—rather than two separate pathways. The social causation hypothesis posits that people living in poverty are more likely to develop mental health problems as a result of the numerous risks to which they are exposed (Lund et al., 2011), such as the chronic stress of poverty, unemployment and poor access to health services (Lund et al., 2010). The social drift or social selection hypothesis shows how people with a mental illness are more at risk of drifting into poverty due to economic vulnerability, reduced productivity, increased health expenditure, and not being able to secure or maintain employment (Lund et al., 2011). The Social Determinants of Health Final Report in 2008 was one of the first high-level initiatives to explicitly highlight the role of social determinants in shaping population mental health (World Health

Organization, 2008), and made a specific link between mental illness and, for example, employment. The report highlighted two arguments critical to understanding the social drivers of mental health (World Health Organization, 2008). Firstly, it focused on the complexity of the relationship between social factors and mental health outcomes. Specifically, it described how exposure to risk to mental health starts before birth, persists throughout the life course, and through a combination of environmental and biological mechanisms is passed on to the next generation (World Health Organization, 2008). Understanding child and adolescent development is essential to understanding the antecedents of later mental illness. A life course perspective encourages us to focus on how the determinants of health operate synergistically or in an additive manner across early childhood, childhood, adolescence, adulthood, and old age, and how they might exert their influence either now (during the exposure), or later (following exposure). This perspective aligns with the imperatives of neuroethics to think comprehensively about maximizing human mental capital for the good of the individual and society (United Kingdom Government Office for Science, 2008).

In a recent paper Lund et al. (2018) provide guidelines for optimizing the SDGs to address mental health. The paper shows how current knowledge about the social determinants of mental health—from the level of the individual to the level of the community and beyond—map onto key SDG targets. For instance, rates of trauma and distress—which lead to mental health disorders—could be brought down if environmental disasters and humanitarian crises were prevented, or at least better systems to mitigate their effects were established (SDGs 13 and 16). The review then examines all the specific evidence for the most established types of social determinants in different domains of human environment, and reflects on how the SDGs—as broad as they are—could be used a springboard from which to address the specific causes of mental health problems.

Education, occupation and mental illness

In mental health, there are numerous examples of how a variety of social outcomes as well as social factors are linked with mental health status. In education, there is evidence of an association between educational attainment and common mental disorders in both HIC and LMIC (Allen, Balfour, Bell, & Marmot, 2014; Andermann, 2016; Armstrong, 1994; Kokko, Pulkkinen, & Puustinen, 2000; Lund et al., 2010; Neighbors et al., 2007). It should also be noted however that some studies from HIC have found no such association (Jaffee, 2002; Jokela et al., 2010; Marmot, Shipley, Brunner, & Hemingway, 2001). The pathway from mental illness to low educational attainment, is as follows: mental health disorders, or even subclinical mental health problems, increase the likelihood that individuals will become disengaged from education (Henry, 2010; Herbig, Dragano, & Angerer, 2013; Waghorn & Chant, 2005). In addition, the path from low attainment to mental health problems may be related to feelings of hopelessness and disengagement arising from educational difficulty or dropout which then results in mental health problems (Benjet et al., 2012; Fergusson, Horwood, & Woodward, 2001; Herbig et al., 2013).

Occupation is also an important social determinant of wellbeing. Some jobs create risk of mental disorder, including those characterized by high levels of job demands (especially emotional demands), as well as insecure jobs (Stansfeld, Rasul, Head, & Singleton, 2011). As much as stressful employment may contribute to increased mental health risk, employment is also a significant contributor to good mental health. For people experiencing mental health problems, for instance, engaging in personally meaningful and socially valued occupations is an important aid to better coping (Doroud, Fossey, & Fortune, 2015). Subjective evaluation of one's socio-economic position has also been shown to contribute to the burden of disorder and distress (Adler, Epel, Castellazzo, & Ickovics, 2000; Twenge & Campbell, 2002). Low socioeconomic position has also been shown to be associated with low self-esteem (Twenge & Campbell, 2002), and low self-esteem is in turn associated with poorer mental health (Sowislo & Orth, 2013). Socioeconomic position also has a buffering effect on stress, with the mental health of married men of lower socio-economic position more greatly impacted by unemployment, than men of higher socioeconomic position (Artazcoz, Benach, Borrell, & Cortès, 2004). A similar pattern emerges among women, with unemployment having a differential effect on mental health depending on socio-economic position (Artazcoz et al., 2004).

Low socio-economic position is linked to a range of mental disorders, including schizophrenia, depressive illness, substance misuse and personality disorders (Dohrenwend et al., 1992; Lund, Stansfeld, & de Silva, 2014). The influence differs depending on when in life it is experienced. Low SES in childhood is associated with a higher risk of internalizing and externalizing disorders, and internalizing symptoms in adulthood (Gilman, 2002). In adulthood, depression is strongly correlated with lower SES within countries, but not across them—suggesting that perceived inequality plays a substantial role (Lorant et al., 2003). Taking action to improve the conditions of daily life from before birth, throughout the life course, will be imperative if population mental health is to be improved and the risk of those mental disorders that are associated with social inequalities is to be reduced (World Health Organization, 2008).

A grounding in neuroethics prompts us to recognize the role of equality in this picture. Individual mental health is influenced substantially by relative position in society, rather than absolute wealth. Evolutionarily, lower mood in relation to social hierarchy is near universal in primate societies, and has been suggested may serve an adaptive function (Hendrie & Pickles, 2009; Rohde, 2001). At the level of individual countries and communities, then, the conditions of daily life of those who are most vulnerable and least well off must be prioritized for intervention. Not only will this ameliorate the impacts of social causes directly linked to poverty, but it may also have a positive impact on the effects of inequality on human mental health (Taylor, Moghaddam, Gamble, & Zellerer, 1987).

Further complicating the picture is the fact that, as much as health outcomes are variable across time depending on inputs from the environment, environmental inputs themselves in constant flux. Factors that are salient contextual determinants of wellbeing in one era, pale in significance in the next, when solutions are found or new, more pressing challenges arrive. These changes usher in a new dawn of mechanisms and mediators to be understood in relation to the brain. Often, when changes and challenges arise, they do so suddenly, and public health must scramble to develop solutions, often at great cost. Thinking prospectively about the social determinants of mental health, then, is imperative if some of these looming challenges are to be pre-empted.

Future threats and the changing global context

Predicting the future is at best a wild and inexact science. Global forecasts for the next 50 years tend to consist of a vivid description of unprecedented, unpredictable and a somewhat messy array of threats to human kind. In terms of health, we posit growing antibiotic resistance and zoonotic outbreaks linked to environmental degradation. In terms of socio-economic outcomes, we imagine a world of ever growing inequality driving ever-increasing conflict, coupled with rapid advances in and the increased automation of jobs previously performed by humans. In terms of the environment, we posit the breakdown of natural systems, catastrophic climate breakdown, and increasing wars over water. Thus, we are at a critical juncture for population mental health, and we need to expand our thinking on the social determinants of mental health to take account of and address future concerns.

Climate breakdown, mental health, and the idea of planetary health

By all accounts the planet is on the edge of an environmental catastrophe—and approaching what has been described as the first human made extinction—the Sixth Extinction (Kolbert, 2014). Despite some notable deniers, the science is clear—glaciers have shrunk and global temperatures have risen markedly in past decades and will continue to rise for decades to come, largely due to greenhouse gases produced by human activity. In the face of the threats just described, mental health will doubtless be challenged. However, even within this plethora of assaults, it is possible to hone in on some which will likely cause the greatest, and most far-reaching consequences.

In late 2018 the Intergovernmental Panel on Climate Change (IPCC) released its latest report and it makes grim reading as it describes how the thriving of humankind over the past 10,000 years has been at the expense of the planet. In this chapter we use the term climate breakdown to describe the reality of what we are facing, rather than the somewhat more benign concept "climate change." In this section, we briefly set the scene, describing current knowledge about the links between climate and human mental health. We turn, then, to an emerging field—Planetary Health—which encompasses in its scope, efforts to understand the emerging interactions between planet, ecology and humankind. Thinking systemically about the planet, embedded systems, and human mental health, we draw out a few examples of growing phenomena—often but not always linked to climate breakdown—which will emerge as determinants of mental health in the future.

Weather conditions linked to climate breakdown have a number of documented effects on health and well-being. For example, heatwaves can result in excess mortality

(Guo et al., 2018) increases in cardiac arrest (Watts et al., 2015), and dehydration and death in infants and children (Kakkad, Barzaga, Wallenstein, Azhar, & Sheffield, 2014). Conflict between individuals has also been shown to be affected by temperature change as a result of heightened levels of aggression within individuals (Hsiang et al., 2017). Children and adolescents are physiologically, immunologically, cognitively and psychologically more vulnerable to adverse climate exposures than adults (Stanberry, Thomson, & James, 2018).

With regard to mental health specifically, climate breakdown will result in up to 40,000 additional suicides across the United States and Mexico by 2050 (Burke et al., 2018). Heatwaves, as well as isolated hot days, have been shown to exacerbate mental disorders (Ding, Berry, & O'brien, 2015; Hansen et al., 2008; Trang, Rocklöv, Giang, Kullgren, & Nilsson, 2016; Williams, Hill, & Spicer, 2016), while the magnitude of negative effect of heat on population mental health may approximate that of unemployment (Berry, Waite, Dear, Capon, & Murray, 2018). Prospectively, people may become anxious at the prospect of climate breakdown (Stokes, Wike, & Carle, 2015); while immediately following extreme events, population mental health deteriorates (Lock et al., 2012; Reacher et al., 2004). Aside from immediate trauma-related reactions to natural disasters, the mechanism of the link between natural disasters and long-term human mental health is not well understood (Ahern, Kovats, Wilkinson, Few, & Matthies, 2005). Hypotheses as to mechanism include reactions to loss and disruption, leading to anxiety and depression (Berry, Bowen, & Kjellstrom, 2010). An additional mechanism may be the impact on community wellbeing and cohesion, both of which could link environmental events and fluctuations to the mental health of people (Berry et al., 2010).

Given these new, and clearly nuanced interactions between planet, climate, and human systems, the need to think systemically about these interactions—and what they mean for humans—has become apparent in the last decade. The term "planetary health" describes an emerging field of study (Horton, 2015) that aims to expand the ways we have today for thinking about and addressing human health to include the natural systems without which human health will collapse. Within planetary health, human sustainability is predicated on the (good) health of the planet, natural diversity, and ecological wellbeing. People exist within natural ecology and therefore flourishing natural systems are a prerequisite for good population health, and that without these, human health will deteriorate. In 2015, the Rockefeller Foundation-Lancet Commission on Planetary Health described in detail the extent to which the ongoing depletion and alteration of Earth's natural systems has already affected human health (Whitmee et al., 2015). As a result of this pressure coupled with long term climate breakdown the natural environment suffers resulting in increasing numbers of natural disasters, number of extreme weather events (frequency as well as severity), land degradation and water depletion, as well as significant increases in urbanization. The impact of these environmental changes causes specific challenges for human physical and mental health. These include food and water insecurity, displacement of people, violence and conflict, loss of culture and community, and over-burdened health systems, among others. Fig. 1 provides a way of conceptualizing the proposed pathway through which human pressure on the environment contributes to population mental health outcomes.

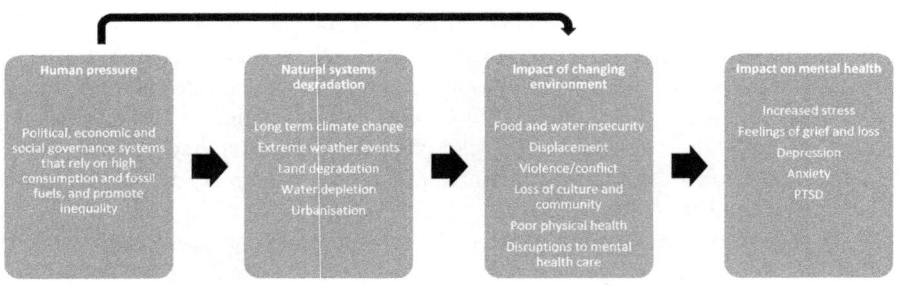

Fig. 1 Pathways from human pressure on the environment to mental health outcomes. Adapted from Berry, H. L., Bowen, K., & Kjellstrom, T. (2010). Climate change and mental health: A causal pathways framework. *International Journal of Public Health*, *55*, 123–32; Berry, H. L., Waite, T. D., Dear, K. B. G., Capon, A. G., & Murray, V. (2018). The case for systems thinking about climate change and mental health. *Nature Climate Change*, *8*, 282; Whitmee, S., Haines, A., Beyrer, C., Boltz, F., Capon, A. G., de Souza Dias, B. F., et al. (2015). Safeguarding human health in the Anthropocene epoch: Report of The Rockefeller Foundation-Lancet Commission on planetary health. *Lancet*, *386*, 1973–2028.

The Planetary Health approach dovetails closely with the SDGs. The SDGs provide a vision, roadmap and indicators for improving human capital and cast a spotlight on what needs to be improved to ensure a habitable planet where all people are able to meet their potential. The SDGs are also useful in their focus on a broad array of threats to human wellbeing (poverty, climate, and poor infrastructure for example).

In the light of this, and having briefly made the case for how mental health is crucially socially determined and how these determinants are increasingly environmental, we now turn to a discussion of seven specific future threats that we would argue are essential to address if we are to make any substantive inroads into improving planetary health, meeting the SDGs and crucially to the prevention of mental illness and the promotion of population mental health.

Inequality

Many of the economic (and resultant health-related) gains of the last century have been driven by unprecedented high levels of "economic growth," driven by an extractive model largely based on fossil fuels together with ever-increasing consumption. One of the consequences of this massive accumulation of capital has been ever increasing levels of inequality. The figures are stark. The US state of California (where it to be considered a country), recently overtook the United Kingdom as the fifth largest economy in the world, and has a higher GDP (by more than $300 billion) than all 54 African countries combined. Country inequity however masks perhaps the more serious inequalities that exist within many countries. In the United States, the richest country in the world, the infant mortality rate in the poorest part of Chicago is worse than that of war torn Syria. The work of Wilkinson (Wilkinson, 1992), and more recently of Piketty (Piketty, 2013), outlines the negative impacts of inequality at the level of population and individual health, as well at the level of country and global governance. Reduced life expectancy (Kondo et al., 2009), poor health (Subramanian & Kawachi, 2004), increased violence and crime (Kennedy, Kawachi, Prothrow-Stith, Lochner, & Gupta, 1998; Nadanovsky & Cunha-Cruz, 2009) have all been linked to income inequality. The same is true for mental disorders with substance use (Galea, Ahern, Tracy, & Vlahov, 2007), suicide (Gunnell, Middleton, Whitley, Dorling, & Frankel, 2003), depression (Ahern & Galea, 2006) and common mental disorders (Weich, Lewis, & Jenkins, 2001) all being associated with income inequality. Social inequalities are associated with increased risk of many common mental disorders (World Health Organization, 2008). Burns has outlined the possible mechanism of how inequality impacts on mental health (Burns, 2015), and outlines the evidence for two mechanisms. The first is the "social defeat" that comes with the shame and resentment that is a by-product of comparing oneself to richer neighbors (Burns, 2015; Chiavegatto Filho, Kawachi, Wang, Viana, & Andrade, 2013). The second is the increased psychosocial vulnerability of people in communities where social capital has been eroded by inequality (Burns, 2015; Mansyur, Amick, Harrist, & Franzini, 2008).

Global climate breakdown while catastrophic in the long term for everybody, may in fact be beneficial for some in the short term. In the wealthy northeast of the United States for instance agricultural yields may improve as a result of milder and less deadly winters, while the hotter Southern states will be affected more negatively (Hsiang et al., 2017). Globally, richer more temperate countries may be less affected. In fact, it is possible that the aggregate economic cost may be reduced but only because poor countries and poor people will experience a disproportionate burden (The Economist, 2017). In trying to understand this disproportionate burden, a useful concept is what the activist Naomi Klein has referred to as "sacrifice zones"—mostly poor remote places where residents, because they lack political power, can be sacrificed to the ravages of (for example) fossil fuel extraction or toxic dumping (Klein, 2015). In the 1970s the US government in fact referred to "national sacrifice areas" where open pit mining was to be allowed. Whether it is tar sand mining in Canada on First Nation land, daily oil spills in the Niger delta, the blasting off of the top of the Appalachian mountains for open caste coal mining, or the development of oil pipelines across Native American land in the United States, the brunt of the "sacrifice" has been borne by poor people, persons of color and women (Mallett, 2015). Increasingly though, even more middle class regions are being "sacrificed" with the advent of (for example) fracking.

As noted earlier, perceived inequality has deleterious impacts on human mental health. Social defeat, however, refers to something slightly different, but also insidious. Social defeat is the depressive reaction shown by social mammals in response to a traumatic loss of social status. It embeds neurologically in young brains (Litvin, Murakami, & Pfaff, 2011), and repeated exposure to social defeat induces long-term changes in neurophysiology in adults, resulting in a depression-like state in animals (although it may have limited applicability to female subjects as the natural phenomena which give rise to it are largely male) (Hollis & Kabbaj, 2014; Keeney & Hogg, 1999). What social defeat in animals suggests—when considered in tandem with perceived inequality—is that perceived aggressions by higher status members of unequal societies will significantly worsen lower status individuals' perceptions of inequality and mental distress. Some of the work which needs to be done to alleviate distress among individuals with lower SES and less social capital, will involve creating "virtuous cycles of opportunity, social inclusion and social cohesion" as well as poverty alleviation (United Kingdom Government Office for Science, 2008). Social capital exists even in unequal and poor societies, and can be leveraged to improve the lives of those upon whom the forces of inequality act with most force.

Gender, climate breakdown, and mental health

The unequal distribution of power between women and men, and the global inequalities which this incurs, bears a significant, twofold relationship to climate breakdown (Denton, 2002). The livelihood of women—particularly women and girls in LMIC—are particularly vulnerable to the risks posed by environmental change (Denton, 2001). Environmental degradation increases women's workloads and decreases their access to resources (Nelson, Meadows, Cannon, Morton, & Martin, 2002). Further, it leads to male out-migration from agricultural areas that leads to dramatic increases in women's work. Following disasters, women are also burdened with caring duties when family members are injured or displaced, which inhibits their agency and ability to participate in remunerated work (Nelson et al., 2002). Chief among the mental health sequelae of climate breakdown is that vulnerable communities will experience disruptions to the social, economic and environmental determinants which influence their health (Fritze, Blashki, Burke, & Wiseman, 2008). Climate breakdown and environmental disasters are likely to fracture social networks, cause mass displacement, and alter community connections through forced migration with women and girls bearing the brunt of this (Fritze et al., 2008).

A singular focus however on women's vulnerability, may risk deflecting attention from gendered inequalities in decision-making (Arora-Jonsson, 2011). Women have less power to negotiate for change, nor influence the scope of global climate breakdown discussions (Denton, 2002). This despite the fact that women (particularly rural women in low-income settings) are key role players and central stakeholders in natural resource management (Denton, 2002). Thus, while women could play a significant role in altering the course of environmental change, they are systematically excluded from political processes pertinent to these concerns (Denton, 2001, 2002). Resolving this issue would include mainstreaming gender perspectives within conservation and natural resource management, and including women—especially poor, rural women—in climate breakdown negotiations (Denton, 2002; Nelson et al., 2002). This would ensure that efforts toward the better administration of natural resources include those most likely to be affected by changes to natural resource allocation and management.

Central to understanding and reacting to both climate breakdown and its sequelae, and the social determinants of mental health in the context of climatic change more broadly, will be a recognition of different levels of vulnerability (Olmos, 2001). Women face barriers in wealth, transport, access to land, income, and other resources, agricultural practices, education, and health services. It is imperative to recognize these layers of vulnerability, and how they impact on women's ability to be resilient to climatic shocks, and participate in efforts at sustainable growth. Efforts to attend to climatic shocks and improve sustainability are incomplete without attention to these gendered influences.

Automation and job losses

Since 2013, four US states have passed laws that allow autonomous cars on the road. The success of driverless cars has simultaneously silenced skeptics, and threatened the livelihoods of millions of professional drivers. It has been estimated that when automated vehicle reach saturation that job losses in the United States could reach 25,000 a month or 300,000 per year (Liberatore, 2017). The success of these vehicles is one example of a far-reaching and fast-emerging problem. As robots and artificial intelligence grow in their capacity to surpass human capabilities, economists are speculating that the employment market will go into crisis (Whitehouse, Rojanasakul, & Sam, 2017). The coming changes—which are gaining speed—could exceed in their impact on human society, the revolution brought about by industrialization in the late 18th and early 19th centuries (Whitehouse et al., 2017). One of the chief drivers of this impact will be the ripples of unemployment that is likely to follow technological innovation. According to a 2013 study 47% of all jobs will disappear in the next 25 years (Frey & Osborne, 2017), and LMIC are likely to be among the most hard hit where many of the existing jobs require low skill and are repetitive—the first jobs likely to go in an era of increased automation. The public health implications of such job losses are considerable, in terms of social unrest but in a more proximal way on the mental health of vulnerable people throughout the world.

Agriculture and suicide

There is a relatively stable and reliable relationship between national GDP, and national suicide rates (Blasco-Fontecilla et al., 2012; dos Santos, Tavares, & Barros, 2016; Yin, Xu, Shao, Li, & Wan, 2016). There are some data that men are more sensitive to the effects of economic fluctuations on their mental health, than are women (dos Santos et al., 2016). Increasingly, we are able to analyze the impact of climate breakdown on individual lives. In 2013, an estimated one billion people globally were employed in the agricultural sector. Although their share in total employment has declined over the past decade, the total number of workers in agriculture has grown. In 2013, the agricultural sector accounted for 61.3% of total employment in sub-Saharan Africa, 47.2% in South Asia and 40.3% in South-East Asia and the Pacific (International Labour Organization, 2014). In India, it has been estimated that an increase of just 1C on an average day during the growing season is associated with 67 more suicides (Carleton, 2017). A key cause is crop failure. Rising temperatures and little rainfall wreak havoc on fragile stocks, and small-share farmers who do not have the resources or skills to protect themselves against these effects. In 2016, the Indian government launched a $1,3bn insurance scheme to protect farmers against crop failures and reduce farmer suicides. However, India is only one of the many LMIC in which people's livelihoods are heavily dependent on crop yields and livestock. More than 80% of the world's food is still produced by family farmers (FAO, 2014). As crops in LMIC fail due to climate breakdown, heat waves, and water scarcity, communities will experience poverty, food insecurity, and related mental health sequelae. The proportion of distressed populations in need of mental health services will increase. Mental health resources in these contexts are already scarce and overburdened and it is highly likely that in this scenario that the treatment gap will widen further (Breuer, Myer, Struthers, & Joska, 2011; Okasha, 2002).

Water scarcity

Water conflict, or water wars as they are popularly termed, are incidents of conflict or violence in which water was either their trigger of the event, or the cause of it. In the latter, water shortages may be caused by conflict, either the intentional or incidental casualties or targets of violence (Tir & Stinnett, 2012). Climate breakdown for example in the Middle East and the Sahel in Africa in particular drive environmental conditions which place increased stress on already fragile contexts—contexts least capable of withstanding strain (Blue, 2018). If attempts by the Paris agreement to curb global warming do not come to fruition, droughts will become ever more pervasive, particularly in this region (Carrão, Naumann, & Barbosa, 2018). Currently, it appears that institutional agreements between countries are proving successful in ensuring that potential conflict does not evolve into full-blown ward and conflicts. But there is no guarantee in the future that such agreements will prove sufficiently robust in the face of increasing pressure and demands on finite water resources (Tir & Stinnett, 2012). In 2010, more than 100 people were killed when fighting erupted in Parachinar in the Kurram region of Pakistan, as conflict over irrigation water escalated (Pacific Institute, 2018). The Middle East, an epicenter of global conflict is also one of the most water stressed regions in the world. It has been estimated that at current rates of global warming that large portions of the Middle East will be uninhabitable by humans by the end of the century (Pal & Eltahir, 2016). The implications for conflict, mass migration and the consequent impact on population mental health are likely to be profound.

Conflict and displacement

Armed conflict has disastrous humanitarian consequences wherever it occurs. Themnér and Wallensteen estimate that there have been 248 armed conflicts in the world since the end of World War II (Themnér & Wallensteen, 2012), while there are 40 active global conflicts (IRIN, 2018). Burke and colleagues have shown a link between rising temperatures and civil war in Africa, and when combining these data with climate model projections of how temperatures will increase, they project a 54% increase in armed conflict incidence (393,000 battle deaths) in Africa by 2030 (Burke, Miguel, Satyanath, Dykema, & Lobell, 2009). It is unlikely that there is a direct relationship between climate breakdown and violent conflict (SIDA, 2018). To reduce (for example), the complex conflict in Syria to a single factor such as climate related drought (Friedman, 2013) is too simplistic. It fails to consider how the causes of the Syrian conflict are multifactorial and may be due as much to geopolitics, the oppression of the Assad regime, and decades of poor agricultural policies (SIDA, 2018), as it was attributable to climate breakdown induced severe drought. What seems to be clear though is that climate related change can strongly influence or exacerbate conflict with the consequent catastrophic impact on migration and population mental health (SIDA, 2018).

The far-reaching consequences of exposure to violence are well documented. Victims of violence have increased rates of depression, anxiety, post-traumatic stress disorder, and suicidal behavior (Krug, Mercy, Dahlberg, & Zwi, 2002). Child victims often experience enduring effects on their health, and are more likely to have poor educational outcomes, and engage in harmful use of substances and risky sexual behavior as adults (Dubowitz & Bennett, 2007; Mock, Peden, Hyder, Butchart, & Krug, 2008). As climate-breakdown related conflict becomes more common, war-related mental health problems are likely to increase.

Estimates of involuntary migration due to climate breakdown vary (Fritze et al., 2008), and it is difficult to distinguish between economic, social, political and climate breakdown-related motivations for migration. Factors that spur immigration, such as food insecurity, may be related to climate breakdown, even if not explicitly so (Brown, 2008). Nonetheless, mounting evidence suggests that the short-term effects of environmental disasters and the long-term effects of more systematic climate breakdown, affect migration in significant ways (Fritze et al., 2008). It is projected that 200 million people will be displaced due to climate breakdown by 2050 (Brown, 2008; Myers, 2005). Migrants and refugees, living in poverty, displaced by war and land degradation, increasingly seek the security and safety of richer countries across the world.

The negative impact of displacement extends beyond the stress of upheaval and resettlement. Not only is the act of fleeing one's homeland psychologically stressful, but—once a migrant arrives in a new country—social, political and economic factors come into play which may have negative impacts on mental health (Eisenbruch, 1991; Martin, 1994). For instance, in many countries, including Australia, there have been long-standing policies of detainment for refugees. The research on the psychological impacts of refugee life in detention has almost unanimously drawn one conclusion: that detention itself magnifies the suffering—especially psychological suffering—of refugees, resulting in increased rates of depression, and traumatic stress (Laban, Gernaat, Komproe, Schreuders, & de Jong, 2004; Silove, Austin, & Steel, 2007; Steel et al., 2011).

A meta-analysis of studies concerned with refugee mental health (among populations displaced in conflicts, specifically), over the course of 50 years, showed that many post-displacement factors play a significant role in the future mental health outcomes (Porter & Haslam, 2005). Mental health disorders are not necessarily post-traumatic consequences of displacement, but, rather, reflect contextual factors of the receiving context (Porter & Haslam, 2005). As such, material and other forms of support may go some way to alleviate the deleterious impact of forced migration. At present, mental health care provision for refugees is lacking, even in HIC. As more and more people are displaced, a greater proportion of the world's population are likely to suffer migration-related mental health problems, with ever fewer services to address the suffering. Importantly, fragile contexts—those contexts in which political, environmental and economic problems make regions unstable—will not be able to withstand the demographic shock of mass migration (Talbi, 2018).

Habitat encroachment and infectious disease epidemics

The effect of natural systems degradation on physical health will also impact upon mental health and well-being. The link between physical and mental health is clear (Prince et al., 2007). There is however considerably less research on the potential impact of the increasing risk of infectious diseases on mental health. Economic growth, particularly in Africa and Asia is increasingly resulting in habitat loss linked to climate breakdown, overcrowding, deforestation, and encroachment into wildlife territories. This habitat pressure contributes to the promotion of outbreaks of another kind—infectious zoonotic diseases (Quammen, 2012). Zoonotic diseases are infectious diseases caused by a range of disease pathogens including viruses, bacteria, fungi and parasites that are transmitted to humans by animals. Nearly two thirds of all infectious diseases are zoonotic. Included in the list, are malaria, Lyme disease, Ebola, and HIV. While zoonoses are ancient, the largest epidemics of zoonnoses in recent decades, have originated in regions where habitat loss and human encroachment into animal habitats, is most profound (Central Africa and Southeast Asia). The Zika virus epidemic has affected countless children and families in Latin America and the Caribbean, and as Stanberry and colleagues point out while much of the focus has been on the severely affected microcephalic children, many children who were asymptomatic at birth may develop later problems including cognitive and mental health problems (Kapogiannis, Chakhtoura, Hazra, & Spong, 2017). The capacity of poor countries or fragile states to manage zoonotic disease outbreaks will be increasingly challenged by increasing population movement, urbanization, and fragile health systems (Hansen et al., 2017). And when fragile health systems are placed under considerable strain even the most basic provision for mental health care that may have been present will be decimated.

The great leveling or the possibility of equality

In *The Great Leveler: Violence and the History of Inequality from the Stone Age to the Twenty First Century*, Scheidel provides a disconcerting vision of "previous successes" in dealing with periods of extreme inequality (Scheidel, 2017). Scheidel shows how our current levels of global and country inequality are not unique and describes numerous epochs where massive inequality has existed (Scheidel, 2017). He argues however that "the solution" to every instance of massive inequality was not a process of social reorganization or any negotiated process, but rather that inequality has only every successfully been reduced by a great war (e.g., World War I), revolution (e.g., Bolshevik revolution) or catastrophe (pestilence such as Black Plague) (Scheidel, 2017). If this is to be avoided, if it can be avoided, then the path forward in development work, Planetary, and public health, will need to include sustained effort at pre-empting emerging threats, and resolving two conflicting, but interrelated quandaries.

The first: how to ensure that low- and middle-income countries (LMICs) are able to "catch up" economically and developmentally with high-income countries, and in so doing redress significant inequalities. The second: how to do this in the context of climate breakdown and widespread environmental damage on a planet that will simply not be able to sustain high growth for all countries. If poor countries are not able to develop economically and sustainability, while also meeting the health needs of their population, redressing inequalities, and do so without further damaging and already fragile planet then economic and health gains are unlikely to continue. A plethora of political, social and geographic factors have contributed to LMIC lagging economically and developmentally. Rich countries have profited, for example, off the damage done by other nations in the process of performing outsourced industry. Today, rich countries can in many cases afford to comply with emerging environmental legislation that aims to minimize further harm to the planet by taxing and otherwise disincentivising damaging industry. LMIC, on the other hand, are at the stage of their developmental curve, often, where further development will involve a move to more environmentally damaging outputs. The consequence is likely to be a host of social problems including increased mental ill health and a growing burden of disease.

The consequences for human mental health, although seemingly inevitable, may be open to mitigation. However, this mitigation will require urgent action, sustained political will, cooperation and investment. In these concluding points, we foreground key actions that must be taken and considerations that must be made by neuroethicists and many others, if the future attended to by Planetary Health and envisioned in the SDGs, is to come to fruition.

- **Stop destroying the planet**. This is non-negotiable—urgent action is needed. Current treaties and global governance are woefully inadequate. Our existing economic and political systems are depleting the Earth's resources for short-term gains and a rush to extreme acquisition. New innovative political and economic approaches are essential on order to protect the planet's natural systems, and thereby the health and development of humans for generations. We need to substantively change consumption patterns, and use technological solutions to address the drivers of environmental change.
- **Economic development and the growth imperative**. The "growth imperative" so central to 21st century capitalism has been described as a "development myth." The argument is that every increasing growth is inimical to sustainability in that trade competitiveness and promoting consumption are the overriding objectives (Bensimon & Benatar, 2006), rather than ensuring the health, wellbeing or flourishing of populations. Unless innovative ways are found to resolve the quandary of development vs environment, in a fragile global context riddled with environmental challenges we will be entering a period of increases of mental illness on a massive scale (Fugelli, 1993).
- **Governance/system issues**. The Millennium Development Goals marked the first steps toward looking beyond economic development only as a means of tracking human progress. The SDGs should be taken on board as an essential mechanism and template for country and global governance in order to ensure an inclusive, sustainable and healthy future.
- **Mental health** is a primary human health and development priority. Ongoing and increased investment into mental health promotion/prevention is key to improve human capital in the context of a fragile environment. Essential in this regard is that this is not only about psychosocial/behavioral interventions and pharmacological treatment, but also a focus on structural changes to the social and physical environment.
- **Social determinants of mental health**. Research into the social determinants of mental health must more explicitly include climate breakdown and its impact and see it as integral rather than simply being seen as optional. As is apparent, including a gendered lens when

contemplating climate-human population interactions will be imperative if the full scope of impact is to be understood. The manner in which climatic and environmental shifts lead to change at the individual and community level needs to be better understood, and causal and mediational pathways between environment and society need further explication.

- **Infectious disease**. Health system improvements particularly in LMIC is essential in order to better deal with infectious disease outbreaks. When planning health programming in light of predicted future risks, it is essential that planning for mental health is integral, as the mental health burden of morbidity in the wake of illness is considerable. Particularly, the manner in which encroachment on natural habitats, overcrowding, natural disasters and increased contact with wild animals will influence human health, particularly at the level of infectious disease vulnerability.
- **Integration.** Continued integration of mental health into disaster and conflict management programs, including for those with existing mental health problems or particularly vulnerable populations is essential.
- **Health information systems**. Mental health indicators into surveillance systems tracking impact of social and environmental changes
- **Preparing for the world of work of the future:** Ever-increasing numbers of workers will be competing in the global market place for work, and for skills. Mental capital, made possible by positive early development, will be crucial if people are to have the essential skills necessary to compete in the job market of the future—the "disposition to learn" (United Kingdom Government Office for Science, 2008).

Climate breakdown and the social upheavals and inequalities it will engender and worsen, are an unprecedented threat to our sense of who we are, our mental health, and action must be taken to mitigate their effects. Technological advances that are the focus of much neuroethics debate also pose similar challenges to society. Yet, they also offer some solutions—which—if harnessed for the betterment of the many, and distributed more equitably, could facilitate flourishing. We have closed this piece with some recommendations for key actions to alter the trajectory of global mental health. Whether the end course will be one of flourishing or failure will be determined in the years that come, as thinking about the social determinants of mental health incorporates in its vision, a fast changing context of human life, and the imperative of societal redress for human mental health.

References

Adler, N. E., Epel, E. S., Castellazzo, G., & Ickovics, J. R. (2000). Relationship of subjective and objective social status with psychological and physiological functioning: Preliminary data in healthy, White women. *Health Psychology, 19*, 586.

Ahern, J., & Galea, S. (2006). Social context and depression after a disaster: The role of income inequality. *Journal of Epidemiology and Community Health, 60*, 766–770.

Ahern, M., Kovats, R. S., Wilkinson, P., Few, R., & Matthies, F. (2005). Global health impacts of floods: Epidemiologic evidence. *Epidemiologic Reviews, 27*, 36–46.

Allen, J., Balfour, R., Bell, R., & Marmot, M. (2014). Social determinants of mental health. *International Review of Psychiatry, 26*, 392–407.

Andermann, A. (2016). Taking action on the social determinants of health in clinical practice: A framework for health professionals. *Canadian Medical Association Journal, 188*, E474–E483.

Armstrong, S. (1994). Rape in South Africa: An invisible part of apartheid's legacy. *Focus on Gender, 2,* 35–39.

Arora-Jonsson, S. (2011). Virtue and vulnerability: Discourses on women, gender and climate change. *Global Environmental Change, 21,* 744–751.

Artazcoz, L., Benach, J., Borrell, C., & Cortès, I. (2004). Unemployment and mental health: Understanding the interactions among gender, family roles, and social class. *American Journal of Public Health, 94,* 82–88.

Benjet, C., Hernández-Montoya, D., Borges, G., Méndez, E., Medina-Mora, M. E., & Aguilar-Gaxiola, S. (2012). Youth who neither study nor work: Mental health, education and employment. *Salud Pública de México, 54,* 410–417.

Bensimon, C. M., & Benatar, S. R. (2006). Developing sustainability: A new metaphor for progress. *Theoretical Medicine and Bioethics, 27,* 59–79.

Berry, H. L., Bowen, K., & Kjellstrom, T. (2010). Climate change and mental health: A causal pathways framework. *International Journal of Public Health, 55,* 123–132.

Berry, H. L., Waite, T. D., Dear, K. B. G., Capon, A. G., & Murray, V. (2018). The case for systems thinking about climate change and mental health. *Nature Climate Change, 8,* 282.

Blasco-Fontecilla, H., Perez-Rodriguez, M. M., Garcia-Nieto, R., Fernandez-Navarro, P., Galfalvy, H., de León, J., et al. (2012). Worldwide impact of economic cycles on suicide trends over 3 decades: Differences according to level of development. A mixed effect model study. *BMJ Open, 2,* e000785.

Bloom, D. E., Cafiero, E., Jané-Llopis, E., Abrahams-Gessel, S., Bloom, L. R., Fathima, S., et al. (2012). *The global economic burden of noncommunicable diseases.* Program on the Global Demography of Aging.

Blue, C. O. (2018). How water scarcity shapes the world's refugee crisis. *EcoWatch.*

Braveman, P., & Gruskin, S. (2003). Poverty, equity, human rights and health. *Bulletin of the World Health Organization, 81,* 539–545.

Breuer, E., Myer, L., Struthers, H., & Joska, J. A. (2011). HIV/AIDS and mental health research in sub-Saharan Africa: A systematic review. *African Journal of AIDS Research, 10,* 101–122.

Brown, O. (2008). *Migration and climate change.* United Nations Pubns.

Burke, M. B., Gonzalez, F., Baylis, P., Heft-Neal, S., Baysan, C., Basu, S., et al. (2018). Higher temperature increase suicide rates in the United States and Mexico. *Nature Climate Change, 8,* 723–729.

Burke, M. B., Miguel, E., Satyanath, S., Dykema, J. A., & Lobell, D. B. (2009). Warming increases the risk of civil war in Africa. *Proceedings of the National Academy of Sciences, 106,* 20670–20674.

Burns, J. K. (2015). Poverty, inequality and a political economy of mental health. *Epidemiology and Psychiatric Sciences, 24,* 107–113.

Carleton, T. A. (2017). Crop-damaging temperatures increase suicide rates in India. *Proceedings of the National Academy of Sciences,* https://doi.org/10.1073/pnas.1701354114.

Carrão, H., Naumann, G., & Barbosa, P. (2018). Global projections of drought hazard in a warming climate: A prime for disaster risk management. *Climate Dynamics, 50,* 2137–2155.

Chiavegatto Filho, A. D., Kawachi, I., Wang, Y. P., Viana, M. C., & Andrade, L. H. (2013). Does income inequality get under the skin? A multilevel analysis of depression, anxiety and mental disorders in Sao Paulo, Brazil. *Journal of Epidemiology and Community Health, 67,* 966–972.

Cooper, P. J., Tomlinson, M., Swartz, L., Woolgar, M., Murray, L., & Molteno, C. (1999). Postpartum depression and the mother-infant relationship in a South African peri-urban settlement. *The British Journal of Psychiatry, 175,* 554–558.

Denton, F. (2001). Climate change, gender and poverty–academic babble or realpolitik? *Point de Vue, 14*, 1–2.

Denton, F. (2002). Climate change vulnerability, impacts, and adaptation: Why does gender matter? *Gender and Development, 10*, 10–20.

Ding, N., Berry, H., & O'brien, L. (2015). The effect of extreme heat on mental health-evidence from Australia. *International Journal of Epidemiology, 44*, 64. Oxford Univ Press Great Clarendon ST, Oxford OX2 6DP, England.

Dohrenwend, B. P., Levav, I., Shrout, P. E., Schwartz, S., Naveh, G., Link, B. G., et al. (1992). Socioeconomic status and psychiatric disorders: The causation-selection issue. *Science, 255*, 946–952.

Doroud, N., Fossey, E., & Fortune, T. (2015). Recovery as an occupational journey: A scoping review exploring the links between occupational engagement and recovery for people with enduring mental health issues. *Australian Occupational Therapy Journal, 62*, 378–392.

dos Santos, J. P., Tavares, M., & Barros, P. P. (2016). More than just numbers: Suicide rates and the economic cycle in Portugal (1910–2013). *SSM-Population Health, 2*, 14–23.

Dubowitz, H., & Bennett, S. (2007). Physical abuse and neglect of children. *Lancet, 369*, 1891–1899.

Economist, T. (2017). Climate change and inequality: The rich pollute, the poor suffer. *The Economist*, Available from: https://www.economist.com/finance-and-economics/2017/07/13/climate-change-and-inequality.

Eisenbruch, M. (1991). From post-traumatic stress disorder to cultural bereavement: Diagnosis of Southeast Asian refugees. *Social Science & Medicine, 33*, 673–680.

FAO. (2014). *The state of food and agriculture*. Italy: Food and Agricultural Organization of the United Nations.

Fergusson, D. M., Horwood, L. J., & Woodward, L. J. (2001). Unemployment and psychosocial adjustment in young adults: Causation or selection? *Social Science & Medicine, 53*, 305–320.

Fisher, J., Cabral de Mello, M., Patel, V., Rahman, A., Tran, T., Holton, S., et al. (2012). Prevalence and determinants of common perinatal mental disorders in women in low- and lower-middle-income countries: A systematic review. *Bulletin of the World Health Organization, 90*, 139G–149G.

Frey, C. B., & Osborne, M. A. (2017). The future of employment: How susceptible are jobs to computerisation? *Technological Forecasting and Social Change, 114*, 254–280.

Friedman, T. (2013). The scary hidden stressor. *The New York Times*.

Fritze, J. G., Blashki, G. A., Burke, S., & Wiseman, J. (2008). Hope, despair and transformation: Climate change and the promotion of mental health and wellbeing. *International Journal of Mental Health Systems, 2*, 13.

Fryers, T., Jenkins, R., & Melzer, D. (2004). *Social inequalities and the distribution of the common mental disorders*. Psychology Press.

Fryers, T., Melzer, D., & Jenkins, R. (2003). Social inequalities and the common mental disorders. *Social Psychiatry and Psychiatric Epidemiology, 38*, 229–237.

Fryers, T., Melzer, D., Jenkins, R., & Brugha, T. (2005). The distribution of the common mental disorders: Social inequalities in Europe. *Clinical Practice and Epidemiology in Mental Health, 1*, 14.

Fugelli, P. (1993). In search of a global social medicine. *Forum for Development Studies, 1*, 101–108.

Galea, S., Ahern, J., Tracy, M., & Vlahov, D. (2007). Neighborhood income and income distribution and the use of cigarettes, alcohol, and marijuana. *American Journal of Preventive Medicine, 32*, S195–S202.

Garner, A. S., Shonkoff, J. P., Committee on Psychosocial Aspects of Child and Family Health, Committee on Early Childhood, Adoption, and Dependent Care, Section on Developmental and Behavioral Pediatrics. (2012). Early childhood adversity, toxic stress, and the role of the pediatrician: Translating developmental science into lifelong health. *Pediatrics*, *129*, e224–e231.

Gilman, S. E. (2002). Childhood socioeconomic status, life course pathways and adult mental health. *International Journal of Epidemiology*, *31*, 403–404.

Gunnell, D., Middleton, N., Whitley, E., Dorling, D., & Frankel, S. (2003). Why are suicide rates rising in young men but falling in the elderly?—A time-series analysis of trends in England and Wales 1950–1998. *Social Science & Medicine*, *57*, 595–611.

Guo, Y., Gasparrini, A., Li, S., Sera, F., Vicedo-Cabrera, A. M., de Sousa Zanotti Stagliorio Coelho, M., et al. (2018). Quantifying excess deaths related to heatwaves under climate change scenarios: A multicountry time series modelling study. *PLoS Medicine*, *15*, e1002629.

Hansen, A., Bi, P., Nitschke, M., Ryan, P., Pisaniello, D., & Tucker, G. (2008). The effect of heat waves on mental health in a temperate Australian city. *Environmental Health Perspectives*, *116*, 1369.

Hansen, A., Xiang, J., Liu, Q., Tong, M., Sun, Y., Liu, X., et al. (2017). Experts' perceptions on China's capacity to manage emerging and re-emerging zoonotic diseases in an era of climate change. *Zoonoses and Public Health*, *64*, 527–536.

Hendrie, C. A., & Pickles, A. R. (2009). Depression as an evolutionary adaptation: Implications for the development of preclinical models. *Medical Hypotheses*, *72*, 342–347.

Henry, K. L. (2010). Academic achievement and adolescent drug use: An examination of reciprocal effects and correlated growth trajectories. *Journal of School Health*, *80*, 38–43.

Herbig, B., Dragano, N., & Angerer, P. (2013). Health in the long-term unemployed. *Deutsches Ärzteblatt International*, *110*, 413.

Hickel, J. (2017). *The divide: A brief guide to global inequality and its solutions*. London: Windmill Books.

Hollis, F., & Kabbaj, M. (2014). Social defeat as an animal model for depression. *ILAR Journal*, *55*, 221–232.

Horton, R. (2015). Offline: Why the unity of life matters for our planetary health. *The Lancet*, *386*, 323.

Hsiang, S., Kopp, R., Jina, A., Rising, J., Delgado, M., Mohan, S., et al. (2017). Estimating economic damage from climate change in the United States. *Science*, *356*, 1362–1369.

International Labour Organization. (2014). *Global employment trends 2014: Risk of a jobless recovery?* Geneva: International Labour Organization.

IRIN. (2018). *Forgotten conflicts: Drawing attention to the wars we neglect*. Available from: https://www.irinnews.org/in-depth/forgotten-conflicts (Accessed August 1, 2018).

Jaffee, S. R. (2002). Pathways to adversity in young adulthood among early childbearers. *Journal of Family Psychology*, *16*, 38–49.

Jokela, M., Singh-Manoux, A., Ferrie, J. E., Gimeno, D., Akbaraly, T. N., Shipley, M. J., et al. (2010). The association of cognitive performance with mental health and physical functioning strengthens with age: The Whitehall II cohort study. *Psychological Medicine*, *40*, 837–845.

Jones, S. P., Patel, V., Saxena, S., Radcliffe, N., Ali Al-Marri, S., & Darzi, A. (2014). How Google's 'ten things we know to be true' could guide the development of mental health mobile apps. *Health Affairs*, *33*, 1603–1611.

Kakkad, K., Barzaga, M. L., Wallenstein, S., Azhar, G. S., & Sheffield, P. E. (2014). Neonates in Ahmedabad, India, during the 2010 heat wave: A climate change adaptation study. *Journal of Environmental and Public Health*, *2014*, 946875.

Kapogiannis, B. G., Chakhtoura, N., Hazra, R., & Spong, C. Y. (2017). Bridging knowledge gaps to understand how zika virus exposure and infection affect child development. *JAMA Pediatrics, 171*, 478–485.

Keeney, A., & Hogg, S. (1999). Behavioural consequences of repeated social defeat in the mouse: Preliminary evaluation of a potential animal model of depression. *Behavioural Pharmacology, 10*, 753–764.

Kennedy, B. P., Kawachi, I., Prothrow-Stith, D., Lochner, K., & Gupta, V. (1998). Social capital, income inequality, and firearm violent crime. *Social Science & Medicine, 47*, 7–17.

Klein, N. (2015). *This changes everything: Capitalism vs. the climate.* New York: Simon and Schuster.

Kokko, K., Pulkkinen, L., & Puustinen, M. (2000). Selection into long-term unemployment and its psychological consequences. *International Journal of Behavioral Development.*

Kolbert, E. (2014). *The sixth extinction: An unnatural history.* New York: Henry Holt and Company.

Kondo, N., Sembajwe, G., Kawachi, I., Van Dam, R. M., Subramanian, S. V., & Yamagata, Z. (2009). Income inequality, mortality, and self rated health: Meta-analysis of multilevel studies. *BMJ, 339*, b4471.

Krug, E. G., Mercy, J. A., Dahlberg, L. L., & Zwi, A. B. (2002). The world report on violence and health. *Lancet, 360*, 1083–1088.

Krugman, P. (2008). Poverty is poison. *The New York Times.*

Laban, C. J., Gernaat, H. B., Komproe, I. H., Schreuders, B. A., & de Jong, J. T. (2004). Impact of a long asylum procedure on the prevalence of psychiatric disorders in Iraqi asylum seekers in The Netherlands. *The Journal of Nervous and Mental Disease, 192*, 843–851.

Lende, D. H. (2012). Poverty poisons the brain. *Annals of Anthropological Practice, 36*, 183–201.

Levy, N. (2008). Introducing neuroethics. *Neuroethics, 1*, 1–8.

Liberatore, S. (2017). *Self-driving vehicles are set to take 25,000 jobs a MONTH away from Americans with truck drivers being worst hit.* Available from: http://www.dailymail.co.uk/sciencetech/article-4534752/Self-driving-cars-takeover-human-jobs.html. (Accessed August 2, 2018).

Litvin, Y., Murakami, G., & Pfaff, D. W. (2011). Effects of chronic social defeat on behavioral and neural correlates of sociality: Vasopressin, oxytocin and the vasopressinergic V1b receptor. *Physiology & Behavior, 103*, 393–403.

Lock, S., Rubin, G. J., Murray, V., Rogers, M. B., Amlôt, R., & Williams, R. (2012). Secondary stressors and extreme events and disasters: A systematic review of primary research from 2010–2011. *PLoS Currents, 4*, ecurrents.dis.a9b76fed1b2dd5c5bfcfc13c87a2f24f.

Lorant, V., Deliege, D., Eaton, W., Robert, A., Philippot, P., & Ansseau, M. (2003). Socio-economic inequalities in depression: A meta-analysis. *American Journal of Epidemiology, 157*, 98–112.

Lu, C., Black, M. M., & Richter, L. M. (2016). Risk of poor development in young children in low-income and middle-income countries: An estimation and analysis at the global, regional, and country level. *The Lancet Global Health, 4*(12), e916–e922.

Lund, C., Breen, A., Flisher, A. J., Kakuma, R., Corrigall, J., Joska, J. A., et al. (2010). Poverty and common mental disorders in low and middle income countries: A systematic review. *Social Science & Medicine, 71*, 517–528.

Lund, C., Brooke-Sumner, C., Baingana, F., Baron, E. C., Breuer, E., Chandra, P., et al. (2018). Social determinants of mental disorders and the sustainable development goals: A systematic review of reviews. *The Lancet Psychiatry, 5*, 357–369.

Lund, C., de Silva, M., Plagerson, S., Cooper, S., Chisholm, D., Das, J., et al. (2011). Poverty and mental disorders: Breaking the cycle in low-income and middle-income countries. *Lancet*, *378*, 1502–1514.

Lund, C., Stansfeld, S., & de Silva, M. (2014). Social determinants of mental health. In V. Patel, H. Minas, A. Cohen, & M. Prince (Eds.), *Global mental health: Principles and practices*. Oxford University Press. Print ISBN-13: 9780199920181.

Mallett, W. (2015). Naomi Klein's radical guide to the anthropocene. *The New Republic*.

Mansyur, C., Amick, B. C., Harrist, R. B., & Franzini, L. (2008). Social capital, income inequality, and self-rated health in 45 countries. *Social Science & Medicine*, *66*, 43–56.

Marmot, M. (2015). *The health gap: The challenge of an unequal world*. London: Bloomsbury.

Marmot, M., Friel, S., Bell, R., Houweling, T. A., Taylor, S., Commission on Social Determinants of Health. (2008). Closing the gap in a generation: Health equity through action on the social determinants of health. *Lancet*, *372*, 1661–1669.

Marmot, M., Shipley, M., Brunner, E., & Hemingway, H. (2001). Relative contribution of early life and adult socioeconomic factors to adult morbidity in the Whitehall II study. *Journal of Epidemiology and Community Health*, *55*, 301–307.

Marmot, M. G., Smith, G. D., Stansfeld, S., Patel, C., North, F., Head, J., et al. (1991). Health inequalities among British civil servants: The Whitehall II study. *Lancet*, *337*, 1387–1393.

Martin, S. F. (1994). *A policy perspective on the mental health and psychosocial needs of refugees*.

Miller, G. E., & Chen, E. (2013). The biological residue of childhood poverty. *Child Development Perspectives*, *7*, 67–73.

Mock, C., Peden, M., Hyder, A. A., Butchart, A., & Krug, E. (2008). Child injuries and violence: The new challenge for child health. *Bulletin of the World Health Organization*, *86*, 420.

Myers, N. (2005). *Environmental refugees: An emergent security issue*.

Nadanovsky, P., & Cunha-Cruz, J. (2009). The relative contribution of income inequality and imprisonment to the variation in homicide rates among developed (OECD), South and Central American countries. *Social Science & Medicine*, *69*, 1343–1350.

Neighbors, H. W., Caldwell, C., Williams, D. R., Nesse, R., Taylor, R. J., Bullard, K. M., et al. (2007). Race, ethnicity, and the use of services for mental disorders: Results from the National Survey of American Life. *Archives of General Psychiatry*, *64*, 485–494.

Nelson, V., Meadows, K., Cannon, T., Morton, J., & Martin, A. (2002). Uncertain predictions, invisible impacts, and the need to mainstream gender in climate change adaptations. *Gender and Development*, *10*, 51–59.

Okasha, A. (2002). Mental health in Africa: The role of the WPA. *World Psychiatry*, *1*, 32.

Olmos, S. (2001). *Vulnerability and adaptation to climate change: Concepts, issues, assessment methods*. Climate Change Knowledge Network (CCKN).

Pacific Institute. (2018). *Water conflict*. Available from: https://www.worldwater.org/water-conflict/ (Accessed August 1, 2018).

Pal, J. S., & Eltahir, E. (2016). Future temperature in southwest Asia projected to exceed a threshold for human adaptability. *Nature Climate Change*, *6*, 197–200.

Patel, V., & Kleinman, A. (2003). Poverty and common mental disorders in developing countries. *Bulletin of the World Health Organization*, *81*, 609–615.

Piketty, T. (2013). *Capital in the twenty-first century*. Boston, MA: Harvard University Press.

Porter, M., & Haslam, N. (2005). Predisplacement and postdisplacement factors associated with mental health of refugees and internally displaced persons: A meta-analysis. *JAMA*, *294*, 602–612.

Prince, M., Patel, V., Saxena, S., Maj, M., Maselko, J., Phillips, M. R., et al. (2007). No health without mental health. *Lancet*, *370*, 859–877.

Quammen, D. (2012). *Spillover: Animal infections and the next human pandemic.* WW Norton & Company.

Reacher, M., Mckenzie, K., Lane, C., Nichols, T., Kedge, I., Iversen, A., et al. (2004). Health impacts of flooding in Lewes: A comparison of reported gastrointestinal and other illness and mental health in flooded and non-flooded households. *Communicable Disease and Public Health, 7,* 39–46.

Rohde, P. (2001). The relevance of hierarchies, territories, defeat for depression in humans: Hypotheses and clinical predictions. *Journal of Affective Disorders, 65,* 221–230.

Rollins, N. C., Bhandari, N., Hajeebhoy, N., Horton, S., Lutter, C. K., Martines, J. C., et al. (2016). Why invest, and what it will take to improve breastfeeding practices? *Lancet, 387*(10017), 491–504.

Rubin, M., Evans, O., & Wilkinson, R. B. (2016). A longitudinal study of the relations among university students' subjective social status, social contact with university friends, and mental health and well-being. *Journal of Social and Clinical Psychology, 35,* 722–737.

Rubin, M., & Kelly, B. M. (2015). A cross-sectional investigation of parenting style and friendship as mediators of the relation between social class and mental health in a university community. *International Journal for Equity in Health, 14,* 87.

Rubin, M., & Stuart, R. (2018). Kill or cure? Different types of social class identification amplify and buffer the relation between social class and mental health. *The Journal of Social Psychology, 158,* 236–251.

Saksena, P., Hsu, J., & Evans, D. B. (2014). Financial risk protection and universal health coverage: Evidence and measurement challenges. *PLoS Medicine, 11*(9), e1001701.

Scheidel, W. (2017). *The Great Leveler: Violence and the history of inequality from the stone age to the twenty-first century.* Princeton: Princeton University Press.

Shonkoff, J. P., Garner, A. S., Committee on Psychosocial Aspects of Child and Family Health, Committee on Early Childhood, Adoption, and Dependent Care, Section on Developmental and Behavioral Pediatrics. (2012). The lifelong effects of early childhood adversity and toxic stress. *Pediatrics, 129,* e232–e246.

SIDA. (2018). *The relationship between climate change and violent conflict.* Stockholm: Swedish International Development Cooperation Agency.

Silove, D., Austin, P., & Steel, Z. (2007). No refuge from terror: The impact of detention on the mental health of trauma-affected refugees seeking asylum in Australia. *Transcultural Psychiatry, 44,* 359–393.

Sowislo, J. F., & Orth, U. (2013). Does low self-esteem predict depression and anxiety? A meta-analysis of longitudinal studies. *Psychological Bulletin, 139,* 213.

Stanberry, L. R., Thomson, M. C., & James, W. (2018). Prioritizing the needs of children in a changing climate. *PLoS Medicine, 15,* e1002627.

Stansfeld, S. A., Rasul, F., Head, J., & Singleton, N. (2011). Occupation and mental health in a national UK survey. *Social Psychiatry and Psychiatric Epidemiology, 46,* 101–110.

Steel, Z., Momartin, S., Silove, D., Coello, M., Aroche, J., & Tay, K. W. (2011). Two year psychosocial and mental health outcomes for refugees subjected to restrictive or supportive immigration policies. *Social Science & Medicine, 72,* 1149–1156.

Stokes, B., Wike, R., & Carle, J. (2015). *Global concern about climate change, broad support for limiting emissions.* Pew Research Center. [ARP].

Subramanian, S. V., & Kawachi, I. (2004). Income inequality and health: What have we learned so far? *Epidemiologic Reviews, 26,* 78–91.

Talbi, A. (2018). Strong thirsts in fragile countries: Walking the water scarce path of refugees. *The World Bank Water Blog.*

Taylor, D. M., Moghaddam, F. M., Gamble, I., & Zellerer, E. (1987). Disadvantaged group response to perceived inequality: From passive acceptance to collective action. *The Journal of Social Psychology*, *127*, 259–272.

Themnér, L., & Wallensteen, P. (2012). Armed conflicts, 1946–2011. *Journal of Peace Research*, *49*, 565–575.

Tir, J., & Stinnett, D. M. (2012). Weathering climate change: Can institutions mitigate international water conflict? *Journal of Peace Research*, *49*, 211–225.

Trang, P. M., Rocklöv, J., Giang, K. B., Kullgren, G., & Nilsson, M. (2016). Heatwaves and hospital admissions for mental disorders in northern Vietnam. *PLoS ONE*, *11*, e0155609.

Twenge, J. M., & Campbell, W. K. (2002). Self-esteem and socioeconomic status: A meta-analytic review. *Personality and Social Psychology Review*, *6*, 59–71.

United Kingdom Government Office for Science. (2008). *Mental Capital and Wellbeing: Making the most of ourselves in the 21st century*. London: The Government Office for Science.

Waghorn, G., & Chant, D. (2005). Labour force activity by people with depression and anxiety disorders: A population-level second-order analysis. *Acta Psychiatrica Scandinavica*, *112*, 415–424.

Watts, N., Adger, W. N., Agnolucci, P., Blackstock, J., Byass, P., Cai, W., et al. (2015). Health and climate change: Policy responses to protect public health. *Lancet*, *386*, 1861–1914.

Weich, S., Lewis, G., & Jenkins, S. P. (2001). Income inequality and the prevalence of common mental disorders in Britain. *The British Journal of Psychiatry*, *178*, 222–227.

Whitehouse, M., Rojanasakul, M., & Sam, C. (2017). Is your job about to disappear?: QuickTake. *Bloomberg*.

Whitmee, S., Haines, A., Beyrer, C., Boltz, F., Capon, A. G., de Souza Dias, B. F., et al. (2015). Safeguarding human health in the Anthropocene epoch: Report of The Rockefeller Foundation-Lancet Commission on planetary health. *Lancet*, *386*, 1973–2028.

Wilkinson, R. G. (1992). Income distribution and life expectancy. *BMJ*, *304*, 165–168.

Williams, M. N., Hill, S. R., & Spicer, J. (2016). Do hotter temperatures increase the incidence of self-harm hospitalisations? *Psychology, Health & Medicine*, *21*, 226–235.

World Health Organization. (2008). *Social determinants of health*. Geneva: World Health Organization.

Yin, H., Xu, L., Shao, Y., Li, L., & Wan, C. (2016). Relationship between suicide rate and economic growth and stock market in the People's Republic of China: 2004–2013. *Neuropsychiatric Disease and Treatment*, *12*, 3119.

Section B

Global neuroethics

The ethics of neurogenetics research in Africa: Considerations and guidelines

Jantina de Vries
Department of Medicine, University of Cape Town, Cape Town, South Africa

Introduction

In recent years, the application of genomic research methods to psychiatric illnesses has led to the identification of several associated mutations (Schizophrenia Working Group of the Psychiatric Genomics Consortium, 2014). There is some optimism that these insights will allow for the further study of the biological pathways involved in disease causation and progression, including the identification of new drug targets, or evidence that could inform individual patient treatment options. Such progress is exciting against a backdrop of the normally slow evolution of insight into the biological etiology of psychiatric illnesses such as schizophrenia and bipolar disorder. A challenge in this work, and in genomics research in general, is its ongoing focus on people of Caucasian descent, with only a small percentage of studies including non-whites (Popejoy & Fullerton, 2016).

Yet there are good scientific and equity reasons to expand psychiatric genomic research to the African continent. Scientific reasons revolve around the expectation that the inclusion of data from African patients will accelerate the discovery of mutations key to disease causation (Need & Goldstein, 2009). In particular, the expectation is that the greater genetic diversity harbored by Africans reduces the size of the haystack researchers need to sift through to find the idiomatic needle they hope is lost in there (Rosenberg et al., 2010). Equity reasons include a concern that genomic research continues to underrepresent global diversity and falls particularly short in the inclusion of Africans (Popejoy & Fullerton, 2016). The threat is that if genomic research and resultant insights and innovations help improve patient prospects, then it is possible that such improvements are not relevant to or effective for African patients, thus further increasing the global treatment gap. That this is not just a hypothetical risk is becoming increasingly evident. For instance, a recent analysis illustrates how some African Americans have been wrongfully identified as being at risk of developing cardiomyopathy based on genetic data that was not representative of their population subgroup (Manrai et al., 2016). An example pertinent to psychiatric illness could be the development of so-called polygenic risk scores (Belsky & Israel, 2014), which may increasingly become of use in research and treatment. If such scores are not based

Global Mental Health and Neuroethics. https://doi.org/10.1016/B978-0-12-815063-4.00006-X

on representative African data, then there is a risk that discoveries and predictive tests will equally not be relevant to African patients.

A number of recent initiatives has sought to remedy these challenges. These include for instance the African Genome Variation Project (Gurdasani et al., 2015) which sought to develop a detailed characterization of African genetic variation for use as reference data in African genomic studies. Another example is the H3Africa Consortium, which is a collection of African genomic research projects focusing on a range of conditions, including quite a few psychiatric and neurodevelopmental conditions (H3Africa Consortium, 2014). To note, the first round of H3Africa included a research project on schizophrenia in the Xhosa population of South Africa (Dalvie et al., 2015) and on hereditary neurological conditions (Landouré et al., 2016). More recently, H3Africa research includes projects on neurodevelopmental conditions in children, on the effect of maternal stressors on infant gene expression and on the transgenerational epigenetics of post-traumatic stress disorder in survivors of the Rwanda genocide. This research has already led to the identification of novel loci associated with some of these disorders. For instance, research in Mali has identified a novel mutation associated with spastic paraplegia and sensory loss (Guinto et al., 2017) while research in Cameroon has tentatively identified novel loci associated with hereditary hearing loss (Lebeko et al., 2017). Such research has obvious clinical and research relevance not just to African patients but potentially to patients around the world. There is thus a strong case for the expansion of genomic research methods to the African continent. Yet such research raises a number of important ethical challenges that need to be considered.

To some extent, these issues are similar to those described for genomics research on other conditions (De Vries et al., 2011; Nyika, 2009; Wright, Koornhof, Adeyemo, & Tiffin, 2013) and include considerations of informed consent, community engagement, stigma and genetic attribution, ethics review and many others. For this purposes of this chapter, I will highlight three of these challenges, namely issues to do with seeking informed consent, with respecting reciprocity obligations, and with ensuring that international collaboration is conducted in a way that is fair and equitable. But first, I will describe four features of the African research context that impact on research ethics.

Features of the African research context that impact on research ethics

In terms of characteristics of the general LMIC research context that are important for a consideration of ethics, what stands out strongly is the limited access of prospective research participants to good healthcare, education and employment. Low general research and health literacy translate into a greater burden the researcher to explain not only the research project but also the condition under investigation, as well as pertinent features of the research approach. Sub-optimal access to good healthcare

combined with poverty translate into increased emphasis on issues to do with inducement, reciprocity and ancillary care.

Simultaneously, the LMIC research context is often characterized by less-resourced
academic and research institutions, with limited experience in grants management and
limited overall support for investigators. These factors constrain LMIC researchers'
ability to be internationally competitive. Furthermore, the scarcity of healthcare professionals and academic researchers means that LMIC researchers need to develop
broad skills. Often, LMIC researchers are not only researchers—they are also heads
of institutions or departments, full-time clinicians, teachers and tutors, supervisors,
national health policy advisors, members of ethics committees, board members of professional committees and so forth. The luxury of hyperspecialization that researchers
in HICs have—to craft an entire career around psychiatric genomics or bioinformatics
for instance—is simply not available to many LMIC researchers.

A third important feature of the LMIC research context is *therapeutic flexibility*,
where patients access both modern and traditional therapies and have mixed beliefs
about the original cause of illness. In the African context, many conditions including
psychiatric and neurological ones, are attributed to mystical or spiritual origins including bewitchment. Such beliefs are pervasive and unlikely to be displaced by medical
explanations offered during research participation. They impact on various elements
of the research process, including the consent process and processes of community
engagement. Importantly, the association of researchers with practices also associated with witchcraft—for instance, the large-scale collection of blood samples—has
the ability to undermine community trust in research (O'Neill et al., 2016; Peeters
Grietens et al., 2014).

A final feature of the African research context that impacts on research ethics relates to the prominence of solidarity as an organizing principle, impacting on the way
individuals see themselves, and on how they operate in relation to their families and
communities. Described as Ubuntu philosophy in South Africa (Chuwa, 2014) but
known under different names elsewhere, this worldview emphasizes the interrelated-
ness of humans (Eze, 2008).

Taken together, these contextual factors impact on the way in which health research
is conducted in LMICs, and the ethical challenges it raises. In the section below, I will
explore some of the more pertinent among these.

Ethical challenges in conducting genetics research in resource-poor settings

When conducted in resource-poor settings such as those found in many lower- and
middle income countries, neurogenetics research raises a number of ethical concerns
that need to be considered in the design and execution of such research. While many
of these issues are not unique to the research context (i.e., HIC vs LMIC) or the conditions under study (i.e., mental illness vs other conditions), the way that they should be

considered may be different when research is conducted in LMICs and on mental or neurological conditions. In the section below, I will focus on the three currently most prominent ethical considerations pertinent to global neurogenetics research. These relate to considerations of informed consent, respecting reciprocity expectations and ensuring that international research collaborations are fair.

Valid informed consent

As a pillar in the protection of the interests of research participants, considerations of how research projects can seek consent are very important in the research context. In genomics research, a number of challenges have been reported (see for instance Tindana & De Vries, 2016 for a review). One particular concern when working in contexts of poverty is that participants may be induced to participate by benefits or compensation offered through participation. Researchers often offer some reward for participation, which can be in monetary or material form (e.g., some projects offer bars of soap or mobile phone vouchers). This is presented as "compensation" for costs incurred, or "transport money" and is often minimal. Yet what constitutes an appropriate amount of compensation is not clearly defined (Geissler, 2011), with some arguing that under-compensation carries serious risk of harm when working in resource-poor communities (Njue, Kombe, Mwalukore, Molyneux, & Marsh, 2014; Njue et al., 2015).

On the flipside, a decision to participate in research may be rational or strategic, in giving participants access to better healthcare for the duration of the project (Paré Toe et al., 2013; Ravinetto et al., 2015). In many low- and middle income countries in the world, public investment in mental healthcare remains extremely low, with most money being spent on psychiatric hospitals and few funds available for non-hospital based healthcare (World Health Organisation, 2018). Where this makes for poor availability of care generally, the provision of mental healthcare services in rural areas is dismal (Matsea, Ryke, & Weyers, 2018). The implication is that many participants enrolling in research projects on mental and neurological conditions may not have received much care for their illness and some may never have received a full diagnostic assessment, or may not have been explained their diagnosis. Where research concerns robust enrolment methods including, for instance taking a detailed history of a person's illness through structured clinical interviews, then this can in itself be a motivating factor for participation. In this context, inducement thus is not just about the provision of financial or other material incentives, and the risk of inducement needs to be balanced against the risks of harm and exploitation by offering too little.

Another challenge to informed consent may be that *voluntariness* in informed consent could be compromised where participants are enrolled through institutions such as psychiatric hospitals, where patients may not feel they have an opportunity to refuse participation. This could also be an issue where the participant is cared for by their family members, as is not unusual in the African context. In that case, family pressure to participate may compromise an individual's ability to refuse consent to participation. These challenges are not easily dealt with in the research context. One strategy available to participants are so-called "silent refusals" (Kamuya et al., 2015) during which participants constructively draw on the use of silence (or, sometimes, absence) to express dissent (Kawabata & Gastaldo, 2015). Kamuya et al., for instance, describe instances in which participants use silence and body language to indicate that they are uncomfortable with the research process or their participation, when they are unable to say so openly. Participants may also express dissent by repeatedly failing to show up for research appointments, by not answering the phone after the initial interaction, or by indicating that they need to consult others before agreeing. All of these are subtle ways in which participants can express their own will without openly disagreeing with others, and need to be respected as such in the research process. Those involved in recruiting participants need to be trained to recognize and empowered to respect these silent refusals.

In research involving psychiatric patients or patients with otherwise diminished capacity to reason, there are logically concerns about their capacity to consent which have been addressed by developing instruments that assess the individual's capacity to consent as well as their understanding of the information provided during the consent process (Gupta & Kharawala, 2012). Such tools will measure not just what participants understood, but how they appreciate this information, what reasons they give for participation and the extent to which they are able to communicate a choice (Appelbaum & Grisso, 1988; Sturman, 2005). While few such studies have been conducted in the African research context, one recent study stands out. Campbell et al. (2017) found that one such instrument, the UBACC tool developed by the University of San Diego (Jeste et al., 2007), provided a helpful way to identify prospective research participants with unacceptably low levels of understanding in a genomics study in South Africa. This information was combined with iterative learning specifically targeting the areas or topics that participants struggled to comprehend.

In the context of genomics research, one important discussion relates to determining whether and when the use of broad consent is appropriate and ethical (Grady et al., 2015). There is a growing body of evidence that suggests that while there are no a priori reasons not to use broad consent on the African continent (Tindana & De Vries, 2016), participants are concerned about the use of their data and samples in ways that they feel would be exploitative (van Schalkwyk, de Vries, & Moodley, 2012). Similarly, participants are concerned about the possibility that they may be identified when data is shared. What seems most important is that where broad consent is used, it is accompanied by genuine community engagement that seeks to explore and accommodate participants' concerns. The use of broad consent also needs to be accompanied by a governance framework that addresses participant concerns and makes decisions in line with their expectations and to their benefit (Tindana, Molyneux, Bull, & Parker, 2017).

Reciprocity obligations

A second important ethical consideration in the ethics of global neurogenetics research relates to how researchers accommodate reciprocity expectations by participants. While in international bioethics discourse the primary principle under consideration is autonomy, in many non-Western societies including those in African countries, solidarity is an equally important principle that requires recognition and consideration (Ijsselmuiden, Kass, Sewankambo, & Lavery, 2010; Tosam, Chi, Munung, Oukem-Boyer, & Tangwa, 2018). A solidarity-based worldview has several practical implications for research practice, the most obvious of which are reciprocity expectations.

An expectation for reciprocity in research means an—often implicit—expectation that researchers reciprocate participants' efforts by responding to some aspect of their need to ensure that research is beneficial not just to the researcher but also to the participants and their communities (Skovdal & Abebe, 2012). Reciprocity obligations have been discussed, at least to some extent, in the context of ancillary care obligations, where scholars explored the extent to which researchers should care for participants post-enrollment or post-study (Belsky & Richardson, 2004; Merrit, 2011; Pratt et al., 2013; Richardson & Belsky, 2004). They have also been discussed in terms of recruitment and training of research staff (Pearson & Paige, 2012) and in terms of benefits emanating from research (Njue et al., 2014). Reciprocity expectations are often high in vulnerable communities, including patient communities affected by psychiatric or neurodevelopmental disorders in lower and middle income countries. When conducting research with people who have very little, such expectations are not abstract and easily brushed off; rather, they can be the source of deep moral anxiety for researchers and fieldstaff (see Huisman, 2008; Kamuya et al., 2013; Nyambedha, 2008 for examples). In such instances, the mere collection of samples or data without any attempt to empower participants, or to alleviate their plight, can feel exploitative not just to the participants but also to those involved in its execution. Furthermore, respecting reciprocity obligations can play a critical role in building trust and promoting ethical conduct of research.

There are several responses to dealing with this challenge. Nyambedha (2008) and Huisman (2008) both suggest that research could be coupled with interventionist activities (for instance, through linkages with NGOs) or service as well as to include a budgetary provision to deal with private emergencies. Others (see for instance Maiter, Simich, Jacobson, & Wise, 2008; Pearson & Paige, 2012) have advocated for the use of "participatory action research"-inspired research methodologies in which research projects and recruitment strategies are co-designed with members of the researched communities, in an attempt to pre-empt these ethical challenges and design the project budget and recruitment strategies in such a way that participants' direct needs can be accommodated. Although such thinking is advanced primarily in the context of qualitative sociological and anthropological research, it is echoed in philosophical literature that calls for "shared sovereignty" in the design and conduct of health systems research (Pratt & Hyder, 2016b). Another way to recognize the importance of reciprocity is by designing "genuine" community engagement. The emphasis on "genuine" distinguishes it from tokenistic engagement conducted merely to satisfy funder requirements, and ensures that the form of engagement satisfies a number of key criteria (Pratt & de Vries, 2018).

One challenge in respecting reciprocity obligations in international collaborative research is that it requires research to be conducted with meaningful involvement of LMIC researchers at leadership levels. As described by Kiluva-Ndunda (2005), what she calls "tourist researchers" are not in a position to forge the kind of relationships with the researched to understand the social, political and linguistic context of research and to enable them to recognize and respond to participants' needs. Researchers knowledgeable of and involved with communities prior to and during research are arguably in a much better position to understand not only the opportunities for doing research, but also the way in which research can empower the researched.

For neurogenetics research involving patient communities from lower- and middle income countries, the implication is that such research should anticipate participants' reciprocity expectations and design approaches that can reasonably address these. Researchers and fieldstaff involved in participant recruitment should be trained to understand the basis of these expectations, and be empowered to respond to them reasonably and appropriately.

Fairness in international collaboration

A third and final ethical issue of key importance in the design of research projects in neuropsychiatric genetics relates to how to ensure that such collaborations are fair and equitable. Due in part to a long history of extractive relations between high-income and low- and middle income countries (HICs and LMICs respectively) (Van Rinsum & Tangwa, 2004), research conducted in collaboration between researchers from LMICs and HICs continues to be characterized by inequality and the perception of exploitation (Munung, Mayosi, & de Vries, 2017). This is due in part to the fact that researchers and institutions based in HICs continue to project themselves as almost self-evidently superior to researchers and institutions in LMICS.

There are ways in which these challenges could be considered or addressed in the design and conduct of genomics research. Emphasis has been given to ensuring that the design of funding structures and projects actively seek to correct inequality, for instance by prescribing that project funds are fairly distributed between research partners (Pratt & Hyder, 2017, 2018) and by ensuring that partners from LMICs have an equal voice in project deliberations (Pratt & Hyder, 2016a) and that they share sovereignty. Genuine recognition of the added value that LMIC researchers and institutions can contribute, and a real attempt at ensuring LMIC leadership in projects—not just in terms of sample and data collection but crucially in terms of the design, analysis and publication of project data—are identified as essential in this respect (Yakubu et al., 2018).

What is also very important is that the governance framework for neuropsychiatric genetics research is designed to promote equity and fairness. As described earlier, most genetic and genomic research now takes place in the context of open science, with storage, sharing and future unspecified use of resources part and parcel of the way in which research is conducted. In that context, the early development of a governance framework is essential to ensure ethical best practice (Yakubu et al., 2018). Importantly, such a governance framework should include procedural descriptions of where resources will be stored, how and with whom they will be shared and for what purposes. When sharing resources generated in LMICs, the emphasis should be on ensuring equity and fairness (Bull, 2016). This means that projects should consider ways of sharing that promote the interests of participants and institutions in LMICs and that reduce the possibility that sharing could be experienced as extractive or exploitative. Examples of elements of governance frameworks that seek to do just that are extended periods in which samples and data are under (partial) embargo to allow LMIC researchers to gain or maintain a competitive edge in analyzing and publishing findings; ensuring shared sovereignty by populating access committees with individuals from the LMICs in which samples and data were collected; and requiring that proposals for sample or data re-use include a plan for capacity building of LMIC individuals (Bull, 2016). Some of these elements were put into practice in the H3Africa governance framework (de Vries et al., 2015), which is a collective of medical genomics research projects under African leadership (H3Africa Consortium, 2014). The governance documents, including a sample and data sharing policy and guidelines for informed consent in African genomics research, are freely available online and could serve as templates for other African genomics initiatives.[a]

Frameworks to guide researchers

These experiences have recently been translated into a number of frameworks that can help guide researchers operating in this space. In particular, three different frameworks or codes of conduct address issues of perceived exploitation and limited benefit. They are the Global Code of Conduct for Research in Resource-poor Settings,[b] the H3Africa Ethics and Governance Framework for Best Practice in African genomics research and biobanking[c] and the San Code of Ethics.[d]

The Global Code of Conduct for Research in Resource-poor Settings specifically addresses research conducted in international collaborations between individuals in high-income countries (HICs) and low- and middle-income countries (LMICs), and specifically research that is funded by organizations based in HICs. The code responds to concerns that such collaborations could lead to "ethics dumping," defined as "doing research deemed unethical in a scientist's home country in a foreign setting with laxer ethical rules" (Nordling, 2018, p. 17). The code, which is binding for all EU-funded research projects funded under Horizon 2020, operationalises the principles of fairness, respect, care and honesty. The code is an outcome of a detailed analysis of several instances of ethics dumping (Schroeder, Cook, Hirsch, Fenet, & Muthuswamy, 2018) and emphasizes the importance of respecting cultural norms, individuals and institutions in LMICs.

---

[a] https://h3africa.org/consortium/documents (Last accessed 24 July 2018).

[b] http://www.globalcodeofconduct.org/ (Accessed 30 August 2018).

[c] https://h3africa.org/9-news/361-framework-for-african-genomics-and-biobanking (Accessed 30 August 2018).

[d] http://trust-project.eu/wp-content/uploads/2017/03/San-Code-of-RESEARCH-Ethics-Booklet-final.pdf (Accessed 30 August 2018).

The H3Africa Ethics and Governance Framework for Best Practice in African Genomics Research sets out what should be considered best practice in genomics research conducted in Africa. It is the result of a lengthy process of engagement with a wide range of stakeholders from the African continent, as well as with selected stakeholders based in HICs (Yakubu et al., 2018). Stakeholders from the African continent include African researchers, members of local and national ethics committees from over 30 African countries, national policy makers from some African countries as well as representatives of some African Academies of Science. Stakeholders from non-African countries include members of funding organizations and selected researchers. The Framework identifies a number of core principles that should guide the design and conduct of genomics research, and also offers more specific guidance for some of the ethical challenges outlined in this chapter. Importantly, the Framework emphasizes the need for genuine African intellectual leadership in genomics research, meaning that African researchers are centrally involved in the conception, design, execution, analysis and publication of genomic research projects—and not merely as data collectors and tokenistic authors on papers.

A third code of conduct pertinent to international genomics research is the San Code of Research Ethics which was developed as a direct result of the San's involvement in international collaborative genomics research (Chennells & Steenkamp, 2018). A project conducted by researchers in the United States a couple of years ago involved four elderly San from isolated communities in Namibia, with total disregard for the San Councils from Namibia and South Africa and without involvement of any of the organizations that protect San interests. This project was perceived by the San as being disrespectful, potentially harmful and exploitative with no real benefit or regard for San communities. In response to this experience, the San Council of South Africa working together with the South African San Institute and others developed a San Code of Research Ethics that emphasizes respect, honesty, justice and fairness and care when conducting research involving the San, and also outlines a process for ensuring ethics approval.

Taken together, these three sources offer international researchers fairly comprehensive guidance on how international collaborative genomics research should be conducted. They call attention to similar issues—for instance, the importance of being respectful to cultural, linguistic and organizational differences and ensuring that research responds to the needs of individuals and communities it involves. But most importantly, these codes all renew calls for ensuring that international collaborative research is fair and offers real opportunities for engagement and leadership to stakeholders based in resource-poor countries. They are increasingly receiving recognition—for instance, all three of these codes received wide international coverage and were the topic of several commentaries and editorials in leading journals such as Nature (Nordling, 2018; The Nature Editors, 2018). Importantly, calls for greater considerations of equality are also gradually becoming integrated in journal publication policy decisions, with The Lancet Global Health recently taking a clear stand against parachute research, including in publication of secondary analyses of data (The Lancet Global Health, 2018).

Discussion

In this chapter, I described three of the most prominent ethical challenges that arise in the conduct of genomics research in the African continent, not because these are the only ethical challenges raised by such research, but because they are currently the most controversial and—in my view—most important ones. The first of these relates to challenges in designing consent models that protect the interests of research participants yet enables the broad re-use of samples and data for research. On the continent, protectionist or paternalistic approaches to consent continue to predominate, with decision-makers relying on more specific consent models to protect participants. The perverse side-effect of such an approach is that it obstructs the sharing and re-use of resources for research that could be of benefit to African patients, researchers and the healthcare system. I argued that, first, there are no a priori reasons for why broad consent should not be permissible on the African continent. I then described that where it is used, however, it should be accompanied by a transparent and accountable governance framework and genuine attempts to engage community members (not in the least in the development of the governance framework.

I then described the importance of recognizing the reciprocity expectations that participants and communities may have early on in the research process and designing project budgets and enrolment strategies in such a way that they can be accommodated. When recruiting particularly vulnerable participants—because of poverty, the absence of good healthcare, or their illness—dealing with patient needs is ethically challenging and may be the source of considerable anxiety on the part of research recruitment staff. Recognition of the needs of participants in the short and longer term and considering seriously how these can reasonably be addressed—or justifying persuasively why some needs or expectations cannot be addressed—is important, not in the least because it promotes the long-term trust participants may have in the researchers.

Lastly, I described what I consider to be the main ethical challenge in the conduct of international collaborative genomics research, which is ensuring that it is fair. International collaborative research continues to be taking place in ways that are explicitly or covertly inequitable, with the power balance skewed in favor of institutions and organizations based in Europe and the United States. Not only do those stakeholders have obvious interests in maintaining the status quo, but the development of more egalitarian models of collaboration takes time, resources and commitment and needs to be premised on trust (Harawa et al., 2018; Merson, Guerin, Barnes, Ntoumi, & Gaye, 2018). The role of ethics codes and funding and publication policies are critical in defining best practice for such international collaborative research and is equally relevant to global neurogenetics research. Similarly, the development of transparent and accountable governance frameworks describing where resources will be stored, how they will be shared, with whom and for what purposes is equally important. A key consideration for the design of such governance frameworks is how decisions about sample and data access and re-use could empower researchers in lower- and middle income countries and positively impact on ensuring equality.

References

Appelbaum, P. S., & Grisso, T. (1988). 'Assessing patients' capacities to consent to treatment. *The New England Journal of Medicine*, *319*, 1635–1638.

Belsky, D. W., & Israel, S. (2014). Integrating genetics and social science: Genetic risk scores. *Biodemography and Social Biology*, *60*, 137–155.

Belsky, L., & Richardson, H. S. (2004). 'Medical researchers' ancillary clinical care responsibilities. *British Medical Journal*, *328*, 1494–1496.

Bull, S. (2016). *Ensuring global equity in open research*. Wellcome Trust: London.

Campbell, M. M., Susser, E., Mall, S., Mqulwana, S. G., Mndini, M. M., Ntola, O. A., et al. (2017). Using iterative learning to improve understanding during the informed consent process in a South African psychiatric genomics study. *PLOS ONE*, *12*(11), e0188466.

Chennells, R., & Steenkamp, A. (2018). International genomics research involving the san people. In D. Schroeder, J. Cook, F. Hirsch, S. Fenet, & V. Muthuswamy (Eds.), *Ethics dumping*. Cham: Springer.

Chuwa, L. T. (2014). *African indigenous ethics in global bioethics. Interpreting ubuntu*. Dordrecht: Springer.

Dalvie, S., Koen, N., Duncan, L., Abbo, C., Akena, D., Atwoli, L., et al. (2015). Large scale genetic research on neuropsychiatric disorders in African populations is needed. *eBioMedicine*, *2*, 1259–1261.

De Vries, J., Bull, S., Doumbo, O. K., Ibrahim, M., Mercerau-Puijalon, O., Kwiatkowski, D. P., et al. (2011). Ethical issues in human genomics research in developing countries. *BMC Medical Ethics*, *12*, 5.

de Vries, J., Tindana, P., Littler, K., Ramsay, M., Rotimi, C., Abayomi, A., et al. (2015). The H3Africa policy framework: Negotiating fairness in genomics. *Trends in Genetics*, *31*, 117–119.

Eze, M. O. (2008). What is African communitarianism? Against consensus as a regulative ideal. *South African Journal of Philosophy*, *27*, 386–399.

Geissler, P. W. (2011). Transport to where? *Journal of Cultural Economy*, *4*, 45–64.

Grady, C., Eckstein, L., Berkman, B. E., Brock, D., Cook-Deegan, R., Fullerton, S. M., et al. (2015). Broad consent for research with biological samples: Workshop conclusions. *The American Journal of Bioethics*, *15*, 34–42.

Guinto, C. O., Diarra, S., Diallo, S., Cisse, L., Coulibaly, T., Diallo, S. H., et al. (2017). A novel mutation in KIF5A in a Malian family with spastic paraplegia and sensory loss. *Annals of Clinical Translational Neurology*, *4*, 272–275.

Gupta, U. C., & Kharawala, S. (2012). Informed consent in psychiatry clinical research: A conceptual review of issues, challenges, and recommendations. *Perspectives in Clinical Research*, *3*, 8–15.

Gurdasani, D., Carstensen, T., Tekola-Ayele, F., Pagani, L., Tachmazidou, I., Hatzikotoulas, K., et al. (2015). The African genome variation project shapes medical genetics in Africa. *Nature*, *517*, 327–332.

H3Africa Consortium. (2014). Research capacity. Enabling the genomic revolution in Africa. *Science (New York, NY)*, *344*, 1346–1348.

Harawa, P. P., Mbale, E., Mallewa, M., Dube, Q., Langton, J., Njiram'madzi, J., et al. (2018). Parasitic and parachute research in global health. *The Lancet Global Health*, *6*, e840.

Huisman, K. (2008). "Does this mean you're not going to come visit me anymore?": An inquiry into an ethics of reciprocity and positionality in feminist ethnographic research*. *Sociological Inquiry*, *78*, 372–396.

Ijsselmuiden, C., Kass, N., Sewankambo, K. N., & Lavery, J. (2010). Evolving values in ethics and global health research. *Global Public Health, 5*, 154–163.

Jeste, D. V., Palmer, B. W., Appelbaum, P. S., Golshan, S., Glorioso, D., Dunn, L. B., et al. (2007). A new brief instrument for assessing decisional capacity for clinical research. *Archives of General Psychiatry, 64*, 966–974.

Kamuya, D. M., Theobald, S. J., Marsh, V., Parker, M., Geissler, W. P., & Molyneux, S. C. (2015). "The one who chases you away does not tell you go": Silent refusals and complex power relations in research consent processes in coastal Kenya. *PLoS ONE, 10*, e0126671.

Kamuya, D. M., Theobald, S. J., Munywoki, P. K., Koech, D., Geissler, W. P., & Molyneux, S. C. (2013). Evolving friendships and shifting ethical dilemmas: Fieldworkers' experiences in a short term community based study in Kenya. *Developing World Bioethics, 13*, 1–9.

Kawabata, M., & Gastaldo, D. (2015). The less said, the better: Interpreting silence in qualitative research. *International Journal of Qualitative Methods, 14*, 1609406915618123.

Kiluva-Ndunda, M. M. (2005). Reciprocity in research: A retrospective look at my work with Kilome Women. *Counterpoints, 275*, 221–233.

Landouré, G., Samassékou, O., Traoré, M., Meilleur, K. G., Guinto, C. O., Burnett, B. G., et al. (2016). Genetics and genomic medicine in Mali: Challenges and future perspectives. *Molecular Genetics & Genomic Medicine, 4*, 126–134.

Lebeko, K., Manyisa, N., Chimusa, E. R., Mulder, N., Dandara, C., & Wonkam, A. (2017). A genomic and protein-protein interaction analyses of nonsyndromic hearing impairment in Cameroon using targeted genomic enrichment and massively parallel sequencing. *OMICS, 21*, 90–99.

Maiter, S., Simich, L., Jacobson, N., & Wise, J. (2008). Reciprocity: An ethic for community-based participatory action research. *Action Research, 6*, 305–325.

Manrai, A. K., Funke, B. H., Rehm, H. L., Olesen, M. S., Maron, B. A., Szolovits, P., et al. (2016). Genetic misdiagnoses and the potential for health disparities. *New England Journal of Medicine, 375*, 655–665.

Matsea, T., Ryke, E., & Weyers, M. (2018). Assessing mental health services in a rural setting: Service providers' perspective. *International Journal of Mental Health, 47*, 26–49.

Merrit, M. W. (2011). Health researchers' ancillary care obligations in low-resource settings: How can we tell what is morally required? *Kennedy Institute of Ethics Journal, 21*, 311–347.

Merson, L., Guerin, P. J., Barnes, K. I., Ntoumi, F., & Gaye, O. (2018). Secondary analysis and participation of those at the data source. *The Lancet Global Health, 6*, e965.

Munung, N. S., Mayosi, B. M., & de Vries, J. (2017). Equity in international health research collaborations in Africa: Perceptions and expectations of African researchers. *PLoS ONE, 12*, e0186237.

Need, A. C., & Goldstein, D. B. (2009). Next generation disparities in human genomics: Concerns and remedies. *Trends in Genetics, 25*, 489–494.

Njue, M., Kombe, F., Mwalukore, S., Molyneux, S., & Marsh, V. (2014). What are fair study benefits in international health research? Consulting community members in Kenya. *PLoS ONE, 9*, e113112.

Njue, M., Molyneux, S., Kombe, F., Mwalukore, S., Kamuya, D., & Marsh, V. (2015). Benefits in cash or in kind? A community consultation on types of benefits in health research on the Kenyan coast. *PLoS ONE, 10*, e0127842.

Nordling, L. (2018). Europe's biggest research fund cracks down on 'ethics dumping'. *Nature, 559*, 17–18.

Nyambedha, E. O. (2008). Ethical dilemmas of social science research on AIDS and orphanhood in Western Kenya. *Social Science & Medicine, 67*, 771–779.

Nyika, A. (2009). Ethical and practical challenges surrounding genetic and genomic research in developing countries. *Acta Tropica, 112*, S21–S31.

O'Neill, S., Dierickx, S., Okebe, J., Dabira, E., Gryseels, C., d'Alessandro, U., et al. (2016). The importance of blood is infinite: Conceptions of blood as life force, rumours and fear of trial participation in a Fulani Village in Rural Gambia. *PLoS ONE, 11*, e0160464.

Paré Toe, L., Ravinetto, R. M., Dierickx, S., Gryseels, C., Tinto, H., Rouamba, N., et al. (2013). Could the decision of trial participation precede the informed consent process? Evidence from Burkina Faso. *PLoS ONE, 8*, e80800.

Pearson, A. L., & Paige, S. B. (2012). Experiences and ethics of mindful reciprocity while conducting research in sub-Saharan Africa. *African Geographical Review, 31*, 72–75.

Peeters Grietens, K., Ribera, J. M., Erhart, A., Hoibak, S., Ravinetto, R. M., Gryseels, C., et al. (2014). Doctors and vampires in sub-Saharan Africa: Ethical challenges in clinical trial research. *The American Journal of Tropical Medicine and Hygiene, 91*, 213–215.

Popejoy, A. B., & Fullerton, S. M. (2016). Genomics is failing on diversity. *Nature, 538*, 161–164.

Pratt, B., & de Vries, J. (2018). Community engagement in global health research that advances health equity. *Bioethics, 32*, 454–463.

Pratt, B., & Hyder, A. A. (2016a). Governance of transnational global health research consortia and health equity. *The American Journal of Bioethics, 16*, 29–45.

Pratt, B., & Hyder, A. (2016b). Governance of transnational global health research consortia and health equity. *American Journal of Bioethics, 17*, 1–37.

Pratt, B., & Hyder, A. A. (2017). Fair resource allocation to health research: Priority topics for bioethics scholarship. *Bioethics, 31*, 454–466.

Pratt, B., & Hyder, A. A. (2018). Designing research funding schemes to promote global health equity: An exploration of current practice in health systems research. *Developing World Bioethics, 18*, 76–90.

Pratt, B., Zion, D., Lwin, K. M., Cheah, P. Y., Nosten, F., & Loff, B. (2013). Ancillary care: From theory to practice in international clinical research. *Public Health Ethics, 6*, 154–169.

Ravinetto, R. M., Afolabi, M. O., Okebe, J., Van Nuil, J. I., Lutumba, P., Mavoko, H. M., et al. (2015). Participation in medical research as a resource-seeking strategy in socio-economically vulnerable communities: Call for research and action. *Tropical Medicine & International Health, 20*, 63–66.

Richardson, H. S., & Belsky, L. (2004). The ancillary-care responsibilities of medical researchers: An ethical framework for thinking about the clinical care that researchers owe their subjects. *The Hastings Center Report, 34*, 25–33.

Rosenberg, N. A., Huang, L., Jewett, E. M., Szpiech, Z. A., Jankovic, I., & Boehnke, M. (2010). Genome-wide association studies in diverse populations. *Nature Reviews Genetics, 11*, 356–366.

Schizophrenia Working Group of the Psychiatric Genomics Consortium. (2014). Biological insights from 108 schizophrenia-associated genetic loci. *Nature, 511*, 421–427.

Schroeder, D., Cook, J., Hirsch, F., Fenet, S., & Muthuswamy, V. (Eds.), (2018). *Ethics dumping. Case studies from North-South research collaborations*. Cham: Springer.

Skovdal, M., & Abebe, T. (2012). Reflexivity and dialogue: Methodological and socio-ethical dilemmas in research with HIV-affected children in East Africa. *Ethics, Policy and Environment, 15*, 77–96.

Sturman, E. D. (2005). The capacity to consent to treatment and research: A review of standardized assessment tools. *Clinical Psychology Review, 25*, 954–974.

The Lancet Global Health. (2018). Closing the door on parachutes and parasites. *The Lancet Global Health, 6*, e593.

The Nature Editors. (2018). A welcome framework for research in Africa. *Nature, 556,* 274.

Tindana, P., & De Vries, J. (2016). Broad consent for genomic research and biobanking: Perspectives from low- and middle-income countries. *Annual Review of Genomics and Human Genetics, 17,* 2.1–2.19.

Tindana, P., Molyneux, S., Bull, S., & Parker, M. (2017). 'It is an entrustment': Broad consent for genomic research and biobanks in sub-Saharan Africa. *Developing World Bioethics, 19*(1), 9–17.

Tosam, M. J., Chi, P. C., Munung, N. S., Oukem-Boyer, O. O. M., & Tangwa, G. B. (2018). Global health inequalities and the need for solidarity: A view from the Global South. *Developing World Bioethics, 18*(3), 241–249.

Van Rinsum, H., & Tangwa, G. B. (2004). Colony of genes, genes of the colony: Diversity, difference and divide. *Third World Quarterly, 25,* 1031–1043.

van Schalkwyk, G., de Vries, J., & Moodley, K. (2012). "It's for a good cause, isn't it?"— Exploring views of South African TB research participants on sample storage and re-use. *BMC Medical Ethics, 13,* 19.

World Health Organisation. (2018). *World mental health atlas 2017.* World Health Organisation: Geneva.

Wright, G., Koornhof, P., Adeyemo, A., & Tiffin, N. (2013). Ethical and legal implications of whole genome and whole exome sequencing in African populations. *BMC Medical Ethics, 14,* 21.

Yakubu, A., Tindana, P., Matimba, A., Littler, K., Munung, N. S., Madden, E., et al. (2018). Model framework for governance of genomic research and biobanking in Africa—A content description. *African Academy of Sciences Open Research, 1,* 13. [version 1; referees: Awaiting peer review].

Cosmetic psychopharmacology in a global context

7

Andrea C. Palk, Dan J. Stein
Department of Psychiatry, University of Cape Town, Cape Town, South Africa

Introduction

Psychotropic agents, including alcohol and other anxiolytics, have been used by humans for thousands of years, for both spiritual and medicinal reasons. In the mid-20th century, the serendipitous discovery of antidepressants, antipsychotics, and mood-stabilizing medications, provided a range of new agents. Careful delineation of the basic mechanisms underlying the effects of these agents, and rigorous determination of their clinical efficacy, provided the foundation for the field of psychopharmacology. The growth of psychopharmacology in turn contributed to significant changes in psychiatric practice, together with the development of massive investment by the pharmaceutical industry in this area (Luhrmann, 2001).

Although global mental health has been particularly concerned with health systems and policies, and with task-shifting psychotherapeutic interventions, it has also paid some attention to psychopharmacology. For example, the World Health Organization (WHO) produced a service guidance package on "Improving access and use of psychotropic medicines" in 2005, and, in collaboration with the Gulbenkian Foundation, a document on "Improving access to and appropriate use of medicines for mental disorders" in 2017. These documents drew on a growing evidence-base addressing the efficacy of psychiatric medications in low- and middle-income settings (Barbui, Dua, Kolappa, Saraceno, & Saxena, 2017; Patel et al., 2003).

Neuroethics has also paid attention to developments in psychopharmacology. Peter Kramer's "Listening to Prozac" (Kramer, 1997) emphasized the growing role of medication treatments in psychiatry, and also raised the question of "cosmetic psychopharmacology." This refers to the possibility of using psychotropic agents not only to treat medical disorders, but also to enhance brain and mind function. A range of publications have further addressed this question (Caplan & Elliott, 2004; Degrazia, 2000; Glannon, 2008; Mohamed & Sahakian, 2012; Schermer, Bolt, de Jongh, & Olivier, 2009; Stein, 2012), drawing on a broader literature that has addressed ethical questions regarding human biomedical enhancement in general (Agar, 2005; Buchanan, 2011; Habermas, 2003; Harris, 2007; President's Council on Bioethics & Kass, 2003; Sandel, 2007; Savulescu, ter Meulen, & Kahane, 2011). Most of this work has been from the perspective of ethicists working in high-income countries drawing on a Western philosophical framework.

In this chapter we consider cosmetic psychopharmacology (CP) in a global context. This involves not only looking at how, if at all, CP fits in with global mental health

Global Mental Health and Neuroethics. https://doi.org/10.1016/B978-0-12-815063-4.00007-1

(GMH), but also looking at the ethical status of CP, itself, in more globally relevant terms. Because debates regarding the ethical status of CP have mostly been conducted with reference to a liberal individualist framework, looking at CP in more globally relevant terms requires that our investigation is not limited to this frame of reference. However, its ethical status aside, given the reality of resource scarcities in mental health care, we take one of the main challenges facing the articulation of a globally relevant CP to be its status with regard to macro-level distributive justice concerns.

We commence with an overview of CP, followed by a brief outline of the GMH agenda. Here, we take the distinction between a right to mental health and a right to mental health care to be significant for our purposes. We then discuss distinctions and concerns that inform the ethical status of CP. In particular, we explore the motives for using CP and the kind of value that it confers, as well as the notion of medical necessity and the concern regarding overmedicalization. This is followed by an overview of a relational account, informed by an African moral framework, which predicates moral value on the ability to be both the subject and object of a particular kind of relationship. We then discuss the implications of this relational account for conceptions of mental health and mental health care. We conclude the chapter by discussing the ethical status of CP in terms of the relational account and address the implications for a negative and positive right to mental health as well as a right to mental health care.

Cosmetic psychopharmacology

CP is a form of biomedical or bioenhancement. Bioenhancement refers to the improvement of human physical functioning and capabilities, lifespan, cognition, mood, and even morally relevant traits, through the use of pharmacological, genetic or neural interventions. A distinction is frequently made between the enhancement of normal functioning and the treatment of pathophysiology (Daniels, 2000). Many forms of bioenhancement that have been envisaged are either not yet fully possible or are not known to be safe or effective. Discussions of bioenhancement are therefore somewhat speculative. However, there are some exceptions, one of these being CP.

Cosmetic psychopharmacology, also referred to as psychopharmacological enhancement or mood enhancement, generally entails the use of psychotropic agents, such as selective serotonin reuptake inhibitors (SSRIs) for subthreshold symptoms or simply to feel more emotionally and functionally resilient. Based on his observations of the effects of fluoxetine (Prozac) in his patients, Kramer argued that a subset of "fairly healthy" patients were "not so much cured of illness as transformed" (Kramer, 1997). In particular, Kramer describes witnessing "how poorly patients fared when they were cautious and inhibited, and how the same people flourished once medication had made them assertive and flexible" (Kramer, 1997), indicating the effects that Prozac has on personality, in some cases. Studies indicate that antidepressants are extensively used for various off-label purposes (Stone, Viera, & Parman, 2003; Wong et al., 2017). The increased use of psychopharmacology for so-called cosmetic purposes, in particular, could arguably represent an advance in clinical practice, or it might be criticized as representing overmedicalization (Berghmans, Ter Meulen, Malizia, & Vos, 2011). In terms of the efficacy of CP, meta-analysis of data from various studies that have assessed the effects of various antidepressants in healthy subjects suggest detectible differences in social and emotional processing (Serretti et al., 2010), including increases in "affiliative behaviors" (Tse & Bond, 2002) and "social bonding" (Tse & Bond, 2003). However, any improvements in healthy volunteers must be weighed against the difficulty in differentiating medication from placebo effects, particularly in the case of subtle symptomatic improvement (Quitkin, 1999).

The terms CP or psychopharmacological enhancement are also sometimes applied to the use of psychopharmaceuticals to augment cognitive functioning that falls within the normal range. In its current form, cognitive enhancement entails the off-label use of psychostimulants (nootropics) such as methylphenidate or modafinil to modify specific neurotransmitters, thereby increasing executive functioning such as attention, concentration, alertness or working memory.[a] Due to the complexity of the brain it is unlikely that it will ever be possible to enhance the trait of intelligence as such; rather, it is more feasible to target various mechanisms of cognition (Sahakian & Morein-Zamir, 2015).

For the purposes of this chapter we focus on mood enhancement and use the term CP to refer accordingly. In the absence of universal availability of cognitive enhancement, and for various reasons that we discuss, we take CP to be more justifiable with reference to the aims of GMH than cognitive enhancement. However, while our focus is on CP we do discuss certain ethical implications of cognitive enhancement insofar as it is able to serve as a useful point of comparison. In the next section we introduce GMH, after which we discuss the ethical status of CP.

Global mental health

GMH developed in response to major inequities in access to mental health services between high-income countries (HICs) and low- and middle-income countries (LMICs), referred to as the treatment gap (Kohn, Saxena, Levav, & Saraceno, 2004; Patel, 2012) . Given the pervasive negative impact of mental disorders on human lives, the treatment gap has been identified as a major human rights concern requiring urgent attention (Stein & Illes, 2015). As a result, GMH has been fundamentally focused on establishing more equitable access to mental health care in resource-strained settings through efficient, innovative, cost-effective approaches that are context-sensitive and evidence-based (Stein & Giordano, 2015).

The recent publication of The Lancet Commission on global mental health and sustainable development represents a distinct shift in the GMH agenda, predominantly informed by the endorsement of the sustainable development goals (SDGs) in 2015

---

[a] Studies conducted in various countries indicate that methylphenidate (e.g., Ritalin and Adderall) is used extensively by students and professionals in various contexts for off-label purposes (Beyer, Staunton, & Moodley, 2014; Brito, 2015; Cohen, Segev, Shlafman, Novack, & Ifergane, 2015; Greely et al., 2008).

(Patel et al., 2018). This shift involves a significantly broader conception of GMH, in line with the SDGs more expansive interpretation of mental health and disorder. In particular, the GMH agenda has been broadened from its earlier focus on reducing the treatment gap to a more encompassing focus on "the improvement of mental health for whole populations and reducing the contribution of mental disorders to the global burden of disease" (Patel et al., 2018). This change is justified with reference to the normative claims, presented as principles, that mental health is both a "global public good…[and] a fundamental human right" (Patel et al., 2018) and by recognition of the dimensional, as opposed to categorical, nature of mental health as well as the social and environmental determinants of mental health.

The broadened GMH agenda also references the protection and promotion of well-being and welfare as an explicit aim, positing a "rights-based approach" as the most effective means of achieving this (Patel et al., 2018). In the context of GMH, the appeal to human rights is doing pragmatic work, it rests on the uncontroversial assumption that we have an intuitive understanding of what it means to have a right to something and why this matters.[b] Asserting a right to something also implies, by definition, that the thing in question is either intrinsically or instrumentally good; we would generally not assert a right to something that wasn't considered desirable. In the reconfigured GMH agenda it is important to note that the appeal is made to a fundamental human right to mental health and not a right to mental health *care*, although the latter would be a possible implication of the former. This distinction has been discussed by Daniels in terms of its macro level implications for justice in general health care (Daniels, 1985, 2017); we take it to be relevant for our assessment of CP in this chapter.

Although they are sometimes used interchangeably, the two appeals are distinct; they are generally used for different purposes, having different implications. Asserting a general right to mental health is a much broader claim that is based on the recognition of the multiple social and environmental determinants of mental health (Daniels, 2017). A right to mental health generally asserts both a positive and negative right, both of which imply an entitlement and an ensuing obligation or duty for that entitlement to be met. The positive component would claim that all societal institutions that have a bearing on mental health outcomes have an obligation or duty to foster, sustain or restore mental health, while the negative component would claim that relevant institutions have an obligation to avoid all actions that threaten mental health (Daniels, 1985). The latter claim is therefore a less demanding one.

The right to mental health is contrasted with the narrower claim of a right to mental health care. A right to mental health care is a positive claim that confers a narrowed range of entitlements and obligations that include both the prevention and treatment of illness, disability and disease to restore health or for palliative purposes. Because this claim implies the obligation to treat or prevent, it must address practical prioritization concerns such as how far the claim extends, i.e., what it includes, and how resources should be shared amongst differential or competing needs in the context of limited

---

[b] The implicit normative assumption that generally informs rights-appeals is that all human beings have equal moral worth, generally captured by the notion of human dignity, therefore human beings have an equal moral claim or entitlement to having certain basic needs met.

resources (Buchanan, 2010; Daniels, 1985). The entitlements and obligations conferred by a right to mental health care are therefore relative to the system or context in which they are made (Daniels, 2017). Furthermore, for a claim right to have force and be implementable, it requires a supportive theory of justice applicable to distribution. Because such a theory will be developed out of a particular conception of human value or "the good"—i.e., what is "it" that must be protected, promoted or distributed, and what is the best way of doing so—it must also be relative or sensitive to the values of the context in which it is applied.

The reconfigured GMH agenda references Amartya Sen's "capability approach" (Sen, 1985, 1999), showing recognition that there is a need for some theoretical framework that may serve as a point of departure. The capability approach, generally used not only for the purposes of justice but also to assess development and well-being, posits that justice presupposes freedom with regard to human capabilities that we have reason to value.[c] It differs from the dominant Rawlsian account of justice as it focuses on capabilities to live in certain ways as an end, rather than on primary goods (such as money or liberty) as generalized means to a variety of ends, because it recognizes that individuals differ in their ability to convert primary goods or resources into valuable opportunities (Justice, 1990). According to this view, the focus of justice should be on promoting equal capabilities, with justice in health care prioritizing the removal of limits to human capabilities posed by poor health, disease or disability. This approach is supportive of the GMH recognition of the social determinants of mental health as it also broadens the scope of health substantially, by not attributing moral significance to the cause of reduced capabilities (Sabin & Daniels, 1994).

In this chapter we assess where CP fits in with the three levels of progressively demanding claim rights, i.e., a negative and positive right to mental health and a (positive) right to mental health care, to establish how it relates to GMH. The outcome of this will be dependent on empirical factors concerning CP as well as its ethical status. Relevant empirical factors include the (clinical) efficacy of CP and its ability to improve health outcomes in terms of the capabilities approach. The ethical status of CP would have an obvious bearing on its inclusion in all three levels of rights. Because a rights assertion implies an intrinsic or instrumental good, if CP is shown to be conclusively ethically problematic then this would clearly warrant its exclusion from all three levels of rights. Furthermore, it must be noted that even if CP can be shown to exert a claim on the grounds of a right to mental health or mental health care, this will not necessarily translate into an entitlement to CP that elicits a positive obligation. For this to be the case CP would have to be assessed with reference to relevant criteria, such as need, and an appropriate conception of justice that is contextually informed.

---

[c] In other words, achieving well-being, interpreted as one's personal conception of "the good," requires an enabling "capability set," which Sen interprets as "the actual freedom of choice a person has over alternative lives that he or she can lead…[and in which he or she can] achieve various alternative combinations of functionings, or doings and beings" (Justice, 1990). Sen's approach is a value-neutral one, he does not articulate which capabilities are relevant or important for well-being; he argues that this should be determined by individuals, in accordance with their notions of the good, and through public discourse. Other capability theorists, such as Martha Nussbaum, have given substantive accounts of the capabilities necessary for well-being and justice (Nussbaum, 2000).

Relevant ethical considerations of CP

Depending on the underlying moral theory, bioenhancement is frequently justified with reference to the fact that it is fundamentally aimed at realizing an "absolute good," such as well-being or the ability of persons to determine their lives as they see fit. Ethical concerns are generally articulated either as practical concerns (e.g., bioenhancement is wrong, in practice, to the extent that it will lead to undesirable outcomes) or general moral-status concerns (bioenhancement is intrinsically wrong, or wrong in principle, irrespective of good or bad outcomes) (see Agar, 2015 for a discussion of this distinction). In this chapter we look at CP in both senses.

When addressing the ethical status of bioenhancements, there are certain ethically relevant distinctions that can be helpful in identifying the motivation for using an enhancement, the kind of good that it confers and its impact on others. Firstly, using cognitive enhancement as an example, the motivation for using a cognitive enhancer is distinctly instrumental. A person will generally take a cognitive enhancer as a means to some end, such as being able to study or work more easily or efficiently (Sattler, Sauer, Mehlkop, & Graeff, 2013). While their reasons for wanting to study or work more effectively will vary according to the nature of their ultimate goals, people do not generally use cognitive enhancers to improve their concentration or retention of information simply for the sake of improving it. It is mostly the case that such drugs are used on the basis of beliefs that the improvements they confer are a more effective or easier way of realizing a particular goal. While using a medication treatment in this way is not intrinsically problematic, in contexts characterized by inequity, to the extent that an intervention assists in realizing a person's ultimate goal, where the goal may not have been achieved—or not as easily or successfully achieved—in the absence of the enhancement, the intervention would constitute a distinct instrumental advantage for the individual, and this would have ethical implications. We will return to this point.

In the case of CP, there could be a variety of reasons motivating its use. For example, it could be used for shyness that is not attributable to a social anxiety disorder but nevertheless produces some impact on a person's life where after using CP she feels that she can be "more herself"; for feelings of low self-esteem whereby "feeling better" enables a person to have the courage to make use of opportunities he would otherwise have avoided, which then leads to subsequent improvements in his self-esteem; or, for a sense of malaise that is not associated with a depressive disorder but is informed by "existential" or contextual factors, whereby using CP results in an improvement in mood that then enables the person to make the requisite changes to her situation. Whether these cases are instances of subthreshold symptoms, that may or may not develop into more serious disorders, or examples of existential ailments that are more social in origin is not relevant at this point. What is relevant is the nature of the reasons for using an intervention in such cases.

In all these examples, while CP is fulfilling different aims—alleviating shyness differs from improving self-esteem or ameliorating a sense of malaise—they share a common goal which could be described as "feeling better." Feeling better could be a precursor of states such as well-being, happiness or flourishing, and could therefore be thought of as instrumental in some way. However, the fact that we wouldn't generally ask someone why they wish to feel better, indicates that the state of feeling better is self-explanatory or recognized to be fundamentally desirable.[d] In the case of CP, we could therefore say that its use is aimed at securing well-being, happiness or flourishing for the sake of well-being, happiness or flourishing. The use of CP is therefore associated with the desire to secure an intrinsic or absolute good.

There is an additional distinction, related to the previous point, that has been used to navigate the ethical status of different forms of bioenhancement (Harris, 2007). We can distinguish between a positional and a non-positional good. A positional good is associated with an advantage that depends on distribution. In other words, the more people that have access to this good, the less advantage it confers. Athletic abilities are a clear-cut example of a positional good because success is dependent on being faster or stronger than one's competitors; if others become faster or stronger this will lesson one's advantage. Intelligence is a positional good in certain competitive environments, so that to the extent that a cognitive enhancement enables a person to perform more efficiently and successfully than others, this will confer some degree of competitive advantage.[e] For this reason, many forms of bioenhancement are vulnerable to the criticism that because improvements in human physical and cognitive functioning are both instrumentally and positionally valuable, the goals of enhancement represent highly individualistic, selfish or greedy aspirations that have divisive effects (see Kass, 2003; Sandel, 2007 for such arguments).[f]

Positional goods can be contrasted with non-positional goods, whereby the associated good is independent of the pattern of distribution. In other words, the extent to which such a good is shared or held by others has no impact on its value. CP would be directed at securing a non-positional good because the value associated with an increased sense of well-being is independent of distribution and unaffected by the presence of competition. This is not to say that having higher levels of well-being

[d] While we would never question why someone wishes to feel better, in certain cases we would challenge their conception of feeling better when it is linked to particular undesirable or destructive behaviors by pointing out long term implications. In such cases there would not be any link between feeling better and objective well-being or flourishing. This indicates that feeling better requires a well-established causal link to some level of objective well-being for it to be regarded as an intrinsically good state to be in.

[e] In cases where a stimulant is used off label by a student for the purposes of performing more effectively, his enhanced performance won't necessarily leave anyone immediately worse off. However, to the extent that the student is able to perform better than he would otherwise have, this advantage would be unfair to students who do not have such an advantage.

[f] A positional-good may, of course, be used for non-competitive purposes. For example, if a cognitive enhancement enabled a scientist to discover a cure for cancer, her decision to undergo such an enhancement would be universally advantageous. However, this would be on account of her having chosen to use the advantage of higher intelligence for altruistic, universally beneficial ends. The fact remains that when an ability, like intelligence, is linked to outcomes that are competitive in any way, the *personal* advantage conferred by the ability is inversely proportional to the number of people who have the ability. A response could be to point out that increasing intelligence only appears to be a zero-sum game in individualistic, competitive environments. While this is a valid point, it remains the case that any form of resource scarcity, i.e. a world structured such as ours, will generally result in persons seeking some form of competitive advantage even if this occurs at a collective rather than an individual level, e.g., seeking kin or group advantage.

would not be advantageous for the person in question, rather, that others will not be left worse off. However, if access to an intervention that is associated with well-being is contingent upon shared resources, this complicates matters. These distinctions are relevant for justice-related arguments which generally develop from the concern that bioenhancements will, or could, exacerbate inequities if access to the benefits they confer is contingent upon resources (Buchanan, Brock, Daniels, & Wikler, 2000; Fukuyama, 2002). Given that a global perspective of mental health is focused on reducing inequities, such an objection to enhancement is relevant for our purposes.

A further relevant distinction is one that has frequently been used to navigate the moral status of bioenhancement in general. For purposes related to justice in public and private health insurance coverage, a rough distinction is frequently drawn between disease and health so as to determine "medical necessity" and ensure that, at the very least, the "worst off" receive treatment (Sabin & Daniels, 1994). Such a distinction would be characteristic of a narrow approach to justice in health care of which Norman Daniel's normal function model (NFM) is a paradigmatic example (Daniels, 1985). This account argues that the dictates of justice in health care translate only into an obligation to prevent, treat, and cure disease or dysfunction, where possible, so as to restore health to a level associated with "normal" functioning or "species-typical" functioning (Boorse, 1975; Buchanan et al., 2000). Any treatment of "dysfunction" not attributable to a diagnosable condition would be the responsibility of individuals themselves, or the appropriate societal institutions (Sabin & Daniels, 1994).

While it is undoubtedly true that justice in health care demands some form of distinction between degrees of need, given the complex etiology of many disorders and diseases, the arbitrary and problematic nature of such a distinction as a criterion for medical necessity has been well-recognized (Erler, 2017; Holtug, 2011). What is relevant for our purposes, is that the notion of medical necessity and the NFM have been used to support the contested distinction between treatment and enhancement, which has been developed as a way of navigating the moral status of bioenhancement. These arguments generally refer to a statistically determined threshold for species typical functioning, and suggest that an intervention which raises functioning to this level is a form of treatment, whereas any improvement beyond this threshold is an enhancement (Kahane, Savulescu, & ter Meulen, 2011).[g] The distinction is then used to support a variety of arguments against bioenhancement (see Juengst, 1998; Pellegrino, 2004; President's Council on Bioethics & Kass, 2003).

The important point for our focus is that using the distinction between disease and health, and thus, between treatment and enhancement as a means of navigating the moral status of CP seems both practically and ethically untenable, given the dimensional nature of mental health. However, while the treatment/enhancement distinction is problematic for these reasons, it is relevant insofar as considering CP in a global

---

[g] For example, a human trait such as intelligence would be measured according to the statistical average in a population by utilizing the Intelligence Quotient (IQ). Falling below a particular figure, in this case 70, would result in receiving the classification of being intellectually impaired or disabled. On this account, an intervention that raises a person's IQ to the average of 70, would be viewed as *treating* this impairment whereas an intervention that raises it above 70 would be regarded as an *enhancement* (Kahane et al., 2011).

context requires forming a position on the claim it would exert in health care contexts. This is an issue of prioritization or competing medical needs which are concerns related to fairness or justice, and, which thus require some reference to medical necessity. Furthermore, the issue of medical necessity is connected to what is probably the most serious ethical challenge for CP, in terms of how it relates to GMH. This is the concern that the use of medication treatments for "existential ailments" or symptoms that are not medical in nature, is indicative of "the medicalization of human unhappiness" (Elliott, 1999 in Bjorklund, 2005) or the pathologizing of "problems of living" (Mills & Fernando, 2014).

In fact, these concerns are related to criticisms that have been directed at the GMH movement itself (Cooper, 2016). Many of these criticisms arguably indicate an inadequate understanding of the GMH agenda and the nature of mental disorders and have been effectively dispelled (see the responses of Cohen, 2014; Patel, 2014). However, considering CP in terms of GMH requires some way of responding to these criticisms because so-called cosmetic uses of psychiatric drugs are particularly vulnerable to concerns regarding overmedicalization or over-commercialization.

There are different ways of responding to the overmedicalization concern. An immediate response would be to use an autonomy-based argument in support of the free choice to use CP if it is deemed effective by the person in question. However, such an argument must account for the persuasive power of a pharmaceutical culture and other factors that inhibit genuine choice between various options. Overuse concerns are generally directed at common mental disorders (see Summerfield, 2012) such as depression and anxiety, and are informed by the difficulties, in certain cases, in distinguishing between clinical and non-clinical conditions (Patel, 2014). A similar concern has been raised that if, in certain cases, we cannot reliably distinguish an "existential ailment" from a clinical condition, we may not be able to distinguish between cosmetic and clinical uses of psychopharmacology (Bjorklund, 2005). What is implied in these concerns is that a biomedical intervention is an inappropriate response to a condition that is social in nature or cause. However, this position is informed by the disease/health distinction which is untenable in light of knowledge of the interplay between social and environmental determinants and biology (Patel, 2014). This distinction also doesn't take into account that, regardless of cause, psychiatric drugs are able to modify brain activity and can, in many cases, lead to improvements in behavior or mood (Persson & Savulescu, 2014). Furthermore, if a person experiencing symptoms, that have a deleterious impact on her life and detract from her general well-being, seeks a medication treatment, labeling an intervention that alleviates these symptoms as an inappropriate use of medication simply because her symptoms are not indicative of an underlying diagnosable disorder seems counter-intuitive.

The tendency to distinguish between a social and clinical condition and appropriate social and clinical solutions may be indicative of a normative judgment that is motivated by an implicit bias towards interventions that are subject- and effort-driven, as opposed to those in which one considers oneself to be the passive object of an intervention. On this distinction, the former would be associated with non-medication treatments that produce behavioral changes attributable to individual effort and ongoing involvement. These "active" interventions would be distinguished from "passive" medication treatments whereby changes would require minimal individual effort (Focquaert & Schermer, 2015). While this distinction disregards the fact that the act of seeking an intervention, implies a non-passive process, it may be informed by deeper authenticity concerns. This would refer to the belief that any improvements or changes to mood or personality would be attributable to the medication, as opposed to originating from the person's volitions or their "self" and would thus be inauthentic in some way. However, if we view the self as divisible in this way, a counter-response could be to point out that even minor symptoms could be regarded as forms of "internal psychological constraint" (Cooper, 2016), and thus by alleviating such symptoms, a medication could enable the "authentic self" to be more present. While the scope of this chapter prevents a full exposition of this matter, the overuse concern remains a problem for CP.

As mentioned above, with few exceptions, the ethical status of bioenhancement has been informed by insights drawn from the Western philosophical tradition, and, in particular, by a liberal individualist framework. This has resulted in the debate perhaps being framed in an overly narrow way. Generally, the ethical status of bioenhancement is articulated in terms of potential benefits vs. harms, autonomy vs. its limits, and its implications for justice and injustice, with reference to properties internal to individuals such as autonomy, authenticity, self-esteem and pleasure. While few arguments are framed in such simplistic terms, more sophisticated arguments are frequently reducible to these fundamental oppositions. Looking at the implications of bioenhancement in such highly individualized terms has resulted in the neglect of alternative values and perspectives that may be useful for infusing fresh insights into the debate. Ultimately, a global perspective on CP, and other globally focused concerns, will not be truly global if it is informed by such a narrowed perspective (Graness, 2015). In light of this, we supplement the observations made in this section with insights from a relational account that draws on an African moral framework.

A relational account of moral value and its implications for justice

Thaddeus Metz's relational account of moral status is located in a more communitarian framework (Metz, 2016). This account draws upon what is common to the normative insights and values that characterize sub-Saharan worldviews, so as to develop a "moral principle" that can serve as an alternative to the dominant Western tradition (Kigongo, 2002; Metz, 2016).[h] Normative moral theories, including rights appeals and theories of justice, are developed out of a particular conception of the source or nature of moral status or worth. The relational account lies between theories which ascribe moral value to some quality intrinsic to human individuals, and those that associate it

---

[h] Metz's aims are modest; his account is not presented as the definitive interpretation of African moral values and norms, nor is it posited to be more justifiable than Western theories or even unique to Africa. Rather, the aim is to show that certain valuable ideas, that are characteristic of an African moral framework, have been neglected in the dominant tradition and that continuing this neglect represents an injustice (Metz, 2016).

with a collective or group, such as a particular "way of life" (Metz, 2016). While some sub-Saharan theorists associate moral status with the latter (Ake, 1987) the relational account contests such an interpretation, drawing upon the work of various African theorists in support of an account of moral status that is not dependent purely upon group membership or internal to the individual but is concerned with being with, and "relating to others", in a particular kind of way (Metz, 2016). On this account:

> *moral status is constituted by some kind of interactive property between one entity and another...something warrants moral consideration only if (and because) it can or does exhibit certain attitudes towards, or have a causal effect on another being (Metz, 2016)[i]*

Metz identifies two ways of relating to others, prevalent in the work of various African theorists, that exemplify the idea of "we" as opposed to "I." "Identifying with others" refers to a subjective feeling of "togetherness," "cooperation" and "compatible ends", while "exhibiting solidarity with others" implies acting with "good will" and "pro-attitudes" or care, in accordance with a shared conception of the good (Metz, 2007, 2017). In other words, this conception prizes relations that are "communal or harmonious" as opposed to discordant (Metz, 2016).[j] Another way of describing this kind of way of relating to others is found in the Ubuntu ethic, a prevalent guiding ideal in southern African thought (Metz, 2007). The sentiment that the Ubuntu ethic aims to capture is encapsulated by the well-referenced slogan: "a person is a person through other persons" as well as Mbiti's interpretation, "I am because we are" (Mbiti, 1990), and Tutu's formulation, "my humanity is caught up, is inextricably bound up in yours" (Tutu, 1999). In short, one is a real person, self or human being insofar as one positively relates to others.

These ideas support the normative claim that because this relational capacity is constitutive of human moral value, it should serve as an ideal. This kind of way of relating or capacity warrants respect in its own right and not as a means to some end; this is how we *should* relate to others (Metz, 2016). This claim is reflected by the succinct formulation of Mbiti's insight that "what is right is what connects people together; what separates people is wrong" (Verhoef & Michel, 1997). In terms of social justice, rather than grounding human rights on an appeal to an individualistic conception of human

---

[i] Elsewhere, Metz describes this as the capacity for being able to be the "subject or object" of a particular kind of modal relationship characterized by "sharing" (Metz, 2012). As Metz points out, this account is able to tell us why animals or those with diminished intellectual abilities have moral status in a way that accounts grounded on the autonomy of persons cannot. While being able to be the subject of a certain kind of shared relationship requires a particular level of intellectual functioning, being the object of such a relationship does not (Metz, 2012).

[j] These ideas find support in certain positions, located in the Western tradition, that have been developed as alternatives to the dominant moral theories that are informed by a liberal individualist framework. The ethics of care has roots in feminist theory and was developed out of the recognition that relationships are characterized by reciprocal dependence and a need for care (Gilligan, 1993; Noddings, 1984). MacIntyre draws on Aristotelian insights to criticize modern moral philosophy and liberal individualism as having led to a distorted view of the self and morality. In particular, he argues that "the self has to find its moral identity in and through its membership in communities" (MacIntyre, 1981). Sandel has also criticized Rawlsian Liberalism for neglecting the way that selfhood is formed through numerous social connections (Sandel, 1998).

dignity, which reduces to autonomy or self-determination, in this framework, persons possess intrinsic human worth or dignity by way of their capacity for "being both a subject and an object of a communal relationship" (Metz, 2016). This account has intuitive appeal as it captures something significant with respect to why negative rights violations are so morally problematic. As Metz points out, murder or rape undoubtedly disregard the ability of the other to determine their own ends, in a Kantian sense, however there is more to what makes murder or rape bad, over and above their disregard for the autonomous determination of the self. Such violations are also deeply problematic in terms of the intense, intentional ill will and discord that motivates them, as well as the way in which they respectively eradicate or impair relations with others (Metz, 2017).

The relational account is also congruent with the "capabilities" approach as exemplified by both Sen (Sen, 1985) and Nussbaum (Nussbaum, 2000). In terms of resource distribution, the relational account identifies the fulfillment of needs as the object of distribution, but it focuses on those needs that enable the fulfillment of a capacity to relate to others, in the stipulated way, as the highest good. Rather than the traditional focus on the fulfillment of needs that are directed at personal, self-determined ends, this would include not only basic needs but also all those resources that support the capacity of people "to engage in harmonious relationships [of identification and solidarity] with each other" (Metz, 2016). The pattern of distribution that is suggested as most appropriate to the relational account is a balanced approach that recognizes the importance of meeting both the needs of the worst off, so as to ensure a "decent minimum," and those needs associated with fostering potential, so as to recognize the value of exceptional human flourishing (Metz, 2016).[k] While the relational principle, and the normative ideas that are drawn from it, does not constitute a complete moral theory, as a particular representation of an alternative, more communitarian worldview, it is both valuable and relevant to our focus in this chapter.[l] In the following section we discuss the implications of the relational account for mental health.

The implications of a relational account for conceptions of mental health and its care

The relational account has implications for the fundamental question upon which an account of justice in health care is built: why is health, and by implication treating illness and impairment related to health, a special kind of good (Metz, 2010)?

---

[k] Here, Metz uses the analogy of how resources are allocated in the context of a family. An ideal familial distribution is equitable, everyone receives a roughly similar share of resources. However, there is also a tendency to allocate more resources to those with urgent needs (e.g., the worst off) as well as those who show potential in some area. For example, in a family where a child has a disability, he should receive a larger share of resources so as to enable him to reach a particular level of functioning. However, on this view, channeling all of the resources towards him would be wrong. A child who shows particular promise or talent should also receive a larger share of resources so as to enable her to actualize her potential (Metz, 2016).

[l] The scope of this article does not permit us to present an exhaustive account of Metz's argument. For a full exposition of his approach, see Metz (2007, 2012).

Answering these questions with reference to mental health draws firstly upon the empirical claim that mental illness negatively impacts social functioning in some way. We can take this claim to be self-evident as mental disorders are, by definition, associated with some degree of impaired social functioning or with some form of impact on personal relationships (Kessler et al., 1997; Kessler, Foster, Saunders, & Stang, 1995; Kessler, Walters, & Forthofer, 1998).

With this in mind, on the relational account, health in general, and mental health specifically, is morally significant because mental disorders have the potential to subvert personhood understood in the relational sense (Metz, 2010). In other words, mental disorders have the potential to isolate persons to the extent that their ability to fully engage with others in shared relationships, characterized by a sense of identification and solidarity, is compromised. This not only gives us a plausible account of what is threatened in the case of mental disorders, it can also tell us why certain cases warrant more urgent attention than others in a way that is not fully captured by traditional approaches (Metz, 2010). For example, as Metz points out, regarding healthcare as a special good simply on account of its ability to reduce suffering leads to problematic conclusions in the case of illness that doesn't confer suffering but is nevertheless not desirable. A comatose patient may not be suffering but his being in a coma is undoubtedly a bad thing for him. In addition, the position that healthcare is a special good because it supports a person's ability to autonomously pursue their own ends, also fails to capture a significant way in which illness impacts the person (Metz, 2010).

We can apply these insights to the justice-related challenge of prioritizing competing medical needs in mental health care that will be relevant to our discussion of CP. Firstly, if moral status inheres in a particular way of relating to others, as both an object and subject of identification and solidarity, then the *ability* or *capacity* to do so is the object of focus. Broadly construed, the purpose of a mental health care system would be to intervene in cases where this ability or capacity is compromised due to any mental health-related causes. In terms of prioritization, on this account, health needs would be situated on a continuum. The most serious impacts on the ability to be both a subject and object of a relationship (i.e., where life itself is threatened) would be located at one end of the continuum and regarded as most urgent. Life-threatening cases aside, as an individual will always be capable of being an object of such a relationship, the focus would generally be on degrees of ability to be a subject of such a relationship. The continuum would thus move from the most extreme impacts on this relational ability through to the least extreme.

Applying this approach to psychiatric disorders specifically, the continuum would move from psychotic disorders such as schizophrenia and bipolar disorders, at the extreme end, to subthreshold symptoms at the opposite end. Placing psychotic disorders at one end of the spectrum and subthreshold symptoms at the other end is relatively unproblematic in terms of our intuitions regarding the stark differences between impacts on relational capacities. The rest of the continuum would comprise all the common mental disorders, assessed with reference to the degree to which symptoms and behavior impact relational abilities.

In terms of specific treatment interventions, the relational account would seemingly lend support to the use of medication treatments for psychiatric disorders, to the extent that such interventions could effectively target and alleviate symptoms associated with an impaired ability to relate to others in the stipulated way. While such treatments produce variable results (Cascade, Kalali, & Kennedy, 2009), their general tendency is arguably to enhance pro-social behaviors (Siegel & Crockett, 2013). For example, the administering of SSRIs, is associated with increases in both fair cooperation (Crockett, 2009; Tse & Bond, 2002) and aversion to harming others (Crockett, Clark, Hauser, & Robbins, 2010). These findings are clear-cut in the case of psychosis and may well be seen in common mental disorders as well as postulated in subthreshold cases.

These points aside, while it is by no means complete, this account of what is threatened in cases of mental disorder is a worthwhile alternative to traditional approaches that are framed with reference to individualist conceptions, which are themselves incomplete. It also accords with the intuition that certain kinds of needs have a stronger claim than others. Furthermore, it emphasizes the interpersonal effects of mental disorders and therefore highlights a valuable concern that is frequently neglected by an individualist framework. Having sketched out a very basic conception of the kinds of good that mental health and mental health care are concerned with, in the following section we bring the various considerations that have been addressed in this chapter together and discuss the ethical status of CP and its relationship to GMH in terms of the three levels of claim rights.

The ethical status of CP and implications for the three levels of claim rights

While our focus in this chapter has been on CP, rather than on cognitive enhancement, we can now articulate why we take CP to be more ethically justifiable than cognitive enhancement in terms of the GMH agenda. Once again, this is not to say that cognitive enhancement is intrinsically morally problematic, rather, it is to say that it would have to be justified in terms of a narrow claim to an individualistic good, such as the autonomy of individuals to determine their lives and secure their own well-being as they see fit. Such a claim is a product of a liberal individualist paradigm and therefore could not claim universal endorsement. Furthermore, in the absence of universal availability and equitable access, it is difficult to see how cognitive enhancement could be justified with reference to a more widespread claim, such as its ability to improve overall well-being. In fact, for the reasons discussed, it is possible that the advantages conferred by cognitive enhancement could worsen existing inequalities with regard to human capabilities. In this regard, cognitive enhancement would be less congruent with the spirit of the GMH focus on improving well-being and capabilities for "whole populations" (Patel et al., 2018).

Support for the conclusion that CP is more ethically justifiable than cognitive enhancement could also be drawn from the relational account. If cognitive enhancement was used with the intention of securing personal ambitions and advantage at the expense of other individuals, this would be indicative of a lack of good will and failure to identify with the goals of others. In addition, to the extent that using such an intervention would lead to divisive outcomes, it would not be in the spirit of the value accorded to relationality. Therefore, both the motives for using cognitive enhancement as well as its consequences for relationships would be relevant considerations.

CP seems more ethically justifiable, and thus more congruent with the conception of mental health as an absolute good, which supports the claim of a right to mental health. Firstly, there would be a causal link between the motives for using CP and a state of well-being. Secondly, because the value of CP is non-positional, it would not leave others worse off. On the contrary, by reducing the impact of the symptoms that caused the person to sufficiently problematize her behavior or mental state and seek a medication treatment, CP could improve the quality of relations with others. Support for this conclusion would rest on the empirical claim that subthreshold symptoms, such as shyness, low-esteem or a general sense of malaise have some degree of impact on the quality of relationships with others, which seems an uncontroversial claim to make.

However, while it seems that a relational account would lend support to CP, a possible response could be that in such cases where symptoms are socially manifested, resorting to an individualistic way of addressing these symptoms overrides the opportunity to address and overcome them relationally. Of course, a medication treatment and a relational "solution" need not, and should not, be mutually exclusive, it may be that the improvement of mood is an enabling factor to addressing the nature of these symptoms with others. However, this response aside, a preference for a non-medical solution brings us back to the overmedicalization or overuse concern. Hypothetically, if a medication treatment were to produce improvements in mood with no negative side effects, and this concern remained, then it would indicate a deeper normative assumption. However, the fact that this concern may be informed by particular normative beliefs does not necessarily negate it, it simply shows that the concern is more complex than it may initially seem. The scope of this chapter limits further discussion of this matter; however, it remains a challenge for CP that will continue to elicit discussion. This point aside, in terms of a negative right to mental health, it seems that CP confers a sufficiently valuable good to exert a claim that society should, at least, refrain from actions that prevent individuals from using CP to improve their mental well-being, particularly where that is constituted by the quality of their relations.

We can then turn to the more demanding positive right to mental health which is the justice-related claim that certain active or positive measures should be taken to support the conditions for, and promotion of, mental health. Both the capabilities account and the relational account lend ostensive support to CP. On a capabilities account, where ability to relate to others is a capability that is supportive of an individual's conception of the good, it seems that CP is justified to the extent that the symptoms that caused the individual in question to seek a medication treatment impact this capability. Further support is provided by the relational account which regards the capability to relate to others, in the stipulated way, as its guiding ideal. On this account, society has a duty to put measures in place that are relevant to, and supportive of, this capability to relate at all levels, from most serious to least serious. Tentative support for this claim could be drawn from the ideas that inform balanced distribution which accounts both for meeting the needs of the worst off and for the realization of human potential or flourishing. However, it is important to note that whether CP is included as one of the means of supporting relational capabilities will depend on the deeper normative beliefs regarding the moral status of psychopharmacological interventions, mentioned above. This will be informed by values that are relative to context. Where medical treatments are regarded as morally neutral, however, it would seem that CP could exert a claim on the basis of a positive right to mental health, and that, where possible, societal institutions should support this option.

Finally, we turn to the most demanding claim which is a right to mental health care. As mentioned, the entitlement to mental health care is relative to system and needs, and thus, would be informed by the availability of resources and other contextual factors. A right to CP could be compatible with an entitlement to it, in the mental health care context, on the grounds of preventative measures. If the extent to which subclinical symptoms progress to clinical conditions is shown to be sufficiently serious to warrant active intervention, then this could justify an entitlement to some allocation of resources for this purpose. Given the GMH emphasis on cost-effectiveness and sustainable development, an argument could be made that preventing subthreshold symptoms from progressing to threshold levels could reduce the higher social and economic costs associated with the latter (Chisholm et al., 2016). Cross-sectional studies that assess the cost-efficiency of treatment for subthreshold symptoms could be helpful here. However, it may be that given the presence of more urgent and serious needs, the claim that CP exerts will remain at the broader and less demanding level of ensuring that societal institutions are structured in such a way that they not only refrain from impeding individuals from using CP but also, where possible, actively support this option.

Conclusion

In this chapter we have attempted to discuss CP in a more globally relevant way. Firstly, we looked at the ethical implications of CP with reference to a moral framework that is more reflective of a relational worldview. While the relational account does not claim to be the definitive interpretation of African normative insights it can claim to more accurately capture the basis of such insights than an individualistic account. Secondly, we looked at CP in terms of how it relates to GMH concerns. This involved looking at how CP fits in with three levels of progressively demanding negative and positive rights to mental health and mental health care respectively. GMH originated from the desire to reduce the burden and suffering associated with untreated mental disorders, however, it has broadened its focus to mental health and well-being in general. It is in the latter area that CP would relate to GMH. However, the urgency of the former is such that the place for CP in a GMH agenda will remain limited and contingent upon contextual factors. We contend that the bioenhancement debate in general will benefit from further discussions of its relevance in light of global needs and alternative moral frameworks.

Acknowledgment

We would like to thank Professor Thaddeus Metz for reading over this chapter and providing helpful input.

References

Agar, N. (2005). *Liberal eugenics: In defence of human enhancement*. Malden, MA: Blackwell.

Agar, N. (2015). Moral bioenhancement and the utilitarian catastrophe. *Cambridge Quarterly of Healthcare Ethics: CQ: The International Journal of Healthcare Ethics Committees*, *24*(1), 37. https://doi.org/10.1017/S0963180114000280.

Ake, C. (1987). The African context of human rights. *Africa Today*, *34*(1), 5.

Barbui, C., Dua, T., Kolappa, K., Saraceno, B., & Saxena, S. (2017). Mapping actions to improve access to medicines for mental disorders in low and middle income countries. *Epidemiology and Psychiatric Sciences*, *26*(5), 481–490. https://doi.org/10.1017/S2045796016001165.

Berghmans, R., Ter Meulen, R., Malizia, A., & Vos, R. (2011). Scientifc, ethical, and social issues in mood enhnancement. In J. Savulescu, R. H. J. Ter Meulen, & G. Kahane (Eds.), *Enhancing human capacities* (pp. 153–165). Chichester, West Sussex: Blackwell Publishing.

Beyer, C., Staunton, C., & Moodley, K. (2014). The implications of methylphenidate use by healthy medical students and doctors in South Africa. *BMC Medical Ethics*, *15*, 20. https://doi.org/10.1186/1472-6939-15-20.

Bjorklund, P. (2005). Can there be a 'cosmetic' psychopharmacology? Prozac unplugged: The search for an ontologically distinct cosmetic psychopharmacology. *Nursing Philosophy*, *6*(2), 131–143. https://doi.org/10.1111/j.1466-769X.2005.00213.x.

Boorse, C. (1975). On the distinction between disease and illness. *Philosophy & Public Affairs*, *5*(1), 49–68.

Brito, G. V. (2015). Evidence for the off-label use of methylphenidate for cognitive enhancement in healthy individuals. *Value in Health*, *18*(3), https://doi.org/10.1016/j.jval.2015.03.734.

Buchanan, A. (2010). The egalitarianism of human rights. *Ethics*, *120*(4), 679–710. https://doi.org/10.1086/653433.

Buchanan, A. E. (2011). *Beyond humanity?: The ethics of biomedical enhancement. Uehiro series in practical ethics*. Oxford: Oxford University Press.

Buchanan, A. E., Brock, D. W., Daniels, N., & Wikler, D. (Eds.), (2000). *From chance to choice: Genetics and justice*. Cambridge: Cambridge University Press.

Caplan, A., & Elliott, C. (2004). Is it ethical to use enhancement technologies to make us better than well? (the PLoS medicine debate). *PLoS Medicine*, *1*(3), e52. https://doi.org/10.1371/journal.pmed.0010052.

Cascade, E., Kalali, A. H., & Kennedy, S. H. (2009). Real-world data on SSRI antidepressant side effects. *Psychiatry (Edgmont (PA: Township))*, *6*(2), 16.

Chisholm, D., Sweeny, K., Sheehan, P., Rasmussen, B., Smit, F., Cuijpers, P., et al. (2016). Scaling-up treatment of depression and anxiety: A global return on investment analysis. *The Lancet Psychiatry*, *3*(5), 415–424. https://doi.org/10.1016/s2215-0366(16)30024-4.

Cohen, A. (2014). A nuanced perspective? *The British Journal of Psychiatry*, *205*(4), 329. https://doi.org/10.1192/bjp.205.4.329.

Cohen, Y., Segev, R., Shlafman, N., Novack, V., & Ifergane, G. (2015). Methylphenidate use among medical students at Ben-Gurion University of the Negev. *Journal of Neurosciences in Rural Practice*, *6*(3), 320–325. https://doi.org/10.4103/0976-3147.158749.

Cooper, S. (2016). Global mental health and its critics: Moving beyond the impasse. *Critical Public Health*, *26*(4), 355–358. https://doi.org/10.1080/09581596.2016.1161730.

Crockett, M. J. (2009). The neurochemistry of fairness: Clarifying the link between serotonin and prosocial behavior. *Annals of the New York Academy of Sciences*, *1167*, 76–86. https://doi.org/10.1111/j.1749-6632.2009.04506.x.

Crockett, M. J., Clark, L., Hauser, M. D., & Robbins, T. W. (2010). Serotonin selectively influences moral judgment and behavior through effects on harm aversion. *Proceedings of the National Academy of Sciences of the United States of America, 107*(40), 17433–17438. https://doi.org/10.1073/pnas.1009396107.

Daniels, N. (1985). *Just health care.* Cambridge: Cambridge University Press.

Daniels, N. (2000). Normal functioning and the treatment-enhancement distinction. *Cambridge Quarterly of Healthcare Ethics, 9*(03), https://doi.org/10.1017/s0963180100903037.

Daniels, N. (2017). Justice and access to health care. In *The Stanford encyclopedia of philosophy.* Metaphysics Research Lab, Stanford University. https://plato.stanford.edu/archives/win2017/entries/justice-healthcareaccess. [Accessed 24 October 2018].

Degrazia, D. (2000). Prozac, enhancement, and self-creation. *The Hastings Center Report, 30*(2), 34–40. https://doi.org/10.2307/3528313.

Elliott, C. (1999). Prozac and the existential novel: Two therapies. In C. Elliott & J. Lantos (Eds.), *The last physician: Walker Percy and the moral life of medicine* (pp. 59–69). Durham, NC: Duke University Press.

Erler, A. (2017). The limits of the treatment-enhancement distinction as a guide to public policy. *Bioethics, 31*(8), 608–615. https://doi.org/10.1111/bioe.12377.

Focquaert, F., & Schermer, M. (2015). Moral enhancement: Do means matter morally? *Neuroethics, 8*(2), https://doi.org/10.1007/s12152-015-9230-y.

Fukuyama, F. (2002). *Our posthuman future: Consequences of the biotechnology revolution.* New York: Picador.

Gilligan, C. (1993). *In a different voice: Psychological theory and women's development.* Cambridge, Mass: Harvard University Press.

Glannon, W. (2008). Psychopharmacological enhancement. *Neuroethics, 1*(1), 45–54. https://doi.org/10.1007/s12152-008-9005-9.

Graness, A. (2015). Is the debate on 'global justice' a global one? Some considerations in view of modern philosophy in Africa. *Journal of Global Ethics, 11*(1), 126–140. https://doi.org/10.1080/17449626.2015.1010014.

Greely, H., Sahakian, B., Harris, J., Kessler, R. C., Gazzaniga, M., Campbell, P., et al. (2008). Towards responsible use of cognitive-enhancing drugs by the healthy. *Nature, 456*(7223), 702–705. https://doi.org/10.1038/456702a.

Habermas, J. (2003). *The future of human nature.* Cambridge: Polity.

Harris, J. (2007). *Enhancing evolution: The ethical case for making better people.* Princeton, NJ: Princeton University Press.

Holtug, N. (2011). Equality and the treatment-enhancement distinction. *Bioethics, 25*(3), 137–144. https://doi.org/10.1111/j.1467-8519.2009.01750.x.

Juengst, E. (1998). What does 'enhancement' mean? In E. Parens (Ed.), *Enhancing human traits* (pp. 29–47). Washington: Georgetown University Press.

Justice, S. A. (1990). Means versus freedoms. *Philosophy & Public Affairs, 19*(2), 111–121.

Kahane, G., Savulescu, J., & ter Meulen, R. (2011). Preface. In J. Savulescu, R. ter Meulen, & G. Kahane (Eds.), *Enhancing human capacities* (pp. 3–18). London: Wiley-Blackwell.

Kass, L. R. (2003). Ageless bodies, happy souls: Biotechnology and the pursuit of perfection. *New Atlantis (Washington, DC)*, (1), 9.

Kessler, R., Berglund, P., Foster, C., Saunders, W., Stang, P., & Walters, E. (1997). Social consequences of psychiatric disorders. II. Teenage parenthood. *American Journal of Psychiatry, 154*(10), 1405. https://doi.org/10.1176/ajp.154.10.1405.

Kessler, R., Foster, C., Saunders, W., & Stang, P. (1995). Social consequences of psychiatric disorders, I: Educational attainment. *American Journal of Psychiatry, 152*(7), 1026. https://doi.org/10.1176/ajp.152.7.1026.

Kessler, R. C., Walters, E. E., & Forthofer, M. S. (1998). The social consequences of psychiatric disorders. III. Probability of marital stability. *The American Journal of Psychiatry*, *155*(8), 1092–1096. https://doi.org/10.1176/ajp.155.8.1092.

Kigongo, J. (2002). The relevance of African ethics to contemporary African society. In A. T. Dalfovo (Ed.), *Ethics, human rights, and development in Africa* (pp. 51–65). Washington, DC: Council for Research in Values and Philosophy.

Kohn, R., Saxena, S., Levav, I., & Saraceno, B. (2004). The treatment gap in mental health care. *Bulletin of the World Health Organization*, *82*(11), 858–866. https://doi.org/10.1590/S0042-96862004001100011.

Kramer, P. D. (1997). *Listening to Prozac*. New York, NY: Penguin Books.

Luhrmann, T. M. (2001). *Of two minds: An anthropologist looks at American psychiatry* (1st ed.). New York: Vintage Books.

MacIntyre, A. (1981). *After virtue* (3rd ed.). London: Duckworth.

Mbiti, J. S. (1990). *African religions & philosophy* (2nd ed.). Oxford: Heinemann.

Metz, T. (2007). Toward an African moral theory. *Journal of Political Philosophy*, *15*(3), 321–341. https://doi.org/10.1111/j.1467-9760.2007.00280.x.

Metz, T. (2010). African and Western moral theories in a bioethical context. *Developing World Bioethics*, *10*(1), 49–58. https://doi.org/10.1111/j.1471-8847.2009.00273.x.

Metz, T. (2012). An African theory of moral status: A relational alternative to individualism and holism. *Ethical Theory and Moral Practice*, *15*(3), 387–402. https://doi.org/10.1007/s10677-011-9302-y.

Metz, T. (2016). An African theory of social Justice: Relationship as the ground of rights, resources and recognition. In G. Biosen & M. Murray (Eds.), *Distributive Justice debates in political and social thought* (pp. 171–190). New York: Routledge.

Metz, T. (2017). Ancillary care obligations in light of an African bioethic: From entrustment to communion. *Theoretical Medicine and Bioethics*, *38*(2), 111–126. https://doi.org/10.1007/s11017-017-9404-1.

Mills, C., & Fernando, S. (2014). Globalising mental health or pathologising the global south? Mapping the ethics, theory and practice of global mental health. *Disability and the Global South*, *1*(2), 188–202. ISSN: 2050-7364.

Mohamed, A. D., & Sahakian, B. J. (2012). The ethics of elective psychopharmacology. *The International Journal of Neuropsychopharmacology*, *15*(4), 559–571. https://doi.org/10.1017/S146114571100037X.

Noddings, N. (1984). *Caring, a feminine approach to ethics & moral education*. Berkeley: University of California Press.

Nussbaum, M. C. (2000). *Women and human development: The capabilities approach. The John Robert Seeley lectures*. Cambridge: Cambridge University Press.

Patel, V. (2012). Global mental health: From science to action. *Harvard Review of Psychiatry*, *20*(1), 6–12. https://doi.org/10.3109/10673229.2012.649108.

Patel, V. (2014). Why mental health matters to global health. *Transcultural Psychiatry*, *51*(6), 777–789. https://doi.org/10.1177/1363461514524473.

Patel, V., Chisholm, D., Rabe-Hesketh, S., Dias-Saxena, F., Andrew, G., & Mann, A. (2003). Efficacy and cost-effectiveness of drug and psychological treatments for common mental disorders in general health care in Goa, India: A randomised, controlled trial. *The Lancet*, *361*(9351), 33–39. https://doi.org/10.1016/S0140-6736(03)12119-8.

Patel, V., Saxena, S., Lund, C., Thornicroft, G., Baingana, F., Bolton, P., et al. (2018). The lancet commission on global mental health and sustainable development. *The Lancet*, https://doi.org/10.1016/s0140-6736(18)31612-x.

Pellegrino, E. (2004). Biotechnology, human enhancement, and the ends of medicine. *Dignity*, *10*(4).

Persson, I., & Savulescu, J. (2014). Against fetishism about egalitarianism and in defense of cautious moral bioenhancement. *The American Journal of Bioethics, 14*(4), 39–42. https://doi.org/10.1080/15265161.2014.889248.

President's Council on Bioethics, & Kass, L. (2003). *Beyond therapy: Biotechnology and the pursuit of happiness.* Washington, DC: The President's Council on Bioethics.

Quitkin, F. M. (1999). Placebos, drug effects, and study design: A clinician's guide. *The American Journal of Psychiatry, 156*(6), 829–836. https://doi.org/10.1176/ajp.156.6.829.

Sabin, J., & Daniels, N. (1994). Determining "medical necessity" in mental health practice. *Hastings Center Report, 24,* 5–13.

Sahakian, B. J., & Morein-Zamir, S. (2015). Pharmacological cognitive enhancement: Treatment of neuropsychiatric disorders and lifestyle use by healthy people. *The Lancet Psychiatry, 2*(4), 357. https://doi.org/10.1016/S2215-0366(15)00004-8.

Sandel, M. J. (1998). *Liberalism and the limits of justice* (2nd ed.). New York: Cambridge University Press.

Sandel, M. J. (2007). *The case against perfection: Ethics in the age of genetic engineering.* Cambridge, MA: Belknap Press of Harvard University Press.

Sattler, S., Sauer, C., Mehlkop, G., & Graeff, P. (2013). The rationale for consuming cognitive enhancement drugs in university students and teachers (research article). *PLoS One, 8*(7), e68821. https://doi.org/10.1371/journal.pone.0068821.

Savulescu, J., ter Meulen, R. H. J., & Kahane, G. (Eds.), (2011). *Enhancing human capacities.* Chichester, West Sussex, UK: Wiley-Blackwell.

Schermer, M., Bolt, I., de Jongh, R., & Olivier, B. (2009). The future of psychopharmacological enhancements: Expectations and policies. *Neuroethics, 2*(2), 75–87. https://doi.org/10.1007/s12152-009-9032-1.

Sen, A. (1985). *Commodities and capabilities. Professor Dr. P. Hennipman lectures in economics.* New York: North-Holland.

Sen, A. (1999). *Development as freedom.* Oxford: Oxford University Press.

Serretti, A., Calati, R., Goracci, A., Di Simplicio, M., Castrogiovanni, P., & De Ronchi, D. (2010). Antidepressants in healthy subjects: What are the psychotropic/psychological effects? *European Neuropsychopharmacology, 20*(7), 433–453. https://doi.org/10.1016/j.euroneuro.2009.11.009.

Siegel, J. Z., & Crockett, M. J. (2013). How serotonin shapes moral judgment and behavior. *Annals of the New York Academy of Sciences, 1299,* 42–51. https://doi.org/10.1111/nyas.12229.

Stein, D. J. (2012). Psychopharmacological enhancement: A conceptual framework. *Philosophy, Ethics, and Humanities in Medicine, 7,* 5. https://doi.org/10.1186/1747-5341-7-5.

Stein, D. J., & Giordano, J. (2015). Global mental health and neuroethics. *BMC Medicine, 13*(1), https://doi.org/10.1186/s12916-015-0274-y.

Stein, D. J., & Illes, J. (2015). Beyond scientism and skepticism: An integrative approach to global mental health. *Frontiers in Psychiatry, 6,* 166. https://doi.org/10.3389/fpsyt.2015.00166.

Stone, K., Viera, A., & Parman, C. (2003). Off-label applications for SSRIs. *American Family Physician, 68*(3), 498–504.

Summerfield, D. (2012). Afterword: Against "global mental health". *Transcultural Psychiatry, 49*(3–4), 519–530. https://doi.org/10.1177/1363461512454701.

Tse, W. S., & Bond, A. J. (2002). Serotonergic intervention affects both social dominance and affiliative behaviour. *Psychopharmacology, 161*(3), 324–330. https://doi.org/10.1007/s00213-002-1049-7.

Tse, W. S., & Bond, A. J. (2003). Reboxetine promotes social bonding in healthy volunteers. *Journal of Psychopharmacology*, *17*(2), 189–195. https://doi.org/10.1177/026988110301 7002007.

Tutu, D. (1999). *No future without forgiveness*. New York: Random House.

Verhoef, H., & Michel, C. (1997). Studying morality within the African context: A model of moral analysis and construction. *Journal of Moral Education*, *26*(4), 389–407. https://doi. org/10.1080/0305724970260401.

Wong, J., Motulsky, A., Abrahamowicz, M., Eguale, T., Buckeridge, D. L., & Tamblyn, R. (2017). Off-label indications for antidepressants in primary care: Descriptive study of prescriptions from an indication based electronic prescribing system. *BMJ*, *356*, j603. https://doi.org/10.1136/bmj.j603.

Some ethics of deep brain stimulation

Joshua August Skorburg, Walter Sinnott-Armstrong
Philosophy Department and Kenan Institute for Ethics, Duke University, Durham, NC,
United States

Introduction

In an oft-cited case report, Schüpbach et al. (2006) describe Patient 1, a 38-year-old female journalist, married with one child, who had Parkinson's disease (PD) with severe dyskinesias. Six months after undergoing deep brain stimulation (DBS), her motor symptoms significantly improved. But after 18 months of stimulation: "she was no longer able to work, had a loss of inspiration and a taste for her work and for life in general," and she said, "Now I feel like a machine, I've lost my passion. I don't recognize myself anymore." (Schüpbach et al., 2006, p. 1812).

In contrast, patients in Klein et al.'s (2016) qualitative study, who underwent DBS for obsessive-compulsive disorder (OCD) or treatment resistant depression (TRD) report that after stimulation: "I'm me without depression" (Patient F3) or "back to sort of a baseline … back to yourself" (Patient F2) (Klein et al., 2016, p. 144).

These studies (and many others like them) have sparked a vast literature about the ethical issues raised by DBS. The examples cited here raise a number of questions: How should we think about the changes that patients report post-DBS? Does DBS ever really turn patients into new people or return them to their old selves? What ethical issues are likely to arise as DBS technology progresses?

This chapter addresses these questions in three sections. In section "Clinical uses of DBS," we review the recent clinical literature on DBS. In section "DBS and threats to identity," we consider whether DBS poses a threat to personal identity. In section "Surveys of judgments of identity change" we argue for engagement with recent psychological work examining judgments of when identity changes.

Clinical uses of DBS

In this section, we review recent research on deep brain stimulation (DBS) for Parkinson's disease (PD) and then psychiatric conditions, including obsessive-compulsive disorder (OCD) and treatment resistant depression (TRD). We conclude with a brief discussion of next-generation DBS technologies.

DBS and PD

In general, DBS involves a surgically implanted battery-operated device which delivers electrical stimulation to a specific brain region. An electrode is inserted through

Global Mental Health and Neuroethics. https://doi.org/10.1016/B978-0-12-815063-4.00008-3

a small opening in the skull and situated within a specific brain region. A pulse generator, which is about the size of a stopwatch, is implanted near the collarbone. An insulated wire connecting the electrode and the pulse generator is then passed under the skin of the head, neck, and shoulder (National Institute of Neurological Disease and Stroke, 2017).

The first commercially marketed DBS devices were introduced by Medtronic in the 1970's to treat chronic pain. Benabid, Pollak, Louveau, Henry, and De Rougemont's (1987) paper later demonstrated the efficacy of thalamic stimulation for tremors associated with PD. In the United States, DBS was approved for treatment of PD in 2002. As of 2012, over 40,000 patients had been treated with DBS (Gardner, 2013). Today, PD, dystonia, and tremor are the three main indications for DBS therapy (Munhoz et al., 2016)

Areas in the basal ganglia and thalamus are the main targets, with the subthalamic nucleus (STN) and globus pallidus internus (GPi) being the most common (Liu et al., 2014). Other targets include the ventral intermediate nucleus of thalamus, ventral oral anterior/posterior nucleus of thalamus, and zona incerta (Hariz, Blomstedt, & Zrinzo, 2013).

In most cases, DBS therapy is used for PD patients whose symptoms can no longer be adequately controlled with medication. There is some debate, however, about whether DBS ought to be used earlier in the disease course, with some evidence suggesting that the severity of later-term symptoms can be reduced, and disease progression slowed (Hacker et al., 2015; Schüpbach et al., 2013). At any rate, patients undergoing DBS are, on average, around 60 years old, with a mean disease duration of 12 years. This targeted population accounts for less than 2% of all PD patients (Hickey & Stacy, 2016).

Since the early 2000's a number of large-scale, randomized, controlled clinical trials have demonstrated the efficacy of DBS for PD and various movement disorders (e.g., Macerollo & Deuschl, 2018; Okun et al., 2009). These studies consistently find that patients receiving DBS (compared to patients receiving only medication) have significantly better quality of life outcomes, reduced duration and severity of motor symptoms, and increased mobility. A recent review of the effects of DBS of non-motor symptoms for PD patients concludes, "overall, cognitive function generally remains stable," but "after surgery, decreased verbal fluency is consistently reported and apathy possibly worsens" (Kurtis, Rajah, Delgado, & Dafsari, 2017, p. 9).

Apathy has an estimated prevalence of between 15% and 70% among PD patients, depending on disease severity and the diagnostics used. Pagonabarraga, Kulisevsky, Strafella, and Krack (2015) classify apathy into four subtypes: (1) reward deficiency syndrome, (2) emotional distress, (3) executive dysfunction, and (4) autoactivation deficit. According to their review, most studies do not find significant increases in apathy post-DBS (compared to non-surgical PD treatment), so long as recommended post-operation medication regimens are followed. Still, while some patients report an improvement in apathy symptoms after STN-DBS, others report worsening symptoms.

DBS and OCD

Other clinical applications for DBS include neuropsychiatric conditions such as obsessive-compulsive disorder (OCD). People with OCD suffer from either obsessions (unwanted, intrusive thoughts), compulsions (repetitive actions to reduce anxiety), or both. Among patients with treatment-refractory OCD, DBS has been explored as a last-resort alternative to ablative neurosurgery. DBS targeting the ventral capsule and ventral striatum for OCD represented the first FDA approval (under a humanitarian device exemption) for a psychiatric disorder (Nuttin, Cosyns, Demeulemeester, Gybels, & Meyerson, 1999).

Kisely et al. (2014) conducted a review and meta-analysis of research using DBS for intractable OCD. In five studies, symptoms reduced in patients who received active (as opposed to sham) treatment. However, one third of patients reported serious adverse effects relating to the surgical operation or the stimulation. A larger but less restrictive meta-analysis by Alonso et al. (2015) found that the percentages of subjects with a clinically significant reduction in symptom severity varied widely from 10% to 61.5%. These mixed results underscore that the targets of DBS for OCD are not yet well understood (compared to DBS for PD). While DBS does appear to reduce symptoms for treatment-refractory OCD, these results must "be tempered by the fact that, in terms of clinical significance, this represents partial, rather than full, remission" and "the procedure was associated with significant adverse effects" (Kisely et al., 2014, p. 3539).

DBS and TRD

Treatment resistant depression (TRD) has been the other main psychiatric indication for DBS therapy. The prevalence of major depression is estimated at 14.6% in high-income countries (Kessler & Bromet, 2013). "Treatment resistant depression" usually refers to the estimated 30% of patients who do not respond to multiple stages of antidepressant medications or electroconvulsive therapy.

Malone et al. (2009) conducted the first open-label trial of DBS for TRD. In the first randomized clinical trial, Dougherty et al. (2015) targeted the ventral capsule/ventral striatum and failed to observe a significant difference between the active and sham DBS conditions during the blinded phase. Bergfeld et al. (2016) targeted the ventral anterior limb of the internal capsule (vALIC) for TRD and classified 10 of 16 patients as "responders" to vALIC-DBS because their depressive symptoms significantly improved: "responder" scores were significantly lower on the 52-point Hamilton Depression Rating Scale during active DBS ($M = 13.6$) compared to sham DBS ($M = 23.1$). Most of the reported adverse side effects due to stimulation were transient (e.g., headache, agitation, disinhibition, etc.) and tolerated by patients, or resolved by lowering the voltage. More recently, Holtzheimer et al. (2017) failed to observe a significant difference between active and sham DBS for TRD.[a] This variation in efficacy could be due to a number of factors, including difficulty in finding the precise place to implant electrodes, and differences in stimulation optimization strategies.

---

[a] For a recent overview, see also Bari et al. (2018). Thanks to Dan Stein for calling these sources to our attention.

The future of DBS

The big picture remains fuzzy. Hariz et al. (2013) report that over 40 brain regions have now been identified as DBS targets for more than 30 different clinical disorders, but despite more than a quarter of century of modern DBS, spanning dozens of clinical applications in which dozens of different brain areas have been targeted, the clinical use of DBS is evidence based in only three conditions (PD, dystonia, and tremor) and only in three targets (the STN, the GPi, and the Vim). Furthermore, even in its most common application over the last 25 years (i.e., PD), with tens of thousands of operated patients, several issues are still not settled: What is the best target for DBS in PD? What is the mechanism of action of DBS? What is the effect of DBS on nonmotor symptoms, axial symptoms, and impulsivity? Which is the best target for the tremor: Vim, caudal zona incerta, or STN? When should we offer DBS in the course of PD? (Hariz et al., 2013, p. 1789).

As the academic cliché goes (higher quality and higher powered) future research is needed.

Efficacy might be improved by new versions of DBS. The interventions described in this section have all been "open-loop" in the sense that the DBS device provides a more or less constant level of electrical stimulation. Newer "closed-loop" DBS uses a single device to both monitor brain signals and deliver variable electrical current. Electrical markers of neuropsychiatric symptoms could be used to tailor the delivery of stimulation, presumably more accurately and efficiently. Patients might even be able to control the level of stimulation without help from a doctor. Such devices raise potential ethical challenges that we will consider in following sections (for a review, see Goering, Klein, Dougherty, & Widge, 2017).

DBS and threats to identity

In a pioneering article on neuroethics, Roskies (2002, p. 500) noted that "in investigating the brain, we investigate the self," and she raised questions such as "is personal identity a brain-based notion?" and "will certain medical or technological therapies change *who we are*?" Others have asked similar questions about drugs, such as Prozac (Kramer, 1993), but DBS raises Roskies's questions specifically about surgical brain interventions. In this section, we review ethical theorizing about DBS with a special focus on its implications for self and identity.

One of the most-cited discussions about the ethical implications of DBS is Schüpbach et al. (2006). Consistent with results reported above, the researchers found that in a population of 29 patients undergoing STN-DBS for PD, most reported improvements in motor symptoms, activities of daily living, and quality of life. However, Schüpbach et al. also found that various forms of social adjustment did not improve, and some significantly worsened. For example, marital conflicts were reported in 17 of the 24 married couples. Over half were unable to return to professional activities after surgery. Two-thirds expressed feelings of strangeness and unfamiliarity with themselves, saying things like "I don't feel like myself anymore," and "I haven't found myself again after the operation" (p. 1813).

Similarly, the case report quoted at the start describes a patient whose motor handicap improved 75% but who "was no longer able to work, had a loss of inspiration and a taste for her work and for life in general" and said, "I don't recognize myself anymore" (Schüpbach et al., 2006, p. 1812). This passage and others like it probably explain why Synofzik and Schlaepfer (2008, p. 2) argue that the question about whether DBS alters the self "seems to be one of the fundamental ethical questions."

Neuroethicists have extensively considered how DBS might affect identity (Focquaert & DeRidder, 2009; Glannon, 2009; Schechtman, 2010; Schermer, 2009); agency (Baylis, 2013; Lipsman & Glannon, 2013) autonomy (Goddard, 2017), and authenticity (Kraemer, 2013a, 2013b). Many of these accounts are nuanced and combine these different themes, but they agree that the kinds of changes brought about by DBS (e.g., apathy, estrangement) must be carefully weighed against the benefits (e.g., improved mobility, reduced tremor).

A recurrent worry is that the kinds of changes brought about by DBS are philosophically quite profound (e.g., no longer feeling like a genuine author of one's desires and actions) but not captured by existing clinical assessment tools. In this section, we will consider one illustration of this worry and then a reply.

Witt, Kuhn, Timmermann, Zurowski, and Woopen (2013, p. 501) echo the common refrain that "DBS may change the patient's identity." They dub this the "change-of-identity thesis" (CIT) and correctly note that "the CIT figures prominently in the current debate on the ethical implications of DBS." Of course, in order to evaluate CIT, we first need to get clear on what is meant by "identity." No small challenge. To do this, Witt and colleagues begin by marking Schechtman's (2007) distinction between questions of *re-identification* and questions of *characterization* in the personal identity literature in philosophy.

Reidentification questions concern quantitative identity: What makes X at T_1 the same as Y at T_2, such that $X = Y$? This issue is not what is in question in cases of DBS. Nobody doubts that the person after the operation is quantitatively identical with the person before the operation. This patient still owns the same home, has the same bills to pay, and is married to same person as before the operation. It is widely accepted that if DBS threatens identity, it does not do so in this quantitative sense.

Instead, DBS potentially threatens identity in the sense of characterization. Characterization questions roughly concern qualitative identity: What makes X who they are? What gives them their distinctive personality?

Not all characteristics matter, so another distinction is needed. Within characterization, the authors further distinguish between *core* and *periphery* attitudes. One attitude is closer to the core than another attitude if and only if the first is "more important for and more distinctive of the person" (p. 503). For example, attitudes about soft drinks are usually more peripheral than attitudes about religion. A patient does not become a new person if all that changes are peripheral attitudes. A person changes in the relevant sense, on their view, only when their core attitudes change.

But which attitudes are core? After rejecting competitors, Witt and colleagues settle on a *foundational function* account. Much as a house's foundation supports its walls, some of our core attitudes support other attitudes. Roughly, if a person's foundational core attitudes change enough, then they change as a person. Below, we will consider how morality might play this role of a foundational core attitude.

On this view, the ethical permissibility of DBS hinges on the extent to which DBS threatens these foundational core attitudes and also on how these threats trade off against potential benefits. Thus, to determine when DBS is morally permissible, we need some way to measure foundational core attitudes. For this purpose, Witt et al. advocate "longitudinal studies combining a philosophical investigation of the concept of "personal identity," semi-structured interviews of patients and their caregivers, and validated quantitative test instruments." (p. 509). Of course, this proposal is underspecified. For one, it does not address the tradeoffs mentioned above. Moreover, it is hard to design and execute longitudinal studies and well-validated psychometrics, especially for hard to reach clinical populations like DBS candidates. Still, we agree that a growing body of empirical research can help to make progress on these issues.[b]

Before introducing this empirical literature, we should consider an opposing view on the change-of-identity thesis (CIT). Baylis (2013), for example, criticizes CIT on three grounds: CIT is *false* because it misconstrues identity as static and essentialist instead of relational and narrative. CIT is *misdirected*, because the real threat to identity (understood relationally) is discriminatory attitudes toward individuals with motor and other disabilities. CIT is also *trivial*, insofar as any experience integrated into a personal narrative could be potentially threatening. None of this denies that DBS raises ethical issues. Instead, Baylis thinks that the issues should be framed in terms of threats not to identity but instead to *agency*—that is, being able to "meaningfully contribute to the authoring of her own life…to the cyclical and iterative process of projecting, defending and revising a self-narrative" (p. 525).

It is beyond the scope of this chapter to adjudicate between the "essentialist" and "relational" accounts of identity invoked here. Still, the fact that these views of identity may be irreconcilable motivates another argument against CIT.

A general skepticism about neuroethicists' ability to converge on an operative definition of identity (among other issues) leads Müller, Bittlinger, and Walter (2017) to argue that the philosophical debates about identity change are what actually pose a threat to DBS patients. On their telling, CIT often relies on cherry-picked interpretations of DBS case reports that are used to support controversial metaphysical accounts of personal identity. This characterization of the literature is controversial (Nyholm, 2017), but their central claim is that metaphysical interpretations of CIT are "inappropriate for ethical analysis of personality changes after brain interventions" and also for revisions of law and medical practice.

For example, if ethicists, lawyers, and clinicians truly regarded patients who presented personality changes after DBS as new persons, as CIT seems to suggest, then advance directives of the (pre-DBS) patient must be disregarded. Because advance directives are "effective legal instruments that allow patients to exercise their autonomy," a controversial metaphysical account of identity which would deprive patients

---

[b] For further discussion of some of these difficulties, see De Haan, Rietveld, Stokhof, and Denys (2017), esp. pp. 22 ff.

of this right "would harm them and restrict their liberty. In this sense the personal identity debate is a threat to patients" (p. 2).

We raise these questions about CIT not to resolve them once and for all, but rather, to highlight that these complex issues will not be solved without meaningful collaboration between philosophers, scientists, and clinicians. Witt and colleagues call for more nuanced psychometrics. Despite their criticisms of Witt et al., Müller et al. (2017) nonetheless agree that, "existing personality tests are insufficient to investigate all aspects of personality changes, feelings of self-estrangement and psychosocial adaptation problems, and new standardized psychometric instruments need to be developed" (pp. 10–11). Baylis calls for more nuanced philosophical analysis. We call for both better scientific assessments and more rigorous philosophical analysis, as well as increased collaborations between these camps.

In the following sections, we will illustrate how psychologists and philosophers can work together to make some progress on disputes about CIT and the ethics of DBS.

Surveys of judgments of identity change

When does one person become another person? This question appears, on the surface, to be descriptive rather than evaluative. We would seem to be able to identify the same person without knowing which person is good or bad. That assumption has come under fire recently in ways that will clarify the debate over CIT and illuminate ethical issues surrounding DBS.[c]

The essential moral self

In a series of studies, Strohminger and colleagues explored lay intuitions about identity change. Surprisingly, aside from a few off-handed citations (e.g., Nyholm, 2017; Nyholm & O'Neill, 2016; Pugh, Maslen, & Savulescu, 2017), this research has not received the attention it deserves in the neuroethics literature.

In an early study, Strohminger and Nichols (2014) conducted a number of experiments where participants read vignettes about a character undergoing different kinds of changes. For example, in one experiment, a character named Jim underwent a "partial brain transplant" following a car accident. Participants were asked to imagine that it is the near future, and neuroscience has advanced to the point that brain tissue can be grown in a lab and then transplanted into patients. The key outcome measures were questions about Jim like "to what extent are they the same as before?" or "do you agree that they are the same person as before?"

There were five between-subjects conditions in the experiment: a "control" condition in which Jim's personality and behavior are described as being exactly the same after the transplant; an "agnosia" condition in which Jim is exactly the same as before, except he lacks the ability to recognize objects; an "apathy" condition in which he is exactly the same as before, except that he has lost his desires; an "amnesia" condition

---

[c] Parts of this section draw from and expand upon Earp, Skorburg, Everett, and Savulescu (2019).

where he is exactly the same as before, but he no longer has pre-transplant memories; finally, a "morality" condition in which Jim loses his moral conscience but is otherwise exactly the same as before. Participants rated the extent to which they agreed with the statement: "The transplant recipient is still Jim."

Surprisingly, Strohminger and Nichols found that when Jim lost his moral conscience, he was judged to be more of a different person than in any other condition. One reason this result might seem surprising is that moral conscience plays little role in philosophical discussions of personal identity. Instead, many philosophers claim that *memories* determine personal identity, so they might have predicted that the amnesia condition would produce judgements of greater identity change. Future work in philosophy should explore the extent to which morality and memories are related to the core, foundational attitudes discussed above.

Although less than morality, the apathy and amnesia conditions (there was no significant difference between them) did produce the second-largest judgements of identity change. The effect of apathy could help to make sense of the journalist case in Schüpbach et al. (2006). When people lose their desires and become apathetic, these results suggest that they are perceived as more of a different person than when they lose other cognitive abilities (such as the ability to recognize everyday objects). Moreover, in a free response follow-up question, 23% of participants spontaneously volunteered that the desires in the apathy condition give a person their identity (while 61% of participants said this about morality). We will have more to say below about the connections among apathy, morality, identity, and DBS.

In another experiment, Strohminger and Nichols (2014) asked participants to imagine that they were meeting an old friend whom they had not seen in years and then to indicate the extent to which a variety of changes would impact their friend's identity. Importantly, Strohminger and Nichols included not only basic cognitive traits (e.g., attention span, planning, etc.) and moral traits (e.g., generous, cruel, etc.), but also personality traits (shy, artistic, etc.). This is worth flagging in the present context because neuroethicists in the CIT debate (e.g., Northoff, 2004) often distinguish between *personality* and *identity*, claiming that changes to the former brought about by DBS do not entail changes to the latter. In any case, consistent with previous results, Strohminger and Nichols find that changes to moral traits scored higher in terms of impact on identity than every other kind of trait, including major changes to cognition and personality.

Some of the vignettes in these studies are admittedly far-fetched (involving, e.g., magic pills, time-travel, and reincarnation). Nonetheless, as Strohminger and Nichols (2014) point out, these results seem relevant for non-sci-fi cases: "disruptions of identity due to medical syndromes and their treatments are likely pervasive; our work suggests that they will be particularly dramatic for outcomes that affect moral faculties" (p. 169). DBS provides a crucial case.

The result that moral traits are perceived as essential to personal identity has now been replicated many times. Strohminger and Nichols (2014) find this effect in real-life cases of patients with frontotemporal dementia. Heiphetz, Strohminger, Gelman, and Young (2018) find that like adults, 8- to 10-year-olds also judge that people change more when their moral beliefs change. Other studies have explored the causal relations among these identity-conferring moral traits (Chen, Urminsky, & Bartels, 2016), their role in social relationships (Heiphetz, Strohminger, & Young, 2017), and their bearing on debates in the philosophy of personal identity (Prinz & Nichols, 2016).

Direction of change

Strohminger and Nichols (2014, p. 169) also speculated that had Phineas Gage's injury (the tamping rod shot through his skull) merely eliminated his memory for how to lay down railroad ties, it seems likely his friends would have seen the same old Gage shining through beneath his impairment." But Gage didn't just lose his memories. Before the accident, Gage was kind and hard-working, but after the accident, he was reported to have become cruel and impulsive. So much so that "he was no longer Gage". This story is probably inaccurate (Macmillan, 2000), but it has long been treated as a paradigmatic case of identity change (e.g., Damasio, 1994).

Kevin Tobia (2015) uses Gage's story to reveal another surprising and important feature of judgements about personal identity. In one condition, participants saw the standard case of Phineas Gage, where he was kind before the accident, but cruel afterwards. That is, Gage *deteriorated*. In another condition, holding the magnitude of the change constant, participants saw a case where Gage was cruel before the accident, but kind afterward. That is, Gage *improved*. In both conditions, Tobia asked participants to judge whether Phineas Gage was the same person as before the accident.

The results indicated that Gage was less likely to be judged as identical to his pre-accident self when the change was in a "bad" direction (deteriorating from kind to cruel) than when the change was in a "good" direction (improving from cruel to kind) even when the amount of change was the same. These results suggest that judgments of identity change are not solely a function of the *magnitude* of the change, but are also importantly related to the *direction* of the change. When people are perceived as deteriorating (and especially when they are perceived to deteriorate morally), they are judged to be more of a different person than when they improve or change in a positive direction.

Some ethics of DBS

The psychological research on the moral self and the direction of change reveals how people actually make judgments of personal identity. Because those common judgments might be dismissed as mistaken, surveys cannot settle the metaphysical issue of when identity really does change.

Nonetheless, this scientific research can guide "an explication of what we mean when judging that someone has become 'another person'" (Witt et al., 2013, p. 501), which is a central task for neuroethicists in debates about DBS. In this section, we will discuss some lessons of the psychological research for personal identity and the ethics of DBS.

Two modest proposals

Our first proposal is to do more experiments. Neuroethicists involved in the CIT debate should adapt research paradigms from the moral self literature to explore what affects our judgments of personal identity after DBS. Scenarios about brain transplants could easily be replaced with scenarios about DBS. In addition to measures of changes to morality, apathy, memory, and personality, new experiments could include other measures of concern to neuroethicists, such as core or periphery attitudes. One precedent in this direction is Klein et al. (2016), which asked about responsibility, identity, privacy, security, and enhancement after closed-loop DBS. Future research should also include measures of moral beliefs, motivations, emotions, actions, etc. This research would benefit neuroethics by supplementing a priori theorizing about identity change with data about what people actually think about identity change. It would also benefit psychological research on identity change by testing theories with consequential, real-life scenarios.

Our second proposal is to build more nuanced psychometrics to assess the kinds of changes DBS patients undergo. This need is recognized by each side of the CIT debate, as we saw in section "Clinical uses of DBS." Because people tend to see moral traits as identity-conferring, as the moral self research shows, measuring changes to moral functioning pre- and post-DBS should be a priority for neuroethicists concerned with identity changes brought about by DBS and other forms of neurostimulation. While this suggestion is modest, conducting the actual work is much more ambitious. Developing and validating new measures involves multiple, iterative processes.

Importantly, this proposed research will need to be sensitive to cross-cultural differences in conceptions of the self and moral values. Future work on the ethics of DBS would also do well to engage the vast literature in psychology which has studied how these conceptions vary across cultures. For example, classic studies in cultural psychology have explored differences between independent versus interdependent conceptions of the self (e.g., Markus & Kitayama, 1991) and differences between individualistic and collectivistic cultures (e.g., Triandis, 1989). In a recent review of this research program, Markus and Kitayama (2010, p. 421) note that the study of cultural influence on self-concepts "has led to the realization that people and their sociocultural worlds are not separate from one another." Thus, the potential threats to identity posed by DBS (or other interventions) should be understood with reference to specific cultural contexts. What might seem like a trivial aspect of the self in one cultural context could be quite profound in another cultural context.

Another growing body of recent research has looked at cultural variation in moral values specifically (see Graham, Meindl, Beall, Johnson, & Zhang, 2016 for a review). Insofar as morality is perceived to be especially important for identity, then we would also expect perceived identity changes to vary as a function of sociomoral context. Again, what might seem like a minor change to a patient's moral functioning in one cultural context could be perceived quite differently in another.

As DBS technology continues to advance and spread, and as indications for DBS continue to proliferate, these cultural considerations about the self and morality will become increasingly important. It should be noted that in terms of neurostimulatory techniques, DBS is among the most expensive and invasive. We do not think this makes the ethical issues any less pressing in a global context, however. Other techniques, such as transcranial magnetic stimulation (TMS) or transcranial direct-current stimulation (TCDS), which are cheaper and less invasive, may raise some of the same concerns considered here. While the present chapter is a contribution to the growing literature about the ethics of DBS specifically, the ethical issues we raised and the empirical evidence we presented should be applicable to less expensive neurotechnologies which may be more likely than DBS to spread around the globe.

Cases of DBS

The moral self literature also throws new light on the case reports in our introduction. Schüpbach et al. (2006) and Klein et al. (2016) highlight the importance of distinguishing between DBS for motor indications (PD) and psychiatric indications (OCD or TRD). The patients from Klein et al. (2016) underwent DBS for OCD or TRD. One reported "I'm me without depression." Another claimed to be "back to sort of a baseline … back to yourself." In contrast, the journalist described in Schüpbach et al. (2006) received DBS for PD and reported that she had "lost her passion," and "didn't feel like herself anymore." Why does one patient feel more like her real self while the other feels more like a new person? Perhaps because the latter deteriorates in motivation. The moral self literature suggests that people tend to view deterioration as more disruptive to identity than improvements and changes to moral functioning and desires (such as losing passions, becoming apathetic, etc.) as more disruptive to identity than changes to basic cognitive or perceptual faculties.

The journalist who received DBS for PD changed in the ways and the direction that reduce judgments of identity persistence, whereas the patients who received DBS for OCD and TRD did not change in those ways, since they improved in motivation. They are now energetic instead of lethargic and exhibit a range of emotions instead of blunted affect. Thus, the moral self research may help to explain this contrast in personal identity judgments after DBS (cf. Nyholm & O'Neill, 2016, p. 650).

Although these cases distinguish judgments about personal identity by patients who receive DBS, judgments by other people matter, too. In a standard PD case, the motor benefits (e.g., reduced tremor) are thought to outweigh the cognitive, motivational, and affective costs (e.g., apathy and decreased verbal fluency) *for the patient*. The case reports often leave unclear how these changes affect others, including children and elderly dependents. Imagine how young children are affected if a parent goes in for surgery and what returns seems to be a different person (or if the same happens to a care-giver for an elderly person with dementia). These changes are bound to produce confusion and dismay. They loved this parent (or caregiver) and had learned how to deal with that individual. Now they have to relearn a lot, and they might not understand why or how the change happened. Dependents can be hurt even more if the parent (or caregiver) becomes morally worse or apathetic. The dependent used to trust their parent (or caregiver), but now they find that the new person is untrustworthy. The patient's apathy can be contagious. Lethargy can also signal lack of love, for example, if the new person refuses to play or talk with the dependent.

Apathy post-DBS might even lead to violations of moral duties, for example, if the new person breaks promises or neglects the dependent. These particular concerns do not arise with DBS for TRD in the same way—much the reverse. When a depressed parent becomes happier and less lethargic, their kids may benefit. The same applies to DBS for OCD if it has no side effects like apathy.

In any case, the point here is that DBS sometimes does have negative effects on dependents and close others, such as family and friends. Neuroethicists and doctors should take into consideration these effects of DBS on people other than the patient. They need to ask: Should doctors should insert DBS when they know that the family will be harmed? Should they wait until kids get old enough to understand and cope better? Should doctors inform patients before surgery of these possible negative side effects on their loved ones?

Closed-loop DBS

Additional questions arise for closed-loop DBS if the patient controls the level of stimulation. Should parents be encouraged to reduce or turn off their DBS when around their children? It might actually be preferable for the parent as well as the child for the patient to feel genuinely excited about going to their child's basketball game, even if it meant that the tremors would return for a while.

More generally, neuroethicists need to ask how much control patients should have. The values of autonomy or freedom speak in favor of letting patients adjust their DBS devices as they wish. However, mistakes as well as intentional abuses are likely, if turning devices higher produces mania or euphoria. Should doctors enable patients to control the level of stimulation after DBS for PD? For TRD? For OCD? As DBS technology progresses, these questions about user control will become increasingly important.

Culture and context

These questions all arise in a particular cultural context, and that matters. In some but far from all cultures, alternative resources are readily available to reduce harms to dependents after a DBS patient becomes apathetic. This context might affect our answer to the question of whether a particular patient with PD should be treated with DBS.

Classical issues in biomedical ethics are also raised in interesting ways in the context of DBS. For example, culture can influence expectations about the doctor's role. In some cultures, a doctor works for the patient and is supposed to do whatever is in the best interest of the individual patient without concern for the patient's family or friends (except to the extent that their welfare affects the patient). In other cultures, a doctor works for society and is expected to do what is in the interest of society as a whole or at least all significantly affected parties, including the patient's family and friends. In these and other ways, cultures differ on how much value they place on individual autonomy when it conflicts with social welfare. Those differences are bound to affect answers to questions about the ethics of DBS.

More questions

We have asked only a small sample of the ethical questions raised by DBS. Here are a few more: Which policies should hospitals adopt about which patients should get DBS? When should doctors and lawyers respect advance directives given before inserting DBS if the patient has different values and even seems like a new person after

DBS? Should we allow DBS trials in the developing world if DBS is likely to turn the patient into a different person (in addition to the usual risks)? Should patients in developed countries have the "right to try" DBS before official approval, despite the risk that the person after DBS might wish that the stimulator had not been inserted? Should prisons be allowed to offer inmates reduced sentences if they consent to insertion of DBS aimed at reducing their violent tendencies? Many of these questions regard far-out fictions, perhaps fortunately. Nonetheless, we need to get prepared to answer these and many more ethical questions about what DBS makes possible.

References

Alonso, P., Cuadras, D., Gabriëls, L., Denys, D., Goodman, W., Greenberg, B. D., et al. (2015). Deep brain stimulation for obsessive-compulsive disorder: A meta-analysis of treatment outcome and predictors of response. *PLoS One*, *10*(7), e0133591.

Bari, A. A., Mikell, C. B., Abosch, A., Ben-Haim, S., Buchanan, R. J., Burton, A. W., et al. (2018). Charting the road forward in psychiatric neurosurgery: Proceedings of the 2016 American Society for Stereotactic and Functional Neurosurgery workshop on neuromodulation for psychiatric disorders. *Journal of Neurology, Neurosurgery, and Psychiatry*, *89*(8), 886–896.

Baylis, F. (2013). "I am who I am": On the perceived threats to personal identity from deep brain stimulation. *Neuroethics*, *6*(3), 513–526.

Benabid, A. L., Pollak, P., Louveau, A., Henry, S., & De Rougemont, J. (1987). Combined (thalamotomy and stimulation) stereotactic surgery of the VIM thalamic nucleus for bilateral Parkinson disease. *Stereotactic and Functional Neurosurgery*, *50*(1–6), 344–346.

Bergfeld, I. O., Mantione, M., Hoogendoorn, M. L., Ruhé, H. G., Notten, P., van Laarhoven, J., et al. (2016). Deep brain stimulation of the ventral anterior limb of the internal capsule for treatment-resistant depression: A randomized clinical trial. *JAMA Psychiatry*, *73*(5), 456–464.

Chen, S. Y., Urminsky, O., & Bartels, D. M. (2016). Beliefs about the causal structure of the self-concept determine which changes disrupt personal identity. *Psychological Science*, *27*(10), 1398–1406.

Damasio, A. (1994). *Descartes' error*. Putnam Publishing.

De Haan, S., Rietveld, E., Stokhof, M., & Denys, D. (2017). Becoming more oneself? Changes in personality following DBS treatment for psychiatric disorders: Experiences of OCD patients and general considerations. *PLoS One*, *12*(4), e0175748.

Dougherty, D. D., Rezai, A. R., Carpenter, L. L., Howland, R. H., Bhati, M. T., O'Reardon, J. P., et al. (2015). A randomized sham-controlled trial of deep brain stimulation of the ventral capsule/ventral striatum for chronic treatment-resistant depression. *Biological Psychiatry*, *78*(4), 240–248.

Earp, B. D., Skorburg, J. A., Everett, J. A., & Savulescu, J. (2019). Addiction, identity, morality. *AJOB Empirical Bioethics*, *10*(2), 136–153.

Focquaert, F., & DeRidder, D. (2009). Direct intervention in the brain: Ethical issues concerning personal identity. *Journal of Ethics in Mental Health*, *4*, 1–7.

Gardner, J. (2013). A history of deep brain stimulation: Technological innovation and the role of clinical assessment tools. *Social Studies of Science*, *43*(5), 707–728.

Glannon, W. (2009). Stimulating brains, altering minds. *Journal of Medical Ethics*, *35*(5), 289–292.

Goddard, E. (2017). Deep brain stimulation through the "lens of agency": Clarifying threats to personal identity from neurological intervention. *Neuroethics, 10*(3), 325–335.

Goering, S., Klein, E., Dougherty, D. D., & Widge, A. S. (2017). Staying in the loop: Relational agency and identity in next-generation DBS for psychiatry. *AJOB Neuroscience, 8*(2), 59–70.

Graham, J., Meindl, P., Beall, E., Johnson, K. M., & Zhang, L. (2016). Cultural differences in moral judgment and behavior, across and within societies. *Current Opinion in Psychology, 8*, 125–130.

Hacker, M. L., Tonascia, J., Turchan, M., Currie, A., Heusinkveld, L., Konrad, P. E., et al. (2015). Deep brain stimulation may reduce the relative risk of clinically important worsening in early stage Parkinson's disease. *Parkinsonism & Related Disorders, 21*(10), 1177–1183.

Hariz, M., Blomstedt, P., & Zrinzo, L. (2013). Future of brain stimulation: New targets, new indications, new technology. *Movement Disorders, 28*(13), 1784–1792.

Heiphetz, L., Strohminger, N., Gelman, S. A., & Young, L. L. (2018). Who am I? The role of moral beliefs in children's and adults' understanding of identity. *Journal of Experimental Social Psychology, 78*, 210–219.

Heiphetz, L., Strohminger, N., & Young, L. L. (2017). The role of moral beliefs, memories, and preferences in representations of identity. *Cognitive Science, 41*(3), 744–767.

Hickey, P., & Stacy, M. (2016). Deep brain stimulation: A paradigm shifting approach to treat Parkinson's disease. *Frontiers in Neuroscience, 10*, 173. https://doi.org/10.3389/fnins.2016.00173.

Holtzheimer, P. E., Husain, M. M., Lisanby, S. H., Taylor, S. F., Whitworth, L. A., McClintock, S., et al. (2017). Subcallosal cingulate deep brain stimulation for treatment-resistant depression: A multisite, randomised, sham-controlled trial. *The Lancet Psychiatry, 4*(11), 839–849.

Kessler, R. C., & Bromet, E. J. (2013). The epidemiology of depression across cultures. *Annual Review of Public Health, 34*, 119–138.

Kisely, S., Hall, K., Siskind, D., Frater, J., Olson, S., & Crompton, D. (2014). Deep brain stimulation for obsessive-compulsive disorder: A systematic review and meta-analysis. *Psychological Medicine, 44*(16), 3533–3542.

Klein, E., Goering, S., Gagne, J., Shea, C. V., Franklin, R., Zorowitz, S., et al. (2016). Brain-computer interface-based control of closed-loop brain stimulation: attitudes and ethical considerations. *Brain-Computer Interfaces, 3*(3), 140–148.

Kraemer, F. (2013a). Me, myself and my brain implant: Deep brain stimulation raises questions of personal authenticity and alienation. *Neuroethics, 6*(3), 483–497.

Kraemer, F. (2013b). Authenticity or autonomy? When deep brain stimulation causes a dilemma. *Journal of Medical Ethics, 39*(12), 757–760.

Kramer, P. D. (1993). *Listening to Prozak: The landmark book about anti-depressants and the remaking of the self.* Penguin Books.

Kurtis, M. M., Rajah, T., Delgado, L. F., & Dafsari, H. S. (2017). The effect of deep brain stimulation on the non-motor symptoms of Parkinson's disease: a critical review of the current evidence. *npj Parkinson's Disease, 3*, 16024.

Lipsman, N. I. R., & Glannon, W. (2013). Brain, mind and machine: What are the implications of deep brain stimulation for perceptions of personal identity, agency and free will? *Bioethics, 27*(9), 465–470.

Liu, Y., Li, W., Tan, C., Liu, X., Wang, X., Gui, Y., et al. (2014). Meta-analysis comparing deep brain stimulation of the globus pallidus and subthalamic nucleus to treat advanced Parkinson disease: a review. *Journal of Neurosurgery, 121*(3), 709–718.

Macmillan, M. (2000). *An odd kind of fame: Stories of Phineas gage*. Cambridge, MA: MIT Press.

Malone, D. A., Jr., Dougherty, D. D., Rezai, A. R., Carpenter, L. L., Friehs, G. M., Eskandar, E. N., et al. (2009). Deep brain stimulation of the ventral capsule/ventral striatum for treatment-resistant depression. *Biological Psychiatry, 65*(4), 267–275.

Macerollo, A., & Deuschl, G. (2018). Deep brain stimulation for tardive syndromes: Systematic review and meta-analysis. *Journal of the Neurological Sciences, 389,* 55–60.

Markus, H. R., & Kitayama, S. (1991). Culture and the self: Implications for cognition, emotion, and motivation. *Psychological Review, 98*(2), 224–253.

Markus, H. R., & Kitayama, S. (2010). Cultures and selves: A cycle of mutual constitution. *Perspectives on Psychological Science, 5*(4), 420–430.

Müller, S., Bittlinger, M., & Walter, H. (2017). Threats to neurosurgical patients posed by the personal identity debate. *Neuroethics, 10*(2), 299–310.

Munhoz, R. P., Picillo, M., Fox, S. H., Bruno, V., Panisset, M., Honey, C. R., et al. (2016). Eligibility criteria for deep brain stimulation in Parkinson's disease, tremor, and dystonia. *Canadian Journal of Neurological Sciences, 43*(4), 462–471.

National Institute of Neurological Disease and Stroke. (2017). Retrieved from: https://www.ninds.nih.gov/Disorders/All-Disorders/Deep-Brain-Stimulation-Parkinsons-Disease-Information-Page.

Northoff, G. (2004). The influence of brain implants on personal identity and personality—A combined theoretical and empirical investigation in neuroethics. In T. Schramme & J. Thome (Eds.), *Philosophy and psychiatry* (pp. 326–342). Berlin: Walter de Gruyter.

Nuttin, B., Cosyns, P., Demeulemeester, H., Gybels, J., & Meyerson, B. (1999). Electrical stimulation in anterior limbs of internal capsules in patients with obsessive-compulsive disorder. *Lancet, 354*(9189), 1526.

Nyholm, S. (2017). Is the personal identity debate a "threat" to neurosurgical patients? A reply to Müller et al. *Neuroethics, 1–7.* https://doi.org/10.1007/s12152-017-9337-4.

Nyholm, S., & O'Neill, E. (2016). Deep brain stimulation, continuity over time, and the true self. *Cambridge Quarterly of Healthcare Ethics, 25*(4), 647–658.

Okun, M. S., Fernandez, H. H., Wu, S. S., Kirsch-Darrow, L., Bowers, D., Bova, F., et al. (2009). Cognition and mood in Parkinson's disease in subthalamic nucleus versus globus pallidus interna deep brain stimulation: The COMPARE trial. *Annals of Neurology, 65*(5), 586–595.

Pagonabarraga, J., Kulisevsky, J., Strafella, A. P., & Krack, P. (2015). Apathy in Parkinson's disease: Clinical features, neural substrates, diagnosis, and treatment. *Lancet Neurology, 14,* 518–531.

Pugh, J., Maslen, H., & Savulescu, J. (2017). Deep brain stimulation, authenticity and value. *Cambridge Quarterly of Healthcare Ethics, 26*(4), 640–657.

Prinz, J. J., & Nichols, S. (2016). Diachronic identity and the moral self. In J. Kiverstein (Ed.), *The Routledge handbook of philosophy of the social mind* (pp. 449–464). New York: Routledge.

Roskies, A. L. (2002). Neuroethics for the new millennium. *Neuron, 35,* 21–23.

Schechtman, M. (2010). Philosophical reflections on narrative and deep brain stimulation. *The Journal of Clinical Ethics, 21*(2), 133–139.

Schechtman, M. (2007). *The constitution of selves*. Cornell University Press.

Schermer, M. (2009). Changes in the self: The need for conceptual research next to empirical research. *The American Journal of Bioethics, 9*(5), 45–47.

Schüpbach, W. M., Rau, J., Knudsen, K., Volkmann, J., Krack, P., Timmermann, L., et al. (2013). Neurostimulation for Parkinson's disease with early motor complications. *New England Journal of Medicine, 368*(7), 610–622.

Schüpbach, M., Gargiulo, M., Welter, M., Mallet, L., Béhar, C., Houeto, J. L., et al. (2006). Neurosurgery in Parkinson disease a distressed mind in a repaired body? *Neurology*, *66*(12), 1811–1816.

Strohminger, N., & Nichols, S. (2014). The essential moral self. *Cognition*, *131*(1), 159–171.

Synofzik, M., & Schlaepfer, T. E. (2008). Stimulating personality: Ethical criteria for deep brain stimulation in psychiatric patients and for enhancement purposes. *Biotechnological Journal*, *3*, 1511–1520.

Tobia, K. P. (2015). Personal identity and the Phineas gage effect. *Analysis*, *75*(3), 396–405.

Triandis, H. C. (1989). The self and social behavior in differing cultural contexts. *Psychological Review*, *96*(3), 506–520.

Witt, K., Kuhn, J., Timmermann, L., Zurowski, M., & Woopen, C. (2013). Deep brain stimulation and the search for identity. *Neuroethics*, *6*(3), 499–511.

Further reading

National Institute of Mental Health. (2017). Retrieved from: https://www.nimh.nih.gov/health/statistics/major-depression.shtml.

Global mental health and the treatment gap: A human rights and neuroethics concern

Karen Herrera-Ferrá
Asociación Mexicana de Neuroética, Atizapán, Mexico

Introduction

Mental health and human rights are both global concerns that have been shaped by two complementary discourses: the human rights of mental health patients, and mental health care as a human right. Both discourses have influenced the development of strategies to better understand and address—at a global scale—the mental health treatment gap.

The mental health treatment gap refers to the discrepancy between the level of mental health treatment that is required and the actual level of mental health that is provided (WHO, 2016a, 2018a). In many ways, then, the mental health treatment gap represents the schism between theory and practice, and between words and action (White & Sashidharan, 2014).

The current persistent and significant global mental health treatment gap has prompted mental health advocates to focus on several implicated factors, including the macroenvironment (which includes political-economic and social determinants) and the microenvironment (which addresses family-community and individual biopsychosocial determinants) (Baingana, al'Absi, Becker, & Pringle, 2015; Kirmayer & Pedersen, 2014; White & Sashidharan, 2014). In these multidisciplinary efforts, mental health has been positioned as an important part of the global human rights agenda, and the promotion of mental health and prevention and treatment of mental disorders have become a priority in and for global public health.

Indeed, several international organizations, including the United Nations (UN) and the World Health Organization (WHO), have called for universal mental health coverage to be legally and socially protected (UN, 2006; WHO, 2018b), and for the framework of human rights to be used to develop international mental health legislation, as stated in the Convention on the Rights of Persons with Disabilities (CRPD), and in the Mental Health Action Plan (UN, 2006; WHO, 2013), among others.[a] Although the UN Universal Declaration of Human Rights (UDHR) (UN, 1948) does not specifically include mental health when addressing to the right to health, the CRPD states

---

[a] International Covenant on Economic, Social and Cultural Rights (ICESCR), International Covenant on Civil and Political Rights (ICCPR), Convention Against Torture and other Cruel, Inhuman or Degrading Treatment or Punishment (CAT), Convention on the Elimination of All Forms of Discrimination Against Women (CEDAW), Convention on the Rights of the Child (CRC, etc., (UN, 2016)).

Global Mental Health and Neuroethics. https://doi.org/10.1016/B978-0-12-815063-4.00009-5

that disabled individuals—including those with mental disabilities—must enjoy all human rights and fundamental freedoms (UN, 2006). This explicitly weaves together the discourses on mental health and human rights, positioning mental health as a focal dimension of human rights (Dhanda & Narayan, 2007; UN, 2016).

The WHO goes further, including the notion of mental health in the definition of "health," and has engaged in multiple efforts to pursue and attain global mental health and mental well-being. The WHO has emphasized that such efforts must appreciate the inequalities of resources and services that shape the reality and disparities of international health (WHO, 2013, 2016a, 2016b). Similar sentiments have been expressed in key collaborative efforts in global mental health, including the Lancet Global Mental Health Group (Horton, 2007), the Global Mental Health Movement (Movement for Global Mental Health, 2019), and more recently, the Lancet Commission on Global Mental Health and Sustainable Development (Patel et al., 2018).

These global endeavors have likely contributed to improved allocation, delivery, and quality of mental health care resources and services. Nevertheless, disparities in mental health care between western, educated, industrialized, rich and developed countries (WEIRD) and low and middle-income countries (LMIC) remain significant. To illustrate, on average 76–85% persons with mental disorders globally do not receive treatment or receive inadequate mental health services (Saxena, Thornicroft, Knapp, & Whiteford, 2007; WHO, 2017a). Although numbers in WEIRD countries are better than in LMIC, they are not particularly encouraging: 35–50% persons with mental disorders in WEIRD countries do not receive treatment (Saxena et al., 2007; WHO, 2017a).

These data reflect both the mental health treatment gap (even though access to mental health services is a human right), and the fact that this gap in the assessment and care of mental illness is not simply restricted to LMIC countries where social determinants of such illness and resource constraints are more obvious (Saxena et al., 2007; WHO, 2017a). It is therefore important to position the mental health treatment gap as a global issue that remains to be tackled successfully, aspiring to achieve the advances that have been made on other global health issues such as maternal-child mortality, malaria, tuberculosis and HIV (WHO, 2016c, 2017b, 2017c, 2017d, 2018c).

The persistence of the mental health treatment gap raises the question of whether other factors are relevant to the ongoing lack of attention to and stigmatization of mental health services. In this chapter I wish to propose that it is crucially important to understand the neurocognitive processes involved in perceiving and evaluating mental health-related concepts, as these may play a key role in decision-making about mental health issues and so contribute (positively or negatively) to the mental health treatment gap. I wish to argue that in order to achieve the vision of the WHO's Mental Health Action Plan 2013–20 (a "*world in which mental health is valued*" (WHO, 2013)), every person must acknowledge and correctly understand the importance and benefits of mental health and mental health-related concepts.

In short, I propose that the way such concepts are understood will influence the value given to mental health-related services and will influence decision-making (e.g., cost/benefit choices) and so to some extent (a) the mental health treatment gap, (b) the human rights of mental health patients and (c) mental health care as a human right.

It is sometimes taken for granted that every stakeholder (from macro to microenvironment agents) equally understands and values mental health-related issues; but more attention need to be paid to neurocognitive processes involved in perceiving and evaluating mental health-related issues. Simply put, to achieve an adequate and equitable global mental health care within a human rights framework, there is a need to address both resource *and* attitudinal barriers. The problem of inadequate mental health care represents a global and multi-disciplinary issue, with the cognitive sciences able to provide a key perspective.

Barriers in and between countries: Resources and attitudes

As discussed earlier, much of current analysis of the mental health treatment gap focuses on factors such as socio-economic considerations, and the role(s) played by governmental and non-governmental institutions in achieving and maintaining global mental health, using public policies and legislation that is supported by a human rights framework (Schulze, 2016). In this light, it would seem evident that an emphasis on human rights is important to any consideration of health, health care and their role in human survival and flourishing (Dhanda & Narayan, 2007). Health care refers to the right to accessible and effective health care, within an integrated system that is supported by political and legal systems (Clapham, 2007; Howell, Mills, & Rushton, 2017), and that helps promote freedom of choice and self-determination (Williams, 2016). More specifically, the provision of services and treatment, and protection from discrimination and violence, can be regarded as instrumental to the human right to life and personal freedoms, especially for vulnerable communities such as mental health patients.

However, even though the availability of mental health *resources* is explicitly a priority as seen in the WHO assertion of: "No health without mental health" (Prince et al., 2007; WHO, 2016a), and that significant advances in brain and cognitive sciences have afforded improved understanding of psychiatric disorders as medical and biological entities, there are persistent attitudinal concerns such as stigmatization, discrimination, and even violence against individuals with mental illness. For example, societal issues are not only relevant given that mental illness often impairs functioning in society, but also because mental illness often leads to stigmatization of affected individuals, their families and their treating institutions (Barnabas, Patel, Farmer, & Lu, 2015; Charlson, Dieleman, Singh, & Whiteford, 2017; Movement for Global Mental Health, 2019; Saxena et al., 2007; White & Sashidharan, 2014; WHO, 2016a, 2016b, 2018a). Biases toward treatment institutions—called "ultimate stigma" (Saxena et al., 2007)—are found in both LMIC and WEIRD countries, as well as within particular communities of some WEIRD countries.

Hence, these *attitudes* towards mental health, psychiatric conditions and their treatment may result in separate and disparate resource allocation between mental health and health in general. As a result, investment in mental health care seems unaffordable

(Prince et al., 2007) or even unnecessary, and compromises the possibility of address-ing mental health care efficiently and diligently within a human rights framework. Thus, social perceptions and evaluations can foster and sustain unfavorable attitudes toward the utilization of available and affordable mental health resources, affecting the type and extent of the mental health treatment gap. Thus, the treatment gap is not only about *availability*, but also about *receptiveness* of resources and services.

Moreover, it is important to be mindful of additional factors that foster attitudi-nal barriers such as (a) the view that socioeconomic determinants of mental distress do not require pharmaceutical intervention and so cannot be framed within a bio-medical model (Howell et al., 2017), (b) the view that it is important to resist the "over-extension of (Western) psychiatric power" within global mental health (Howell et al., 2017), including the utilization of emerging neuroscientific and neurotechno-logical tools and techniques, and (c) the view that a focus by global mental health on evidence-based medicine may undermine an emphasis on sociocultural determinants (Baingana et al., 2015; Bemme & D'souza, 2014; Jain & Orr, 2016; Patel, 2014).

Thus, addressing the mental health treatment gap requires also giving some thought to subtly shaped attitudes that affect the understanding and evaluation of mental health-related issues. This caveat is particularly true when focusing on local health au-thorities (e.g., governments) and society's attitudes to mental health services, as well as on impairments in patients' decision-making regarding whether or not to approach and/or accept mental health treatment. In each case, erroneous attitudes may worsen the treatment gap and ignore human rights.

Mental health care as a need and a human right...and a cognitive process?

Why the lack of resources for mental health services? What do mental health patients understand by "mental health" and "mental illness"? How do mental health patients understand mental health care as a need, or as a priority? How do they link mental health and human rights? How are these questions relevant to global mental health care and the treatment gap? These are concerns that unfortunately—and frequently—I have confronted throughout more than 20 years of private clinical practice, and they raised the further question: What if part of the underlying attitudinal problem involves neurocognitive processes that are involved in conceptualizing the value of mental health?

Concepts, concepts and concepts, but whose perceptions?

First a comprehensive understanding of concepts of "mental health" and "mental ill-ness" as well as of "the need for mental health care" is required. Mental health is defined by the WHO as *"....a state of well-being in which every individual realizes his or her own potential, can cope with the normal stresses of life, can work productively and fruitfully, and is able to make a contribution to her or his community."* (WHO, 2018d).

The Diagnostic and Statistical Manual of Mental Disorders 5th edition (DSM-5)—defines a mental disorder as *"[A] syndrome characterized by clinically significant disturbance in an individual's cognition, emotion regulation, or behavior that reflects a dysfunction in the psychological, biological, or developmental processes underlying mental functioning"* (American Psychiatric Association, 2013), and the ICD-10 refers to *"... the existence of a clinically recognizable set of symptoms or behaviour associated in most cases with distress and with interference with personal functions."* (WHO, 1990). Perception of need in mental health care is, however, not addressed in these documents; despite the fact that from a human rights perspective it is crucial to robustly address mental disorders (Eaton, 2012; Fisk, 2000).

Furthermore, mental health patients' perceptions of "need," "emergency" and "priority" of mental health care, might be biased by cognitive processes characteristic of their own mental illness; these might include self-stigma, self-devaluation, and poor insight (Eaton, 2012; Fisk, 2000; Sadler, 2004). Indeed, disruption of mental health (with resulting distress, impairment and disability) is sometimes not recognized as a mental health issue, and those with mental disorders may not be able to appropriately evaluate the risks and benefits of mental health treatment (Eaton, 2012; Fisk, 2000; Sadler, 2004). Such factors may further contribute to the mental health treatment gap.

While recognition of neurodiversity is consistent with a focus on human rights, there are also important risks of simplistically accepting patients' self-concepts and evaluations. For example, some people with mental health problems do not appropriately perceive the need for mental health care (Ali, Teich, & Mutter, 2015; Dezetter et al., 2015; Meadows & Burgess, 2009; Walker, Cummings, Hockenberry, & Druss, 2015), or do not understand that access to mental health care is an important human right (Vijayalakshmi, Ramachandra, & Redd, 2013). Indeed, there is evidence that some individuals with mental disorders do not recognize mental health care as a human right (Radden, 2012; Saavedra & Uchofen-Herrera, 2016), and rather consider such care to be a choice, an optional support net, or a luxury (Henao, Restrepo, Alzate, & González, 2009; Herrman & Swartz, 2007).

Thus, perceptions of mental health-related concepts—and of needs, rights, and prioritization—may influence the approach of individuals with mental disorders to mental health care, and should be a target of public mental health interventions such as destigmatization and psychoeducation (Eaton, 2012). It is important to be mindful of the neurocognitive processes of decision-making (e.g., cost/benefit choices) and how these are impacted by mental illness; the decision to approach a mental health service, could be delayed or postponed for many reasons (resource and/or attitude) until the need for such care is perceived as a priority.

Perception of priority plays a causal role in the global mental health treatment gap

Decision-making is shaped by the *value* granted to specific stimuli or concepts (Glimcher & Fehr, 2014), in the case of mental disorders, decision-making is shaped by the perceived value of mental health, mental well-being and mental health care as a human right. The value given to these constructs may influence perceptions of need, urgency, and priority, and so will impact decisions about the prioritization of mental health and mental well-being as a human right, and the equitable and prudent allocation of resources. The value of mental health-related concepts is directed by a range of biopsychosocial structures and mechanisms (Glimcher & Fehr, 2014; Todorov, Fiske, & Prentice, 2011), which are in turn impacted by nature and nurture (Evers, 2015; Giordano, 2011). Indeed it is important to more fully delineate the genesis of individual and socio-cultural perceptions and evaluations of mental health-related concepts including need, rights, and priorities.

Accordingly, the *biological* arena includes reference to the brain and different systemic organs (e.g., thyroid gland) and/or systems (e.g., immunologic), including genotype and phenotype, as well as body-states (e.g., hypoxemia, metabolic states, drug-effect, etc.) that are implicated and can alter the normal neurodevelopment and/ or continuous functionality of the brain. The *psychological* arena is for the most part, a neurocognitive adaptation of personal experiences of multiple interactions between the internal (e.g., hunger, fear, metabolism, somatic state, sense perceptions, pain, etc.) and external (e.g., socio-ecological stimuli, etc.) environments. These neurocognitive adaptations and coping mechanisms are the result of multiple factors such as personality, experiences, education, preferences, resilience skills, previous reinforcements, etc., that shape perceptions of mental well-being, mental health, mental illness and the use of neuroscience and neurotechnology as humane. Within the *social* arena, culture, human relationships, roles, gender, age, rituals, beliefs, traditions, trends, global issues, politics, economy, etc., are key.

As such, individual *perceptions* are strongly influenced by internal and external environmental factors and dynamics (that are not unique to LMIC), such as neurodevelopmental issues, poverty, hunger, violence, pain, discrimination, imminent life-threatening health issues, natural disasters, and education and gender equality among others. There is neurocognitive diversity, with a range of perceptions and values given to concepts, including the "need and right" and "urgency and prioritization" of mental health care and well-being. Unfortunately, in environments with long-standing lack of resources, and inadequate socio-legal and economic frameworks, mental health may not be given appropriate value, so further exacerbating the treatment gap. Can we address this vicious cycle? I would argue that this is a question about education and about how to create the conditions that will promote and enhance such awareness.

Education: The bridge in the gap?

Global mental health and human rights expose not only a biomedical concern, but also a social problem, that requires a robust integrative and collaborative approach. Thus, it is necessary to acknowledge the many possible factors that contribute to this binominal issue (health-right, right-health), and the interdisciplinarity required to reduce the global mental health treatment gap within a human rights framework. Notwithstanding the relevance of current endeavors in the macro and micro environment (e.g., top to bottom and bottom to top), a complementary intervention using the cognitive sciences may improve these efforts. The understanding of perceived needs and how this affects the neurocognitive process of decision indicates the importance of re-directing current global, domestic and individual educational strategies. For instance, what are the specific variables selected by the brain in a cost/benefit choice? What are the perceived and expected cost(s) and benefit(s)? What are the perceived affected dimensions? Are the effects of choices perceived as temporal or permanent?, etc.

The brain, as a complex organ, is significantly affected by experience and learning, and will attend to personal preferential values that affect decision-making (Evers, 2015; Glimcher & Fehr, 2014; Todorov et al., 2011). Put differently, the nature via nurture dynamic interrelation, adapts neuronal connectivity in accordance with changes in its internal and external environment (Buchanan, Grindstaff, & Pravosudov, 2013; Evers, 2015; Giordano & Gordjin, 2010; Rese, 2016; Riffell & Rowe, 2016; Sherry, 2006). This means that biopsychosocial interactions impact synaptic connectivity, and contribute to the formation of a variety of patterns of neural activity which might be proactively shaped through correct learning, including of the value of mental health-related concepts.

Given that psychobiological mechanisms underlie attitudinal barriers, education may have a particularly important role and responsibility in addressing the mental health treatment gap. The cognitive sciences could enable educational campaigns that empower patients, diminish stigma, strengthen leadership and governance, provide comprehensive, integrated and responsive mental health and social care, and lead to implementation of strategies for promotion and prevention, and so possibly to improved global mental health consistent with the WHO's Mental Health Action Plan 2013–20 (WHO, 2013). Further research is of course needed to fully validate the claims made here.

Conclusion

As discussed, distinctions in mental health care between LMIC and WEIRD countries come into stark relief when examining accessibility and affordability of health resources and services. The treatment gap is based on a range of factors including resource constraints, lack of political will, and an inadequate understanding and acceptance of mental disorders as medical entities. Importantly, however, the mental health treatment gap in and between countries, is also a human rights concern that is not restricted to LMIC.

Global strategies focused on diminishing structural barriers to mental health services may be enhanced by including the cognitive sciences to address a common barrier found in both, WEIRD and LMIC: The attitudinal barrier. Special attention should be given to the neurocognitive processes related to the perception and evaluation of concepts such as "mental health," "the need for mental health care," and "mental health care as a human right." Such an approach may address the resistance of many stakeholders to acknowledging that mental health care is a key part of health care, and that acknowledgment is key for safe-guarding human rights.

I argue that the value associated with mental health-related concepts may influence the prioritization of resources for mental health, and that the neurocognitive process of decision-making (e.g., cost/benefit choices) related to mental health impacts both the mental health treatment gap and the respect for the human rights of individuals with mental health problems. In addition, I propose the use of current methods in education to harness and leverage global efforts focused on resource allocation, in an attempt to address the mental health treatment gap within a human rights framework. In sum, I advocate that the treatment gap is not only about *availability* but also about *receptiveness* of resources and services and accordingly, both structural and attitudinal barriers must be globally addressed.

Acknowledgments

The author would like to acknowledge Arleen Salles and James Giordano for their valuable comments while preparing this chapter, and Dan Stein for his help, guidance and editing.

References

Ali, M. M., Teich, J. L., & Mutter, R. (2015). The role of perceived need and health insurance in substance use treatment: Implications for the Affordable Care Act. *Journal of Substance Abuse Treatment, 54*, 14–20. https://doi.org/10.1016/j.jsat.2015.02.002.

American Psychiatric Association. (2013). *Diagnostic and statistical manual of mental disorders-V* (5th ed.). Washington, DC: American Psychiatric Publishing.

Baingana, F., al'Absi, M., Becker, A. E., & Pringle, B. (2015). Global research challenges and opportunities for mental health and substance-use disorders. *Nature, 527*(7578), S172–S177. https://doi.org/10.1038/nature16032.

Barnabas, J. G., Patel, V., Farmer, P. E., & Lu, C. (2015). Assessing development assistance for mental health in developing countries: 2007–2013. *PLoS Medicine, 12*(6), e1001834. https://doi.org/10.1371/journal.pmed.1001834.

Bemme, D., & D'souza, N. A. (2014). Global mental health and its discontents: An inquiry into the making of global and local scale. *Transcultural Psychiatry, 51*(6), 850–874. https://doi.org/10.1177/1363461514539830.

Buchanan, K. L., Grindstaff, J. L., & Pravosudov, V. V. (2013). Condition-dependence, developmental plasticity, and cognition: Implications for ecology and evolution. *Trends in Ecology & Evolution, 28*(5), 290–296.

Charlson, F. J., Dieleman, J., Singh, L., & Whiteford, H. A. (2017). Donor financing of global mental health, 1995–2015: An assessment of trends, channels, and alignment with the disease burden. *PLoS ONE, 12*(1), e0169384.

Clapham, A. (2007). *Human rights: A very short introduction*. New York, NY: Oxford University Press.

Dezetter, A., Duhuox, A., Menear, M., Roberge, P., Chartrand, E., et al. (2015). Reasons and determinants for perceiving unmet needs for mental health in primary care in Quebec. *Canadian Journal of Psychiatry, 60*(6), 284–293. https://doi.org/10.1177/070674371506000607.

Dhanda, A., & Narayan, T. (2007). Mental health and human rights. *The Lancet, 370*, 1197–1198.

Eaton, W. (2012). *Public mental health*. New York, NY: Oxford University Press.

Evers, K. (2015). In T. Metzinger & J. M. Windt (Eds.), *Can we be epigeneticaly proactive?*. https://doi.org/10.15502/9783958570238.

Fisk, M. (2000). *Toward a healthy society*. Kansas: University Press of Kansas.

Giordano, J. (2011). *Maldynia: Multi-disciplinary perspectives on the illness of chronic pain*. New York, NY: Taylor-Francis.

Giordano, J., & Gordjin, B. (2010). *Scientific and philosophical perspectives in neuroethics*. New York, NY: Cambridge University Press.

Glimcher, P. W., & Fehr, E. (2014). *Neuroeconomics: Decision making and the brain* (2nd ed.). London: Elseiver.

Henao, S., Restrepo, V., Alzate, A. F., & González, C. M. (2009). Percepción sobre el acceso a los servicios de salud mental que tienen los residentes de tres municipios de Antioquia, 2004–2006. *Revista Facultad Nacional de Salud Pública, 27*(3), 271–281. http://www.scielo.org.co/scielo.php?script=sci_arttext&pid=S0120-386X2009000300004&lng=en&tlng=es.

Herrman, H., & Swartz, L. (2007). Promotion of mental health in poorly resourced countries. *The Lancet, 230*. https://doi.org/10.1016/S0140-6736(07)61244-6.

Horton, R. (2007). Launching a new movement for mental health. *The Lancet, 370*, 806.

Howell, A., Mills, C., & Rushton, S. (2017). The (Mis)appropriation of HIV/AIDS advocacy strategies in Global Mental Health: Towards a more nuanced approach. *Globalization and Health*, https://doi.org/10.1186/s12992-017-0263-3.

Jain, S., & Orr, D. (2016). Ethnographic perspectives on global mental health. *Transcultural Psychiatry, 53*(6), 685–695. https://doi.org/10.1177/1363461516679322.

Kirmayer, L. J., & Pedersen, D. (2014). Toward a new architecture for global mental health. *Transcultural Psychiatry, 51*(6), 759–776. https://doi.org/10.1177/1363461514557202.

Meadows, G. N., & Burgess, P. M. (2009). Perceived need for mental health care: Findings from the 2007 Australian Survey of Mental Health and Wellbeing. *The Australian and New Zealand Journal of Psychiatry, 43*(7), 624–634. https://doi.org/10.1080/00048670902970866.

Movement for Global Mental Health. (2019). *Movement for mental global health*. Retrieved 14 December 2016, from: http://www.globalmentalhealth.org.

Patel, V. (2014). Why mental health matters to global health. *Transcultural Psychiatry, 51*(6), 777–789. https://doi.org/10.1177/1363461514524473.

Patel, V., Saxena, S., Lund, C., Thornicroft, G., Baingana, F., et al. (2018). Lancet commission on global mental health and sustainable development. *The Lancet, 392*(10157), P1553–P1598. https://doi.org/10.1016/S0140-6736(18)31612-X.

Prince, M., Patel, V., Saxena, S., Maj, M., Maselko, J., et al. (2007). No health without mental health. *Lancet, 370*, 859–877.

Radden, J. H. (2012). Recognition rights, mental health consumers and reconstructive cultural semantics. *Philosophy, Ethics, and Humanities in Medicine, 7*, 6. https://doi.org/10.1186/1747-5341-7-6.

Rese, J. E. (2016). Chronic stress, cortical plasticity and neuroecology. *Behavioural Processes, 129*, 105–115.

Riffell, J. A., & Rowe, A. H. (2016). Neuroecology: Neural mechanisms of sensory and motor processes that mediate ecologically relevant behaviors: An introduction to the symposium. *Integrative and Comparative Biology, 56*(5), 853–855. https://doi.org/10.1093/icb/icw109.

Saavedra, J., & Uchofen-Herrera, V. (2016). Percepciones sobre la atención de salud en personas con problemas autoidentificados de salud mental en zonas rurales del Perú. *Revista Peruana de Medicina Experimental y Salud Pública, 33*(4), 785–793.

Sadler, J. (2004). Diagnosis/antidiagnosis. In J. Radden (Ed.), *The philosophy of psychiatry: A companion* (pp. 163–179). New York, NY: Oxford University Press.

Saxena, S., Thornicroft, G., Knapp, M., & Whiteford, H. (2007). Resources for mental health: Scarcity, inequity, and inefficiency. *Lancet, 370*, 878–889.

Schulze, M. (2016). Human rights principles in developing and updating policies and laws on mental health. *Global Mental Health, 3*, e10. page 1 of 7 https://doi.org/10.1017/gmh.2016.5.

Sherry, D. F. (2006). Neuroecology. *Annual Review of Psychology, 57*, 167–197.

Todorov, A., Fiske, S., & Prentice, D. (2011). *Social neuroscience: Toward understanding the underpinnings of the social mind.* New York, NY: Oxford university Press.

UN. (1948). *United Nations universal declaration of human rights.* UN. Retrieved 14 December 2016, from: http://www.un.org/en/documents/udhr/.

UN. (2006). *United nations convention on the rights of persons with disabilities.* Retrieved 8 January 2018, from: http://www.un.org/disabilities/documents/convention/convention_accessible_pdf.pdf.

UN. (2016). *Convention on the rights of persons with disabilities.* Convention on the Rights of Persons with Disabilities (CRPD). Retrieved February 2018, from: https://www.un.org/development/desa/disabilities/convention-on-the-rights-of-persons-with-disabilities.html.

Vijayalakshmi, P., Ramachandra, K., & Redd, K. (2013). Perceived human rights violation in persons with mental illness: Role of education. *The International Journal of Social Psychiatry, 59*(4), 351–364. https://doi.org/10.1177/0020764012437322.

Walker, E. R., Cummings, J. R., Hockenberry, J. M., & Druss, B. G. (2015). Insurance status, use of mental health services, and unmet need for mental health care in the United States. *Psychiatric Services, 66*(6), 578–584. https://doi.org/10.1176/appi.ps.201400248.

White, R. G., & Sashidharan, S. P. (2014). Towards a more nuanced global mental health. *The British Journal of Psychiatry, 204*, 415–417. https://doi.org/10.1192/bjp.bp.113.139204.

WHO. (1990). *International clasification of diseases 10.* World Health Organization. Retrieved February 2018, from: http://www.who.int/classifications/icd/en/bluebook.pdf.

WHO. (2013). *Mental health action plan 2013–20.* WHO. Retrieved 15 December 2016, from: http://apps.who.int/iris/bitstream/10665/89966/1/9789241506021_eng.pdf?ua=1.

WHO. (2016a). *Mental health: Strengthening our response.* WHO. Retrieved 22 January 2017, from: http://www.who.int/mediacentre/factsheets/fs220/en/.

WHO. (2016b). *mhGAP intervention guide.* WHO. Retrieved 15 December 2016, from: http://apps.who.int/iris/bitstream/10665/250239/1/9789241549790-eng.pdf?ua=1.

WHO. (2016c). *HIV progress report 2016.* WHO. Retrieved February 2018, from: http://www.who.int/hiv/pub/WHO_HIV_2016.24.pdf?ua=1.

WHO. (2017a). *WHO: Mental disorders.* Retrieved February 2018, from: http://www.who.int/mediacentre/factsheets/fs396/en/.

WHO. (2017b). *Global tuberculosis report 2017.* Retrieved February 2018, from: http://apps.who.int/iris/bitstream/10665/259366/1/9789241565516-eng.pdf?ua=1.

WHO. (2017c). *Levels and trends in child mortality report 2017.* Retrieved February 2018, from: http://www.who.int/maternal_child_adolescent/documents/levels_trends_child_mortality_2017/en/.

WHO. (2017d). *World malaria report 2017.* WHO. Retrieved February 2018, from: http://apps.who.int/iris/bitstream/10665/259492/1/9789241565523-eng.pdf?ua=1.

WHO. (2018a). *Mental health atlas 2017.* Geneva: WHO. Retrieved 22 January 2017, from: http://apps.who.int/iris/bitstream/10665/178879/1/9789241565011_eng.pdf.

WHO. (2018b). *WHO.* Mental Health. Retrieved February 2018, from: http://www.who.int/mental_health/en/.

WHO. (2018c). *WHO: Maternal mortality.* Retrieved February 2018, from: http://www.who.int/mediacentre/factsheets/fs348/en/.

WHO. (2018d). *World Health Organization*. World Health Organization. Retrieved February 2018, from: http://www.who.int/features/factfiles/mental_health/en/.

Williams, A. R. (2016). Opportunities in reform: Bioethics and mental health ethics. *Bioethics*, *30*(4), 221–226. https://doi.org/10.1111/bioe.12210.

Further reading

DiEuliis, D., & Cabayan, H. (2013). *Topics in the neurobiology of aggression: Implications to deterrence*. Strategic Multilayers (SMA).

DiEuliis, D., & Giordano, J. (2017). *A primer on the neurocognitive science of aggression, decision making, and deterrence*. NSI. Retrieved from: http://nsiteam.com/social/wp-content/uploads/2017/08/A-Primer-on-Neuroscientific-insights_Final.pdf.

Singla, D. R., Kohr, B. A., Murray, L. K., Anand, A., Chorpita, B. F., et al. (2017). Psychological treatments for the world: Lessons from low- and middle-income countries. *Annual Review of Clinical Psychology*, *08*(13), 149–181. https://doi.org/10.1146/annurev-clinpsy-032816-045217.

Steel, Z., Marnane, C., Iranpour, C., Chey, T., & Jackson, J. W. (2014). The global prevalence of common mental disorders: A systematic review and meta-analysis 1980–2013. *International Journal of Epidemiology*, *43*(2), 476–493.

The Lancet. (2018). *The Lancet Commission on global mental health and sustainable development*. Retrieved from: https://www.thelancet.com/commissions/global-mental-health.

Poverty and mental health in post-war countries: The case of Uganda and Sierra Leone

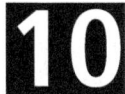

Fabrice Jotterand[a,c], Abdul R. Shour[b], Ronald Anguzu[b]
[a]Center for Bioethics and Medical Humanities, Institute for Health and Equity, Medical College of Wisconsin, Milwaukee, WI, United States, [b]Public and Community Health Program, Institute for Health and Equity, Medical College of Wisconsin, Milwaukee, WI, United States, [c]Institute for Biomedical Ethics, University of Basel, Basel, Switzerland

Introduction

The impact of environmental factors on brain development in children and adolescents has become a growing research focus in recent years. Low socioeconomic status (SES) has been linked to adverse health outcomes, mental disorders, and low academic achievements (Katsnelson, 2015) (chapter in this volume by Tomlinson). Studies have demonstrated that living in poor conditions impacts the neurological and behavioral development of children negatively affecting; (1) cognitive abilities, leading to poor academic attainment (Hair, Hanson, Wolfe, & Pollak, 2015; Luby et al., 2013); (2) brain structure, in particular the hippocampus and the amygdala—brain regions associated with memory, emotions, decision making, attention, speech, and motivation (Barch et al., 2016; Brito & Noble, 2014; Jednoróg et al., 2012; Luby et al., 2013; Noble et al., 2015); and (3) overall mental, emotional and behavioral health with potential higher risks of mental disorders and antisocial behavior (Hackman, Farah, & Meaney, 2010; Luby et al., 2013; van Goozen, Fairchild, & Harold, 2008). Another factor investigated with regard to brain development is the effects of exposure to community violence or crime, e.g., physical violence, shootings, use of drugs and stabbings (Fowler, Tompsett, Braciszewski, Jacques-Tiura, & Baltes, 2009; Saxbe et al., 2018). Saxbe et al. (2018) report that community violence exposure leads to (1) deficiency in cognitive and emotional development (Heleniak, King, Monahan, & McLaughlin, 2018; McCoy, Raver, & Sharkey, 2015); (2) low school attainment (Borofsky, Kellerman, Baucom, Oliver, & Margolin, 2013); and (3) post-traumatic stress disorder (PTSD) (Fowler et al., 2009). In their study, they point out that these negative outcomes "are associated with brain structure and function, making community violence a potentially meaningful correlate of neural characteristics" (Saxbe et al., 2018).

Research on the impact of adverse events on brain development has mostly focused on first-world countries like the United States or countries in the Western world. This chapter will focus specifically on two African countries, Uganda and Sierra Leone. These two countries are among the poorest in the world and have been plagued by

Global Mental Health and Neuroethics. https://doi.org/10.1016/B978-0-12-815063-4.00010-1

civil wars and political violence. The combination of poverty and violence represents a tremendous challenge in the development of strategies to address the ongoing mental health crisis in Uganda and Sierra Leone. As this chapter outlines, to address the mental health issues in these countries requires not only access to good mental health care services but also interventions at the socioeconomic level, given that determinants of health are multifactorial. The aim of our analysis is twofold: first, we investigate particular mental health needs and challenges in the light of the aftermath of civil unrest, political violence and continuous economic and political difficulties in Uganda and Sierra Leone. Second, we examine how neuroethics can help develop strategies to address the mental health crisis that has not been adequately assessed and addressed in Uganda and Sierra Leone. In particular, we address the question of how to improve access to new neuroscientific knowledge and treatment options relevant to the impact of poverty and violence.

Mental health in the African continent

Mental and behavioral disorders are conditions characterized by alterations in thinking, mood or behavior associated with personal distress and impaired functioning (World Health Organization, 2014). According to the World Health Organization (WHO), mental disorders contribute 14% to the global burden of disease (Whiteford et al., 2013). Globally, the highest proportion (56.7%) of disability-adjusted life-years (DALYs) is attributable to mental disorders (Whiteford et al., 2013) with mental illness accounting for 32.4% of years lived with disability (YLDs) (Vigo, Thornicroft, & Atun, 2016). In addition, there is an imbalance in how research efforts are conducted. It is estimated that 90% of clinical neuroscience research focuses on 10% of the global population living in high income countries—the 90:10 research gap (Henrich, Heine, & Norenzayan, 2010; Saxena, Paraje, Sharan, Karam, & Sadana, 2006). For this reason, there is an urgent need for mental health research in Low- and Middle-Income Countries (LMIC) as these countries have tremendous mental health challenges and needs. To this end, the United Nations set specific goals outlined in the Sustainable Development Goal (SDG) 3 document which aims at a one third reduction in mortality from non-communicable diseases through prevention, treatment and promotion of mental health and wellbeing by 2030 (United Nations, 2016). Similarly, the Common African Position is to reduce the incidence of non-communicable diseases, including mental health disorders, as a priority of the African Union (African-Union, 2014).

In the light of these considerations, this chapter focuses on Uganda and Sierra Leone in an attempt to provide a framework that will help guide the development of strategies to improve mental health. These countries have a history of civil war, political violence, poverty and a lack of health care resources. Taken together, these factors constitute a tremendous challenge and a human tragedy that cannot be ignored.

Uganda

Socio-political context

Uganda experienced two civil wars between 1981 and 2006. A 5-year armed conflict in central Uganda between 1981 and 1986, followed by two decades of war in Northern Uganda lead by the Lord's Resistance Army from 1986 to 2006. Both conflicts involved child soldiers (Amone-P'Olak et al., 2013). These wars were both preceded by several years of political turmoil beginning in 1971. The majority of the population in the war-affected areas was exposed to atrocities and suffered the consequences without access to appropriate resources (Ovuga, Boardman, & Wasserman, 2005). Individuals in these war-torn areas experienced torture, overwhelming fear, helplessness and isolation (Amone P'Olak, 2009; Amone-P'Olak, Garnefski, & Kraaij, 2007). Civilians of northern Uganda faced forced conscription and abduction into armed guerilla groups resulting in psychological trauma (Pham, Vinck, & Stover, 2009). It is well established that the experience of war and its aftermath may have long-term mental health effects with psychosocial outcomes such as depression, anxiety, psychotic symptoms, prosocial behavior, behavioral problems or somatic complaints (Amone-P'Olak et al., 2013).

The burden of mental health

The World Health Organization (WHO) has recognized in the last decade the significant contribution of mental, neurological and substance abuse disorders to the disease burden globally, with at least one in every four persons experiencing some form of mental disorder at some point in their life (World Health Organization, 2001). In addition, evidence suggests a relationship between poverty levels and poor mental health (Flisher et al., 2007). Uganda, a low-income country with one third (31%) of its population (39 million) living below the poverty line (UBOS, 2015), is facing a tremendous challenge as the result of the emergence of social, political and civil strife coupled with the spread of infectious disease such as HIV/AIDS, malaria, diarrheal and respiratory tract infections. Mental disorders have become a major problem postwar, contributing 13% of the disease burden (Ministry of Health, 2011). According to Uganda's Ministry of Health, incident mental health cases account for about 1% of all new outpatient health cases. In this national hospital outpatient survey of healthcare seeking clinic attendees, the highest incident of mental health conditions per 100 outpatients were epilepsy 6 per 100 outpatients and approximately 1 per 100 outpatients for; anxiety disorders; depression; mania; schizophrenia; alcohol or drug abuse and other forms of mental illness (Ministry of Health, 2011). The amplitude of the problem faced by Ugandan mental health services can be summarized by a brief overview of the most prevalent mental disorders affecting the country:

(a) Epilepsy is a disease of the brain characterized by enduring predisposition to epileptic seizures (Fisher, 2017; Fisher et al., 2014). The prevalence of epilepsy is higher in developing countries and Uganda has an estimated epilepsy burden of 3% in the general population (Kaiser, Asaba, Leichsenring, & Kabagambe, 1998; Uganda Ministry of Health, 2010; World Health Organization, 2017). Several risk factors are considered associated with epilepsy. In infants, a major risk factor is febrile seizures due to conditions such as malaria, bronchopneumonia and measles (Duggan, 2010). Other neglected tropical diseases such as onchocerciasis (eye and skin disease) and neurocysticercosis (infection of the nervous system) are common causes of seizures in certain geographical locations of sub-Saharan Africa including Uganda (Kaiser et al., 1996; Kilian, Kipp, Kasoro, & Burnham, 1994; Ovuga, Kipp, Mungherera, & Kasoro, 1992). Insult to the brain caused by problematic labor during birth, neuroanatomical abnormalities, and genetic makeup are also potential risk factors (WHO, 2004). Low socio-economic status, malnutrition and poor access to healthcare services may contribute to the severity of seizures.

(b) Depression: In Uganda, population data on the burden of depression highlights it as a major mental health problem in the country. The WHO estimates the burden of depressive disorders in Uganda at 4.6% (World Health Organization, 2017). For example, data indicates that among school-going adolescents with highly prevalent depressive symptoms (21%), approximately 11% had major depression (Nalugya-Sserunjogi et al., 2016). Over 90% of people who inflict harm to themselves or commit suicide manifest clinical depression (UBOS, 2011). In two rural districts of Uganda (Adjumani and Bugiri), overall prevalence of depression was 17.4%, with a higher level in the Adjumani district where people experienced the armed insurgency from the northern region and live in poor living conditions depending mostly on agriculture for their livelihood. The district of the Adjumani also has a higher refugee populations from armed conflict in neighboring South Sudan and the Democratic Republic of Congo (Ovuga et al., 2005).

(c) Posttraumatic stress disorder (PTSD): two civil wars in the last four decades have affected the mental health of those exposed to atrocities. Several studies conducted in post-conflict northern Uganda revealed that exposure to stressful events during the war or following the experience of war atrocities increased the risk of occurrence of PTSD, in addition to anxiety and depressive symptoms (Pfeiffer & Elbert, 2011; Roberts, Ocaka, Browne, Oyok, & Sondorp, 2008; Weierstall, Schalinski, Crombach, Hecker, & Elbert, 2012). Child victims of the abduction by the Lord's Resistance Army of warlord Joseph Kony in northern Uganda developed symptoms of PTSD (Annan, Blattman, Mazurana, & Carlson, 2011). This disorder was also observed among women (Roberts et al., 2008).

(d) Alcohol and substance abuse: Evidence suggests that societal conflicts may lead to unplanned urbanization (Büscher, Komujuni, & Ashaba, 2018) and may negatively impact behavior (Namagembe et al., 2010; Swahn, Palmier, Kasirye, & Yao, 2012) via increased alcohol consumption and drug use in Uganda (Tumwesigye & Kasirye, 2005; Tumwesigye, Kyomuhendo, Greenfield, & Wanyenze, 2012).

In concluding this brief overview, populations affected by the common mental health conditions and those in need of mental health care are predominantly from lower socioeconomic backgrounds. This reinforces evidence that barriers to accessing health services perpetuates the vicious circle of insecurity, risk or occurrence of civil unrest, poverty and violence (Conti & Burton, 1994; Kigozi, Ssebunnya, Kizza, Cooper, & Ndyanabangi, 2010).

Unique challenges

In addition to the burden of specific mental health conditions, Uganda faces the challenge of a high refugee population. The West Nile region shares international borders with South Sudan and the Democratic Republic of Congo (DRC), two countries that experienced ongoing decades of armed conflict resulting in a large influx of refugees into Uganda (Bayer, Klasen, & Adam, 2007). Similarly, in the Western and South West regions, refugees have sought safety in Uganda following the Rwanda genocide of 1994 and the subsequent political violence. In the Gulu district, a post-conflict setting in northern Uganda, war abducted adolescents have manifested signs of PTSD, major depression and generalized anxiety (Okello, Onen, & Musisi, 2007). Likewise in the West Nile region, Sudanese refugees have also demonstrated PTSD symptoms (Karunakara et al., 2004; Neuner et al., 2004; Peltzer, 1999).

Organization of mental health services

The Government of Uganda, through its Ministry of Health is mandated with policy formulation, planning, resource mobilization, standard setting, capacity building and co-ordination of interventions to address mental health conditions (MoH, 2015). Through private-public partnerships, there are several interventions implemented that are intended to address the high burden of mental health problems in Uganda (Molodynski, Cusack, & Nixon, 2017). This includes the integration of mental health care into HIV care and treatment and primary health care (Mugisha, Ssebunnya, & Kigozi, 2016). A community strategy, which includes health education and promotion to increase community awareness, was developed to increase access to primary and referral mental health services. Increasing the total number of functional mental health units is aimed at improving community access to and provision of essential mental healthcare.

Despite government efforts to alleviate psychosocial needs in war-torn northern Uganda, current health service delivery is still inadequate. The National Health Policy is comprised of the Uganda Minimum Healthcare Package (UMHCP) which includes mental health service provision (Kirunga Tashobya, Ssengooba, & Oliveira Cruz, 2006; MoH, 2015; Uganda Ministry of Health, 2014). Specifically, mental health services are provided through a decentralized referral health system organized in terms of catchment and general out- and in-patient health service areas at regional and district levels (World Health Organization, 2006). The financing is disproportionately allocated to the National Mental Hospital (Butabika) and regional referral hospitals with mental health units which also provide access to no-cost medication for mental health conditions (MoH, 2016). The country comprises only one National Mental Hospital and few public regional referral hospitals (Ministry of Health, 2011); these are resourced by a variety of mental health professionals including psychiatrists, general practitioners, clinical officers, clinical psychologists, nurses, social workers and occupational therapists (MoH, 2016). Policy efforts in Uganda to make access more equitable, has seen mental health being incorporated into primary health care. However, evidence from one survey in rural Uganda shows that such integration has not been effectively implemented (Kigozi et al., 2010).

Sierra Leone

Socio-political context

Over the course of the 11 years of civil war (1991–2002) in Sierra Leone, Human Rights Watch reported in 2004 that an estimated 50,000 people were murdered, and over 20,000 children and adolescents were involved with armed groups as perpetrators and/or victims of violent atrocities (Human Rights Watch, 2004). Women and children experienced posttraumatic stress as a result of having witnessed torture, killings, maiming or public rape during the war and from the loss of loved ones and family members to the scourge of Ebola. In addition, the combination of the civil war, the Ebola epidemic and poor economic outlook resulted in high level of youth unemployment (46%) in West Africa (Human Rights Watch, 2004); this is reflected in Sierra Leone's ranking (180 out of 182) in the Human Poverty Report with a Human Poverty Index of 47.7 (UN Development Program, 2009). Overall, the convergence of these factors affects existing peace and security, and health outcomes. Studies suggest that the 10-year civil war, the recent Ebola crisis and daily socioeconomic stressors such as poverty and high rates of unemployment represent major contributors to the increased prevalence of mental disorders (Akinsulure-Smith & Conteh, 2018). A recent WHO survey in 2012 revealed that the most predominant mental conditions in Sierra Leone included severe depression (4%); psychosis (2%); substance abuse (4%); mental retardation (1%); and epilepsy (1%) (Alemu et al., 2012). These findings led the WHO to advocate for the creation of community based mental health services in the country (Asare & Jones, 2005).

The burden of mental health

The effects of the civil war and Ebola remain key risk factors for anxiety, depression, and posttraumatic stress disorder in Sierra Leone (Helleringer & Noymer, 2015). During the war, civilians were used as protective shields, were abducted or enslaved, tortured and raped (De Jong, Mulhern, Ford, Van Der Kam, & Kleber, 2000). Both the war and the Ebola epidemic stimulated fear and anxiety among the population, due to witnessing of gross human right violations (Shultz, Baingana, & Neria, 2015). In 2008, it was estimated that about 90% of admissions to the Sierra Leone psychiatric hospital were drug-related; this reflects the high level of alcohol consumption and substance abuse (WHO, 2004). According to the United Nations, the production of illicit drugs such as marijuana (locally called "jamba") occurs locally and is transnationally organized for its shipment and sale in other countries. "Highway 10," a West African transit zone, is used by organized criminals to transit large quantities of cocaine from South America to Europe and West Africa. Additionally, studies by WHO reveal that alcohol also represents a significant public health concern in Sierra Leone, with Sierra Leoneans consuming on average 9.7 L of alcohol per capita in 2005, in contrast to 6.2 L per capita for the rest of the African region. Another major issue to consider is the cultural interpretation of mental illnesses, which is commonly considered spiritual or supernatural in nature, and which is associated with help-seeking from traditional healers and/or religious societies. However, this comes with stigmatization and social exclusion for the mentally ill.

In summary, the government of Sierra Leone has recognized that mental health is largely a neglected problem with a high socio-economic burden. However, it is estimated that among the 715,000 people presently suffering from mental illnesses only 2000 receive medical treatment (Alemu et al., 2012).

Systemic challenges to improve access

Although Sierra Leone is moving toward restoring its public health infrastructure (including mental health delivery systems) after the decade-long civil war and Ebola crisis, there are systemic barriers to access to mental health services. The political violence Sierra Leone experienced left its health care system largely dysfunctional with limited resources for providing mental healthcare (Alemu et al., 2012). With a population of over 7,000,000 people, Sierra Leone has only two psychiatrists, two clinical psychologists, and 19 mental health nurses, and only four nurses have a specialty in child and adolescent mental health (WHO, 2005). Sierra Leone has an estimated mental health treatment gap of about 99%, that is to say, formal mental health services are inadequate or inappropriate for the majority of Sierra Leoneans (Yoder, Tol, Reis, & de Jong, 2016). However, little attention has been paid to the potential relationships between trauma and mental health in Sierra Leone's post-war recovery.

Since the end of the civil war, there have been several policy and programmatic initiatives to address the social determinants of mental health and treatment gap in Sierra Leone. The WHO is working with the Sierra Leone Ministry of Health and Sanitation to reduce the treatment gap and to provide quality mental health care at all levels (primary, secondary and tertiary). As a result, a few initiatives have ensued. In 2002, the first "Systematic Needs Assessment on Mental Health and Substance Abuse Survey" took place under the direction of the Ministry of Health and Sanitation (WHO, 2006); this in turn led to the WHO Country Cooperation Strategy (CCS) Sierra Leone (2004–08) which recognized mental health as a priority area. Subsequently, in 2012 a Mental Health Steering Committee was launched under the Ministry of Health and Sanitation and produced a National Mental Health Policy and Plan.

These initiatives led to the establishment of the National Mental Health Coalition, the first national mental health conference (Yoder et al., 2016), the National Mental Health Strategic Plan (2010–15), and the establishment of the Mental Health Users and Families' Association. It is also worth mentioning that the push for better mental health includes a new psychiatric nurse training course at University of Sierra Leone-College of Medicine and the creation of a new program, the Mental Health Leadership and Advocacy Programme launched in 2012, with mental health stakeholders receiving training in public mental health and service development. These various initiatives are good steps in the right direction, but at this point no data is available as to whether there has been a noticeable improvement in mental health outcomes in Sierra Leone.

Neuroethics and the challenge of global mental health

Setting a global agenda

As the previous sections demonstrate, addressing the challenges of mental health in Uganda and Sierra Leone is not just an issue of improving access to mental health services but also a (bio)political one. How and what health care resources should be allocated to mental health presupposes a set of values (political, cultural and moral) shaping the development of policies and guidelines that will affect brain research and

clinical interventions. In addition, as future research on the impact of poverty and violence on child brain development takes place, it is essential to examine carefully how
this type of research can be used ethically in various socio-cultural settings, including
in developing countries plagued by civil war, poverty, and political violence. There are
issues related to disparities in research, the 90:10 research gap (90% of clinical research
focuses on only 10% of the global population, mostly from high income countries), but
also questions concerning where mental health ranks in the order of priorities in health
care despite the increasing global burden of mental disorders—according to the WHO,
20% of the people are affected by a mental disorder in their life and 3 out 4 people suffering from a severe mental disorder do not receive treatment (WHO, 2013).

To address this challenge the WHO established a comprehensive Mental Health
Action Plan 2013–20 that outlines four objectives: (1) "strengthen effective leadership and governance for mental health"; (2) "provide comprehensive, integrated and
responsive mental health and social care services in community-based settings";
(3) "implement strategies for promotion and prevention in mental health"; and
(4) "strengthen information systems, evidence and research for mental health" (WHO,
2013). These four objectives constitute a multidisciplinary approach and reflect the
complexity of mental health research and clinical care. When these objectives are
considered in the context of Uganda and Sierra Leone, for instance, issues of leadership and governance demand an understanding of the historical, socio-cultural and
political backdrop against which mental health should be examined and discussed.
Furthermore, a community-based approach can only take place when there is buy-in
from the community and a correct appreciation of the culture(s) under consideration.
Thus, the successful implementation of interventions to promote healthy mental health
practices and preventative measures requires adaptation to the local context. As mentioned previously, for some segments of the population, a mental illness is understood
in spiritual or supernatural terms. How neuroscientific knowledge is translated and
explained to individuals is key for good community work. Last but not least, neuroscience research and the implementation of novel neurotechnologies (if and when available considering the context of Uganda and Sierra Leone) should reflect the highest
standards of responsible conduct of research and clinical practice.

The current refugee crisis in Europe and North America will pose a tremendous
challenge to European countries like Germany, Spain, Sweden or Italy and the United
States to address the mental health needs of individuals fleeing poverty, physical and
mental abuse and political violence. European countries and the United States are
equipped and prepared (or at least better equipped and prepared) to handle such situations but Uganda is unlikely able to deal with its increasing refugee population
and the mental health issues associated with such flux of persons. The development
of strategies to address such crisis on African soil should carefully contextualize the
nature of these interventions. Such contextualization should always be assessed in
relation to the potential of stigmatization. So while recognizing how living in poverty
and/or being exposed to political, physical or psychological violence may affect overall mental health and brain development, it does not mean that necessarily imply that
such individuals have a "diseased brain" or have acquired an irreversible neurological
deficit (Lipina & Evers, 2017).

The contribution of neuroethics

Neuroethics is often depicted as a field of investigation that analyses the implications of brain research and neurotechnology for ethics and policy (Jotterand & Ienca, 2017). In what follows we argue that the biopolitical dimension of neuroethics must be carefully analyzed in order to make a contribution to global mental health in contexts such as Uganda and Sierra Leone. To this end, it is worth briefly defining biopolitics and its implications for neuroethics before we make the connection with global mental health.

The term biopolitics, popularized by philosopher Michel Foucault in his book *The History of Sexuality, Vol.1* (1980), refers to how political power is used to manage human life. In his work, he refers to biopower to designate the change in thinking and practice regarding political power that happened in the 18th century. Biopolitics signifies that humans as biological entities are managed as political entities, so undermining the mastery of one's body to create the space for interventions at the social level for the regulation of populations and their biological bodies. This paradigm shift established two important points: first, the state has become the ruler over (human) life and an agent of control over populations, and second, human beings are dependent upon particular goals set by political entities. For instance, some neurotechnologies enable the collection, storage and reuse of data that could potentially be used to monitor and control "human social and biological processes" (Jotterand & Ienca, 2017). Recognizing the hypothetical nature of this scenario but also the realities of political divisions, ethnic tensions in countries like Uganda and Sierra Leone, it wouldn't be improbable that these neurotechnologies could be exploited for political gain.

The implication for neuroethics is that the object of neuroscience research (the brain) has become a potential entity for socio-political control. This point has been very well articulated by Stuart Henry and Dena Plemmons who recognize the socio-political context of science. They note that "the politics of conflicting and ideologically shaped interests mediate the outcome of public policies based on scientific research, often with negative impacts on society's most vulnerable populations. Neuroscience and, therefore, neuroethics, are inherently political" (Henry & Plemmons, 2012). What Henry and Plemmons rightly discern is that neuroethics is biopolitical in nature and that the development of public health policies related to mental health can potentially be manipulated to achieve particular ends set by political agents. This is exemplified by bio-political tensions in research involving nodding syndrome, a neurological disorder of childhood onset with no known cause and treatment to date (Anguzu et al., 2018; Colebunders, Suykerbuyk, Jacob, & van Oijen, 2017; Idro et al., 2016; Bemmel, 2016). Policies and public discourse surrounding this mysterious neurological disease in Northern Uganda (Vogel, 2012) have to some extent strained research efforts potentially due to tensions between affected families (Buchmann, 2015), neuroscientists, neuro-practitioners (Musisi, Akena, Nakimuli-Mpungu, Abbo, & Okello, 2013) and political actors, so negatively affecting the national response (Deogratius, David, & Christopher, 2015; Schmutzhard & Winkler, 2015). This point become even more salient when we consider the state of needs and the past political turmoil of countries like Uganda and Sierra Leone. In 2010, a 5-year Mental Health Policy was enacted by the Government of Sierra Leone which sets clear directions for the development of mental health services and the promotion of mental health in the country (Shackman & Price, 2013). However, the implementation of this policy was challenged by myths, based on cultural and religious beliefs common among the indigenous population in Sierra Leone (Alemu et al., 2012). Even with such policy, mental health in Sierra Leone has received little attention and efforts to alleviate issues in the nation's health care systems (Palmer, 2013). Hence, for a long time, the people of Sierra Leone have been accustomed to myths surrounding mental health which negatively impact effective policy implementation. In addition to scarce resources for mental health due to the civil war, such myths are perpetuated by the traditional methods of mental health care which are perceived as solutions to mental health problems in the country (Yoldi, 2012). Neuroscience research has a lot to contribute in addressing these underlying issues by providing mental health capacity building, including knowledge regarding culturally appropriate assessment and treatment of mental illness, advocacy for changes in national mental health policy, and guidelines for funding and training of health professionals and lay individuals (Shackman & Price, 2013).

Now that the biopolitical dimension of neuroethics has been established, we need to demonstrate how neuroethics can contribute to global mental health. In this chapter global health is understood as:

> an area for study, research, and practice that places a priority on improving health and achieving equity in health for all people worldwide. Global health emphasises transnational health issues, determinants, and solutions; involves many disciplines within and beyond the health sciences and promotes interdisciplinary collaboration; and is a synthesis of population-based prevention with individual-level clinical care.
>
> (Koplan et al., 2009, p. 1995)

In particular there is an emphasis on issues such as the protection of human rights; addressing extreme poverty and associated problems such as corruption, malnutrition, and human trafficking (Levy & Sidel, 2013). Global mental health is the application to these principles in the context of addressing neurological and psychological disorders.

Concerns related to vulnerable populations, public policies, justice, and moral guidance, have been addressed by scholars in public health and bioethics so one could make the case that there is no need, in principle, to have a specific "neuroethics" angle. We want to challenge this assumption and argue that neuroethics has a special contribution to make to global mental health. Neuroethics is distinct from bioethics or global health. Its focus is specifically on the implications of progress in neuroscience and neurotechnology, and their implications for brain research and the treatment of neurological disorders. Neuroscience research is increasing our ability to diagnose, treat, and prevent neurological and mental disorders but by the same token challenges human self-understanding and raises ethical and policy issues that requires a distinct and careful analysis, which neuroethics can provide. There is enough evidence to establish a correlation between poverty or SES, community violence and brain structure and function. However, the interpretation of these neuroscientific findings and its implications for the care of this patient population raise its own set of challenges as outlined below.

To press this point further, let's consider an important distinction made by philosopher and neuroscientist, Adina Roskies, concerning neuroethics. She divides neuroethics into *the ethics of neuroscience* and *the neuroscience of ethics* (Roskies, 2002). The former examines the ethical implications raised by the use of neurotechnologies for intervention in the brain in the clinical and social context. The latter is an examination, using the tools of neuroscience and philosophical inquiry, of the nature of moral agency, responsibility, free will, personal identity, etc. The neuroscience of poverty or the neuroscience of community violence are not limited to the ethics of neuroscience, which is, to a certain extent, an extension of research ethics. Issues related to vulnerable population, justice, cost effectiveness, the development of ethical guidelines to influence public policies are, and have already been explored. The implications of community and political violence or war on brain development, however, are relatively new areas of concerns in brain research. As pointed out, some studies have demonstrated that children from lower SES have a higher risk of mental disorders and antisocial behavior (Lipina & Evers, 2017; Luby et al., 2013; van Goozen et al., 2008). Another study showed that exposure to community violence affects areas of the brain involved in cognitive and emotional development in adolescents (Saxbe et al., 2018). It is likely that governments might be interested in using this new knowledge to address social and mental health problems and gain access to neurotechnologies—while countries like Uganda and Sierra Leone are poor it is always perplexing to see how sophisticated weapons are present in conflicts; it is not improbable to think that governments could access neurotechnologies to monitor "human social and neurobiological processes." In addition, political divisions and ethnic tensions could contribute to their misuse. Neuroethics can provide a framework on how these findings can translate into policies and interventions implemented ethically and without stigmatizing individuals or pathologizing poverty as a disease. In addition, as the development of neurotechnological tools follows its course, the nature and boundaries of brain interventions will need to be clearly determined even in the absence of political tensions. Risks and benefits need to be assessed before implementation and vulnerable populations protected from abuse, manipulation or coercion. Finally, questions of how first world countries, where these technologies are developed and becoming increasingly accessible, should have a moral obligation to make them available to countries plagued by poverty, and social and political unrest must be addressed in the geopolitical realities of these countries. These important matters cannot be examined fully in this chapter, but they demonstrate that neuroethics can make a substantive contribution to global mental health through the development of collaborative initiatives (research, scholarship, etc.) and programs between countries from the African continent and first world countries. In addition, as cognitive neuroscientist Martha Farah explains, neuroscience may be uniquely positioned to help develop strategies for people of low SES. She points out that there is "a substantial body of research has revealed association between SES and brain structure and function… neuroscience can be expected to illuminate the processes by which SES become associated with a wide range to important life outcomes and to suggest ways of improving outcomes for people of low SES" (Farah, 2017, p. 62). However, she also stresses that it is too early to make generalizations about "a brain signature and SES or poverty" (Farah, 2017).

Concluding remarks

In conclusion, we would like to offer some recommendations as a way to stimulate further reflections concerning how to improve mental health and access to mental health services in Uganda and Sierra Leone, while recognizing the challenge to meet these needs. As we outline in this chapter, factors such as low socioeconomic status, violence and political unrest contribute to mental disorders and affect brain structure and function. In both countries, children, adolescents and young adults are the most vulnerable and efforts should focus on a prioritization of youth needs, culturally sensitive interventions and capacity building to foster income-generating activities to reduce poverty and its associated mental health risks. In additional, increasing funding should be allocated to support further research initiatives focusing on the long-term impact of poverty and violence on the mental health of the people of Uganda and Sierra Leone as well as the facilitation of access to medications and mental health facilities. Two other important areas in need of improvement should be included: (1) policy development that puts in place robust mental health initiatives that reflect the socio-cultural identity and needs of each country; and (2) the training of current and future mental health professionals. Both countries have a shortage of mental health professionals and therefore efforts should be made to create opportunities for training and continuing education.

The fulfillment of these recommendations will require considerable resources Uganda and Sierra Leone currently do not have. The development of dialogue between global mental health and neuroethics can be a fruitful opportunity to raise awareness initially of the issues surrounding the neuroscience of poverty. The challenge, though, will be how best to improve the mental health of the people of Uganda and Sierra Leone.

Acknowledgment

This project was funded through the Advancing a Healthier Wisconsin Endowment at the Medical College of Wisconsin.

References

African-Union. (2014). *Common Africa Position (CAP) on the post- 2015 development agenda.* In: *22nd ordinary session of the assembly of the union on 31 January 2014.*

Akinsulure-Smith, A. M., & Conteh, J. A. (2018). The Emergence of Counseling in Sierra Leone. (International) (Report). *Journal of Counseling and Development, 96*(3), 327–334. https://doi.org/10.1002/jcad.12206.

Alemu, W., Funk, M., Gakurah, T., Bash-Taqi, D., Bruni, A., Sinclair, J., et al. (2012). *WHO profile on mental health in development (WHO proMIND): Sierra Leone.* Geneva: World Health Organization.

Amone P'Olak, K. (2009). Torture against children in rebel captivity in Northern Uganda: Physical and psychological effects and implications for clinical practice. *Torture, 19*(2), 102–117.

Amone-P'Olak, K., Garnefski, N., & Kraaij, V. (2007). Adolescents caught between fires: Cognitive emotion regulation in response to war experiences in Northern Uganda. *Journal of Adolescence*, https://doi.org/10.1016/j.adolescence.2006.05.004.

Amone-P'Olak, K., Jones, P. B., Abbott, R., Meiser-Stedman, R., Ovuga, E., & Croudace, T. J. (2013). Cohort profile: Mental health following extreme trauma in a northern Ugandan cohort of War-Affected Youth Study (the WAYS study). *Springerplus*, https://doi.org/10.1186/2193-1801-2-300.

Anguzu, R., Akun, P. R., Ogwang, R., Shour, A. R., Sekibira, R., Ningwa, A., et al. (2018). Setting up a clinical trial for a novel disease: A case study of the Doxycycline for the Treatment of Nodding Syndrome Trial—Challenges, enablers and lessons learned. *Global Health Action*, *11*(1), 1431362. https://doi.org/10.1080/16549716.2018.1431362.

Annan, J., Blattman, C., Mazurana, D., & Carlson, K. (2011). Civil war, reintegration, and gender in northern Uganda. *Journal of Conflict Resolution*, https://doi.org/10.1177/0022002711408013.

Asare, J., & Jones, L. (2005). Tackling mental health in Sierra Leone. *BMJ*, *331*(7519), 720.

Barch, D., Pagliaccio, D., Belden, A., Harms, M. P., Gaffrey, M., Sylvester, C. M., et al. (2016). Effect of hippocampal and amygdala connectivity on the relationship between preschool poverty and school-age depression. *American Journal of Psychiatry*, *173*(6), 625–634. https://doi.org/10.1176/appi.ajp.2015.15081014.

Bayer, C. P., Klasen, F., & Adam, H. (2007). Association of trauma and PTSD symptoms with openness to reconciliation and feelings of revenge among former Ugandan and Congolese child soldiers. *Journal of the American Medical Association*, https://doi.org/10.1001/jama.298.5.555.

Bemmel, K. V. (2016). The quest for treatment: The violated body of nodding syndrome in Northern Uganda. *Journal of Peace and Security Studies*, *2*, 16.

Borofsky, L. A., Kellerman, I., Baucom, B., Oliver, P. H., & Margolin, G. (2013). Community violence exposure and adolescents' school engagement and academic achievement over time. *Psychology of Violence*, *3*(4), 381–395. https://doi.org/10.1037/a0034121.

Brito, N. H., & Noble, K. G. (2014). Socioeconomic status and structural brain development. *Frontiers in Neuroscience*, *8*. https://doi.org/10.3389/fnins.2014.00276.

Buchmann, K. (2015). 'These nodding people': Experiences of having a child with nodding syndrome in postconflict Northern Uganda. *Epilepsy & Behavior*, *42*, 71–77.

Büscher, K., Komujuni, S., & Ashaba, I. (2018). Humanitarian urbanism in a post-conflict aid town: aid agencies and urbanization in Gulu, Northern Uganda. *Journal of Eastern African Studies*, *12*(2), 348–366.

Colebunders, R., Suykerbuyk, P., Jacob, S. T., & van Oijen, M. (2017). Nodding syndrome, other forms of epilepsy, and the Nakalanga syndrome most likely directly or indirectly caused by *Onchocerca volvulus*. *Journal of the Neurological Sciences*, *372*, 439–440.

Conti, D. J., & Burton, W. N. (1994). The economic impact of depression in a workplace. *Journal of Occupational Medicine: Official Publication of the Industrial Medical Association*, *36*(9), 983–988.

De Jong, K., Mulhern, M., Ford, N., Van Der Kam, S., & Kleber, R. (2000). The trauma of war in Sierra Leone. *The Lancet*, *355*(9220), 2067–2068.

Deogratius, M. A., David, K. L., & Christopher, O. G. (2015). The enigmatic nodding syndrome outbreak in northern Uganda: An analysis of the disease burden and national response strategies. *Health Policy and Planning*, *31*(3), 285–292.

Duggan, M. B. (2010). Epilepsy in rural Ugandan children: Seizure pattern, age of onset and associated findings. *African Health Sciences*, https://doi.org/10.1097/00000441-192407000-00001.

Farah, M. J. (2017). The neuroscience of socioeconomic status: Correlates, causes, and consequences. *Neuron*, *96*(1), 56–71. https://doi.org/10.1016/j.neuron.2017.08.034.

Fisher, R. S. (2017). The new classification of seizures by the International League Against Epilepsy 2017. *Current Neurology and Neuroscience Reports*, *17*(6), 48.

Fisher, R. S., Acevedo, C., Arzimanoglou, A., Bogacz, A., Cross, J. H., Elger, C. E., et al. (2014). ILAE official report: A practical clinical definition of epilepsy. *Epilepsia*, https://doi.org/10.1111/epi.12550.

Flisher, A. J., Lund, C., Funk, M., Banda, M., Bhana, A., Doku, V., et al. (2007). Mental health policy development and implementation in four African countries. *Journal of Health Psychology*, https://doi.org/10.1177/1359105307076237.

Fowler, P. J., Tompsett, C. J., Braciszewski, J. M., Jacques-Tiura, A. J., & Baltes, B. B. (2009). Community violence: A meta-analysis on the effect of exposure and mental health outcomes of children and adolescents. *Development and Psychopathology*, *21*(01), 227. https://doi.org/10.1017/S0954579409000145.

Hackman, D. A., Farah, M. J., & Meaney, M. J. (2010). Socioeconomic status and the brain: Mechanistic insights from human and animal research. *Nature Reviews Neuroscience*, *11*(9), 651–659. https://doi.org/10.1038/nrn2897.

Hair, N. L., Hanson, J. L., Wolfe, B. L., & Pollak, S. D. (2015). Association of child poverty, brain development, and academic achievement. *JAMA Pediatrics*, *169*(9), 822–829. https://doi.org/10.1001/jamapediatrics.2015.1475.

Heleniak, C., King, K. M., Monahan, K. C., & McLaughlin, K. A. (2018). Disruptions in emotion regulation as a mechanism linking community violence exposure to adolescent internalizing problems. *Journal of Research on Adolescence: The Official Journal of the Society for Research on Adolescence*, *28*(1), 229–244. https://doi.org/10.1111/jora.12328.

Helleringer, S., & Noymer, A. (2015). *Assessing the direct effects of the Ebola outbreak on life expectancy in Liberia, Sierra Leone and Guinea*. Retrieved from: http://currents.plos.org/outbreaks/article/assessing-the-direct-effects-of-the-ebola-outbreakon-life-expectancy-in-liberia-sierra-leone-and-guinea/.

Henrich, J., Heine, S. J., & Norenzayan, A. (2010). The weirdest people in the world? *Behavioral and Brain Sciences*, https://doi.org/10.1017/S0140525X0999152X.

Henry, S., & Plemmons, D. (2012). Neuroscience, neuropolitics and neuroethics: The complex case of crime, deception and fMRI. *Science and Engineering Ethics*, *18*(3), 573–591. https://doi.org/10.1007/s11948-012-9393-4.

Human Rights Watch. (2004). *Human Rights Watch: World Report 2004, World Report 2004*.

Idro, R., Opar, B., Wamala, J., Abbo, C., Onzivua, S., Mwaka, D. A., et al. (2016). Is nodding syndrome an *Onchocerca volvulus*-induced neuroinflammatory disorder? Uganda's story of research in understanding the disease. *International Journal of Infectious Diseases*, *45*, 112–117.

Jednoróg, K., Altarelli, I., Monzalvo, K., Fluss, J., Dubois, J., Billard, C., et al. (2012). The influence of socioeconomic status on children's brain structure. *PLoS ONE*, *7*(8), e42486https://doi.org/10.1371/journal.pone.0042486.

Jotterand, F., & Ienca, M. (2017). The biopolitics of neuroethics. In *Debates about neuroethics*. Cham: Springer.(pp. 247–261). https://doi.org/10.1007/978-3-319-54651-3_17.

Kaiser, C., Asaba, G., Leichsenring, M., & Kabagambe, G. (1998). High incidence of epilepsy related to onchocerciasis in West Uganda. *Epilepsy Research*, https://doi.org/10.1016/S0920-1211(98)00007-2.

Kaiser, C., Kipp, W., Asaba, G., Mugisa, C., Kabagambe, G., Rating, D., et al. (1996). The prevalence of epilepsy follows the distribution of onchocerciasis in a West Ugandan focus. *Bulletin of the World Health Organization*, https://doi.org/10.1371/journal.pntd.0000461.

Karunakara, U. K., Neuner, F., Schauer, M., Singh, K., Hill, K., Elbert, T., et al. (2004). Traumatic events and symptoms of post-traumatic stress disorder amongst Sudanese nationals, refugees and Ugandans in the West Nile. *African Health Sciences, 4*(2), 83–93.

Katsnelson, A. (2015). News feature: The neuroscience of poverty. *Proceedings of the National Academy of Sciences, 112*(51), 15530–15532. https://doi.org/10.1073/pnas.1522683112.

Kigozi, F., Ssebunnya, J., Kizza, D., Cooper, S., & Ndyanabangi, S. (2010). An overview of Uganda's mental health care system: Results from an assessment using the world health organization's assessment instrument for mental health systems (WHO-AIMS). *International Journal of Mental Health Systems, 4*(1), 1. https://doi.org/10.1186/1752-4458-4-1.

Kilian, A. H. D., Kipp, W., Kasoro, S., & Burnham, G. (1994). Onchocerciasis and epilepsy. *The Lancet*, https://doi.org/10.1016/S0140-6736(94)90110-4.

Kirunga Tashobya, C., Ssengooba, F., & Oliveira Cruz, V. (2006). *Health Systems Reforms in Uganda: Processes and Outputs.* https://doi.org/10.1509/jmr.48.6.1074.

Koplan, J. P., Bond, T. C., Merson, M. H., Reddy, K. S., Rodriguez, M. H., Sewankambo, N. K., et al. (2009). Towards a common definition of global health. *Lancet (London, England), 373*(9679), 1993–1995. https://doi.org/10.1016/S0140-6736(09)60332-9.

Levy, B. S., & Sidel, V. W. (2013). International and global health. In *Social injustice and public health*. Oxford University Press. Retrieved from: https://global.oup.com/academic/product/social-injustice-and-public-health-9780199939220?cc=us&lang=en&#.

Lipina, S. J., & Evers, K. (2017). Neuroscience of childhood poverty: Evidence of impacts and mechanisms as vehicles of dialog with ethics. *Frontiers in Psychology, 8*. https://doi.org/10.3389/fpsyg.2017.00061.

Luby, J., Belden, A., Botteron, K., Marrus, N., Harms, M. P., Babb, C., et al. (2013). The effects of poverty on childhood brain development: The mediating effect of caregiving and stressful life events. *JAMA Pediatrics, 167*(12), 1135–1142. https://doi.org/10.1001/jamapediatrics.2013.3139.

McCoy, D. C., Raver, C. C., & Sharkey, P. (2015). Children's cognitive performance and selective attention following recent community violence. *Journal of Health and Social Behavior, 56*(1), 19–36. https://doi.org/10.1177/0022146514567576.

Ministry of Health. (2011). *Annual health sector Performance report financial year 2016/2017.*

MoH. (2015). *Health Sector Development Plan 2015/16–2019/20.* Republic of Uganda.

MoH. (2016). *Annual Health Sector Performance Report 2007–2008.*

Molodynski, A., Cusack, C., & Nixon, J. (2017). Mental healthcare in Uganda: Desperate challenges but real opportunities. *BJPsych International, 14*(4), 98–100.

Mugisha, J., Ssebunnya, J., & Kigozi, F. N. (2016). Towards understanding governance issues in integration of mental health into primary health care in Uganda. *International Journal of Mental Health Systems, 10*(1), 25.

Musisi, S., Akena, D., Nakimuli-Mpungu, E., Abbo, C., & Okello, J. (2013). Neuropsychiatric perspectives on nodding syndrome in northern Uganda: A case series study and a review of the literature. *African Health Sciences, 13*(2), 205–218.

Nalugya-Sserunjogi, J., Rukundo, G. Z., Ovuga, E., Kiwuwa, S. M., Musisi, S., & Nakimuli-Mpungu, E. (2016). Prevalence and factors associated with depression symptoms among school-going adolescents in Central Uganda. *Child and Adolescent Psychiatry and Mental Health*, https://doi.org/10.1186/s13034-016-0133-4.

Namagembe, I., Jackson, L. W., Zullo, M. D., Frank, S. H., Byamugisha, J. K., & Sethi, A. K. (2010). Consumption of alcoholic beverages among pregnant urban Ugandan women. *Maternal and Child Health Journal, 14*(4), 492–500.

Neuner, F., Schauer, M., Karunakara, U., Klaschik, C., Robert, C., & Elbert, T. (2004). Psychological trauma and evidence for enhanced vulnerability for posttraumatic stress disorder through previous trauma among West Nile refugees. *BMC Psychiatry*, https://doi.org/10.1186/1471-244X-4-34.

Noble, K. G., Houston, S. M., Brito, N. H., Bartsch, H., Kan, E., Kuperman, J. M., et al. (2015). Family income, parental education and brain structure in children and adolescents. *Nature Neuroscience*, *18*(5), 773–778. https://doi.org/10.1038/nn.3983.

Okello, J., Onen, T. S., & Musisi, S. (2007). Psychiatric disorders among war-abducted and non-abducted adolescents in Gulu district, Uganda: A comparative study. *African Journal of Psychiatry*, https://doi.org/10.4314/ajpsy.v10i4.30260.

Ovuga, E., Boardman, J., & Wasserman, D. (2005). The prevalence of depression in two districts of Uganda. *Social Psychiatry and Psychiatric Epidemiology*, https://doi.org/10.1007/s00127-005-0915-0.

Ovuga, E., Kipp, W., Mungherera, M., & Kasoro, S. (1992). Epilepsy and retarded growth in a hyperendemic focus of onchocerciasis in rural western Uganda. *East African Medical Journal*, *69*(10), 554–556.

Palmer, L. (2013). *Perceptions of mental health in Sierra Leone—A family doctor's view*. Retrieved from http://www.commonwealthhealth.org/wp-content/uploads/2013/07/Perceptions-of-mental-health-in-Sierra-Leone_CHP13.pdf.

Peltzer, K. (1999). Trauma and mental health problems of Sudanese refugees in Uganda. *The Central African Journal of Medicine*, https://doi.org/10.4314/cajm.v45i5.8465.

Pfeiffer, A., & Elbert, T. (2011). PTSD, depression and anxiety among former abductees in Northern Uganda. *Conflict and Health*, https://doi.org/10.1186/1752-1505-5-14.

Pham, P. N., Vinck, P., & Stover, E. (2009). Returning home: Forced conscription, reintegration, and mental health status of former abductees of the Lord's Resistance Army in northern Uganda. *BMC Psychiatry*, https://doi.org/10.1186/1471-244X-9-23.

Roberts, B., Ocaka, K. F., Browne, J., Oyok, T., & Sondorp, E. (2008). Factors associated with post-traumatic stress disorder and depression amongst internally displaced persons in northern Uganda. *BMC Psychiatry*, https://doi.org/10.1186/1471-244X-8-38.

Roskies, A. (2002). Neuroethics for the new millenium. *Neuron*, *35*(1), 21–23. https://doi.org/10.1016/S0896-6273(02)00763-8.

Saxbe, D., Khoddam, H., Piero, L. D., Stoycos, S. A., Gimbel, S. I., Margolin, G., et al. (2018). Community violence exposure in early adolescence: Longitudinal associations with hippocampal and amygdala volume and resting state connectivity. *Developmental Science*, *21*(6), e12686. https://doi.org/10.1111/desc.12686.

Saxena, S., Paraje, G., Sharan, P., Karam, G., & Sadana, R. (2006). The 10/90 divide in mental health research: Trends over a 10-year period. *British Journal of Psychiatry*, *188*, 81–82.

Schmutzhard, E., & Winkler, A. S. (2015). Nodding syndrome—A critical note and a plea to join forces. *Tropical Medicine & International Health*, *20*(2), 201–204.

Shackman, J., & Price, B. K. (2013). Mental health capacity building in northern Sierra Leone: Lessons learned and issues raised. *Intervention*, *11*(3), 261–275.

Shultz, J. M., Baingana, F., & Neria, Y. (2015). The 2014 Ebola outbreak and mental health: Current status and recommended response. *The Journal of the American Medical Association*, *313*(6), 567–568.

Swahn, M. H., Palmier, J. B., Kasirye, R., & Yao, H. (2012). Correlates of suicide ideation and attempt among youth living in the slums of Kampala. *International Journal of Environmental Research and Public Health*, *9*(2), 596–609.

Tumwesigye, N. M., & Kasirye, R. (2005). Gender and the major consequences of alcohol consumption in Uganda. *Alcohol, Gender and Drinking Problems*, 189.

Tumwesigye, N. M., Kyomuhendo, G. B., Greenfield, T. K., & Wanyenze, R. K. (2012). Problem drinking and physical intimate partner violence against women: Evidence from a national survey in Uganda. *BMC Public Health, 12*(1), 399.

UBOS. (2011). *Uganda demographic and health survey 2011.* Uganda Demographic and Health Survey.

UBOS. (2015). *Population projections 2015–2020.* Uganda Bureau of Statistics.

Uganda Ministry of Health. (2010). *Health sector strategic plan III.* Government of Uganda.

Uganda Ministry of Health. (2014). *Health Sector Strategic Plan 3.* Government of Uganda.

UN Development Program. (2009). Human Development Report—2009 Overcoming Barriers : Human Mobility and Development. *Human Development,* https://doi.org/10.1016/S0883-153X(98)80004-0.

United Nations. (2016). *The sustainable development goals report.* United Nations. https://doi.org/10.18356/3405d09f-en.

van Goozen, S. H. M., Fairchild, G., & Harold, G. T. (2008). The role of neurobiological deficits in childhood antisocial behavior. *Current Directions in Psychological Science, 17*(3), 224–228. https://doi.org/10.1111/j.1467-8721.2008.00579.x.

Vigo, D., Thornicroft, G., & Atun, R. (2016). Estimating the true global burden of mental illness. *The Lancet Psychiatry,* https://doi.org/10.1016/S2215-0366(15)00505-2.

Vogel, G. (2012). *Mystery disease haunts region.*

Weierstall, R., Schalinski, I., Crombach, A., Hecker, T., & Elbert, T. (2012). When combat prevents PTSD symptoms-results from a survey with former child soldiers in Northern Uganda. *BMC Psychiatry,* https://doi.org/10.1186/1471-244X-12-41.

Whiteford, H. A., Degenhardt, L., Rehm, J., Baxter, A. J., Ferrari, A. J., Erskine, H. E., et al. (2013). Global burden of disease attributable to mental and substance use disorders: Findings from the Global Burden of Disease Study 2010. *Lancet (London, England),* https://doi.org/10.1016/S0140-6736(13)61611-6.

WHO. (2004). *Epilepsy in the WHO African Region: Bridging the gap.* World Health Organization. https://doi.org/10.1111/j.1528-1167.2009.02184.x.

WHO. (2005). *Mental health atlas 2005.* World Health Organization Technical report series, 894(894), i–xii, 1–253. https://doi.org/10.1097/01.nmd.0000260057.17679.7a.

WHO. (2006). *WHO Profile on mental health in development (WHO proMIND): Sierra Leone.* Geneva: World Health Organization.

WHO. (2013). *Comprehensive mental health action plan 2013–2020.* WHO. Retrieved 7 August 2018, from: http://www.who.int/mental_health/action_plan_2013/en/.

World Health Organization. (2001). *Mental disorders affect one in four people.* World Health Organisation. https://doi.org/10.1192/bjp.180.1.29.

World Health Organization. (2006). *WHO-AIMS Report: Mental Health System in Uganda.* World Health Organization. https://doi.org/10.1017/CBO9781107415324.004.

World Health Organization. (2014). *WHO mental health gap action programme (mhGAP).* WHO.

World Health Organization. (2017). *Depression and other common mental disorders: Global health estimates.* Geneva: World Health Organization. Licence: CC BY-NC-SA 3.0 IGO.

Yoder, H. N. C., Tol, W. A., Reis, R., & de Jong, J.T.V.M. (2016). Child mental health in Sierra Leone: A survey and exploratory qualitative study. *International Journal of Mental Health Systems, 10*(1), 48. https://doi.org/10.1186/s13033-016-0080-8.

Yoldi, O. (2012). Sierra Leone: Trapped in the shadows of the mind. *Refugee Transitions, 26,* 60–65.

Further reading

Bangirana, P., John, C. C., Idro, R., Opoka, R. O., Byarugaba, J., Jurek, A. M., et al. (2009). Socioeconomic predictors of cognition in Ugandan children: Implications for community interventions. *PLoS ONE*, *4*(11). https://doi.org/10.1371/journal.pone.0007898.

Bradley, R. H., & Corwyn, R. F. (2002). Socioeconomic status and child development. *Annual Review of Psychology*, https://doi.org/10.1146/annurev.psych.53.100901.135233.

Hackman, D. A., & Farah, M. J. (2009). Socioeconomic status and the developing brain. *Trends in Cognitive Sciences*, https://doi.org/10.1016/j.tics.2008.11.003.

Idro, R., Jenkins, N. E., & Newton, C.R.J.C. (2005). Pathogenesis, clinical features, and neurological outcome of cerebral malaria. *The Lancet Neurology*, *4*(12), 827–840. https://doi.org/10.1016/S1474-4422(05)70247-7.

Idro, R., Carter, J. A., Fegan, G., Neville, B. G. R., & Newton, C.R.J.C. (2006). Risk factors for persisting neurological and cognitive impairments following cerebral malaria. *Archives of Disease in Childhood*, *91*(2), 142–148. https://doi.org/10.1136/adc.2005.077784.

Patel, V., & Kleinman, A. (2003). Poverty and common mental disorders in developing countries. *Bulletin of the World Health Organization*, *81*(8), 609–615.

Ssebunnya, J., Kigozi, F., & Ndyanabangi, S. (2012). Developing a national mental health policy: A case study from Uganda. *PLoS Medicine*, https://doi.org/10.1371/journal.pmed.1001319.

Vohr, B. R., Poggi Davis, E., Wanke, C. A., & Krebs, N. F. (2017). Neurodevelopment: The impact of nutrition and inflammation during preconception and pregnancy in low-resource settings. *Pediatrics*, *139*(Supplement 1), S38–S49. https://doi.org/10.1542/peds.2016-2828F.

Section C

Disorders/developmental stages

Interactive role-playing and health-related quality of life assessment in children with neurocognitive sequelae: A global neuroethics research approach

11

Vasiliki Rahimzadeh[a], Gillian Bartlett[b], Cristina Longo[b], Judy Illes[c]
[a]Postdoctoral Fellow, Stanford Center for Biomedical Ethics, Stanford University, Stanford, CA, United States, [b]Department of Family Medicine, McGill University, Montréal, QC, Canada, [c]Neuroethics Canada, Department of Neurology, University of British Columbia, Vancouver, BC, Canada

> *Physicists are perfectly right in stressing the difficulties of research into elementary particles. But they should not resent being told that such research is child's play in comparison with the scientific comprehension of games played by children! The rules of any game are only a conventionally marked path; children "run" along this path very capriciously, violating its borders at every turn, because they possess free will and their choice cannot be predicted. Nothing in the world is more complex or more perplexing than a human being.*
> —**On the Human Being and Being Human, A. Spirkin**

Introduction

In this chapter, we explore the practical and theoretical strengths of role-playing games (RPGs) as a method to understand health-related quality of life (HRQoL) in children with neurodevelopmental and cognitive sequelae (NDCS) resulting from brain cancer. We call attention to proxy reporting in empirical studies and its effects on the body of HRQoL knowledge upon which care strategies in the pediatric NDCS population are largely based. This chapter is among the first to promote the gamification of HRQoL research, and in particular RPGs as an engagement-oriented research and clinical data collection tool for children with NDCS. The theoretical underpinnings of HRQoL through role-playing as they manifest through functional forms of play among children with NDCS are described in depth, including the practical strengths and challenges thereof. In landscaping the history and practice of HRQoL research with children, we echo the observation that the "research community has lacked the expertise, imagination and capability to engage the most disabled (especially children) in research processes that can genuinely capture their experiences and enable positive and emancipatory changes

Global Mental Health and Neuroethics. https://doi.org/10.1016/B978-0-12-815063-4.00011-3

to result (Hodge, 2008)" (Simmons, 2014). The methods and outputs of role-playing can be used as an adjunctive, patient/child-centered information tool for clinical decision-making in the NDCS context in specific. Our intent is to propose an RPG that is amenable to adaptation in HRQoL research and shared decision-making involving neurodiverse children and their families more broadly. Role-playing games as HRQoL research methodology abandon categorical assumptions of vulnerability—including for children with life threatening/limiting disorders—which too often mask children's exclusion from research behind a protectionist bioethical rationality.

We appreciate that brain cancer may not always lead to neuropsychiatric disorders, but significant overlap exists with neurocognitive disorders when depression (Buchbinder et al., 2017), difficulty sustaining peer relationships (Vannatta, Gerhardt, Wells, et al., 2007) and other psychosocial sequelae involving cognitive functioning evolve following cancer diagnosis or during treatment. With game-play as a borderless and ubiquitous, although not socially or socioeconomically-neutral phenomenon, we conclude this chapter with potential applications to other fields of pediatric research inquiry, contexts and populations. Such potential contributions to research methodology in neuroethics and brain and mental health disorders make RPGs truly global in their clinical application across care and research contexts involving children. In the section to follow, we discuss the research-care nexus unique to pediatric oncology, the clinical successes therein, and the accentuated need to improve HRQoL research among children diagnosed with, as well as survivors of childhood cancer.

At the nexus of tumor research, care and survivorship

Brain tumors and other nervous system cancers constitute one of the leading causes of cancer-related death in children (Fitzmaurice, Allen, Barber, et al., 2017), while childhood epilepsy represents the greatest burden of disease post treatment for childhood brain- or other CNS tumor (Feigin, Abajobir, Abate, et al., 2017; Kenborg, Winther, Linnet, et al., 2018). This finding is documented worldwide, although data are most readily available for middle and high income countries (Howard, Davidson, Luna-Fineman, et al., 2017). Evidence-based standards of care are problematized by both the relative rarity of cancer in children, and the stringent regulatory norms of involving vulnerable populations such as neurodevelopmentally disabled children in research. The implications of knowledge lacunas resulting from children's exclusion from research is perhaps best illustrated in oncology. Dosing regimens for many anti-cancer therapies, for example, are extrapolated from studies conducted with adults, and can be highly toxic when administered to children (Feinstein, Morrato, & Feudtner, 2017).

Pediatric oncology is among the few specialties where therapeutic opportunities are afforded through both standard care and participation in clinical research. Survivorship following childhood cancer now exceeds 80% in high-income countries thanks in large part to highly coordinated research networks and international cancer consortia that offer patients opportunities to participate in clinical trials and share trial data (Pui, Gajjar, Kane, et al., 2012). The completion of the Human Genome Project in 2003, as well as subsequent advances in the "omics" disciplines have, in turn, expanded clinical research and translational science opportunities. These include cancers with genetic predispositions to neurodevelopment and other behavioral disorders. The Human Genome Project also had the effect of reconfiguring the very nature of research participation and associated benefit-risk calculi; as research participation increasingly constitutes the collection, analysis, and sharing of children's genomic and associated clinical data, informational risks, in addition to physiological risks, become chief ethical considerations.

The effects of expanding such research opportunities are likewise tangible in the pediatric brain- and CNS tumor field. The involvement of children in clinical and genomic research is at an all-time high (Dufetelle, Jong, & Kaguelidou, 2018; Surun, Dujaric, Aerts, et al., 2018),[a] and clinical databases such as ClinVar and dbGaP make aggregate genomic and associated clinical data involving children available to researchers and clinicians alike. Access to linked genotypic and phenotypic data from children diagnosed with brain and other cancers have already resulted in significant improvements to individual patient diagnosis and care in what scholars define as learning healthcare systems (Institute of Medicine et al., 2007).[b] Indeed, convergence of research and clinical care (Wolf, Amendola, Berg, et al., 2018) are defining attributes of the learning healthcare system "that is designed to generate and apply the best evidence for the collaborative healthcare choices of each patient and provider; to drive the process of discovery as a natural outgrowth of patient care" (Institute of Medicine et al., 2007).

Overall survival at 1 and 2 years post diagnosis, however, remain dismal for children with brain gliomas specifically (Hassan, Pinches, Picton, et al., 2017) despite the advances that learning healthcare systems and broader access to linked clinical data have together ushered in. This situation persists also despite vast improvements in 5-year survival rates for many other pediatric cancers, accentuating the need to optimize HRQoL[c] both during, and post treatment for brain and other tumors of the central nervous system (CNS) (Engelen, 2011).

Of adolescent and young adult cancer survivors, the prevalence of NDCS is highest among those with brain and other CNS tumors (Forrest et al., 2014; Hocking, Hobbie, Deatrick, et al., 2011; Stone, Waern, Khabra, et al., 2017). This population

---

[a] Although participation rates are steadily increasing, nonpublication bias remains a scientific concern. Crockett and colleagues note that among registered phase 3 randomized controlled trials, nearly a third (29%) go unpublished.

[b] Learning healthcare systems are meant to transcend patient populations and geographies, yet some example of such systems specifically geared towards improved learning in pediatric settings have been developed (see for example, Forrest, Margolis, Seid, et al., 2014).

[c] Although not an uncontested construct, HRQoL is generally accepted to encompass "functional effects of a medical condition and/or its consequent therapy upon a patient…[and] is thus subjective and multidimensional, encompassing physical and occupational function, psychological state, social interaction and somatic sensation" (ISOQOL, What is Health-Related Quality of Life Research). The Healthy People 2020 project further clarifies the features of quality of life that make it explicitly health-related: "When quality of life considered in the context of health and disease, it is commonly referred to as HRQoL to differentiate it from other aspects of quality of life. Since health is a multidimensional concept, HRQoL is also multidimensional and incorporates domains related to physical, mental and emotional, and social functioning" (Healthy People 2020, 2019).

has specific difficulties in executive functioning and lowered IQ, among other developmental and behavioral challenges. Studies also report lower HRQoL across several indicators when compared to other pediatric oncology populations (Penn, Shortman, Lowis, et al., 2010; Schulte, Russell, Cullen, et al., 2017; Varni, Burwinkle, Sherman, et al., 2005; Wolfe, Orellana, Ullrich, et al., 2015) and youth with chronic conditions (Barakat, Hobbie, Minturn, et al., 2017; Hobbie, Ogle, Reilly, et al., 2016). Quast et al. attribute these poorer HRQoL outcomes in part to ongoing and additional anti-cancer therapy (Quast, Phillips, Li, et al., 2018).

Precision oncology is furthermore shedding new light on the "omics" etiologies of childhood brain and other cancers and contributing to longer life expectancies as a result (Goudie, Coltin, Witkowski, et al., 2017). Consequently, the population of pediatric brain tumors survivors is growing, albeit not for all children, everywhere (Phillips, Padgett, Leisenring, et al., 2015). Disparities in cancer cure rates between low/middle and high-income countries are cause for grave concern. Whereas "in high-income countries (HIC), 75% of children with cancer are cured…over 80% of the world's children live in [low income countries], in which cancer cure rates often do not exceed 35% (Fitzmaurice et al., 2017; Vannatta et al., 2007). Even more unfortunate is the fact that the gap in survival between children with cancer in LIC versus HIC continues to widen as curative therapies are developed in the latter but not implemented in the former" (Bao, Zheng, Wang, et al., 2009).

The availability of quality data suggesting increases in cancer survivorship is attributable largely to standard reporting and monitoring of global pediatric cancer trends by organizations such as the International Agency for Cancer Research—a specialized subsidiary of the World Health Organization—and the International Classification of Disease Oncology, respectively. Incidence and prevalence data on pediatric brain and other CNS tumors are predominantly reflective of European and North American populations (Storm, Engholm, Mägi, et al., 2017), while comparable data from low and middle-income countries (LMIC) are limited (De Robles, Fiest, Frolkis, et al., 2015; Ezzat, Kamal, El-Khateeb, et al., 2016; Frazier, Piñeros, Fuentes, et al., 2017). The evolving areas of unmet need among children living with NCDS are exacerbated in LMICs that lack specialty care services and resources for longitudinal patient management (Howard et al., 2017). Frazier et al. (2017) highlight such discrepancies in available data across the Global North and South. The authors describe the significance of cancer registries and classification in LMICs towards accurately assessing the burden of disease related to such childhood cancers on a global scale (Bastos, Silveira, Luna, et al., 2017; Frazier et al., 2017). A lack of regional diversity in the clinical genomic databases mentioned earlier further constrain possible inferences into etiologies of childhood cancer across global contexts.

Studies assessing the impacts of NDCS on HRQoL, especially in the face of refractory disease in LMICs, is also markedly scant (Bhat, Goodwin, Burwinkle, et al., 2005; Stone et al., 2017; Tock, Bhat, Szymonifka, et al., 2014). In one of the only systematic reviews of its kind, Macartney et al. note 16 empirical studies investigating HRQoL in pediatric brain cancer survivors, and identified 10 heterogenous HRQoL instruments (Macartney, Harrison, VanDenKerkhof, et al., 2014). The authors note that "[…] while some instruments captured individual symptoms, only three studies explored the relationship between symptoms and HRQL outcomes. Although there is a negative relationship between pain, fatigue, and HRQL reported in the literature, the relationship between other symptoms and HRQL is unknown (Macartney et al., 2014)." Recent studies have since highlighted the need to investigate longitudinal HRQoL factors in this population (de Ruiter, Schouten-van Meeteren, van Vuurden, et al., 2016; Demers, Gélinas, & Carret, 2016), including fatigue (Tomlinson, Zupanec, Jones, et al., 2016), physical activity (Devine, Mertens, Whitton, et al., 2018; Paxton, 2010), and anxiety (Lazor, Tigelaar, Pole, et al., 2017) among others. Schulte et al., in a more recent meta-analysis discovered that survivors of pediatric brain and other CNS tumors experience poor HRQoL up to 25 years following treatment. For this reason, future research is needed to correlate leading NDCS with brain tumor diagnosis to improve prognosis and HRQoL for childhood cancer survivors (Schulte et al., 2017).

The situational vulnerability of children diagnosed with, or survivors of cancer in LMICs is hence compounded. First, a cancer diagnosis is relatively rare when compared to other health conditions, e.g., communicable and chronic diseases that may be more prominent in LMICs. These children are, secondly, further disadvantaged when their home countries are ill-equipped to provide treatment options and follow up on any NDCS that may result from their cancer.

Instrumentalizing and globalizing HRQoL research

While a nascent field of inquiry in the medical humanities, HRQoL research methodology has remained relatively preserved. Armstrong (2009) provides a useful historical analysis of HRQoL as a methodological construct in medical research from 1970 to 2007. He writes about an empirical turn in the early 1990s that made HRQoL "a vague idea into a measurable 'fact'; quality of life made the transition from rhetorical concept to a hard end-point of clinical practice." (Armstrong, 2009). Measurement and quantification of HRQoL stood in stark contrast to the phenomenological and ethnographical research that preceded this empirical turn, and which at its height in the early 1960s and 70s was driven by qualitative health research giants including Glaser, Strauss, Bluebond-Langner and others (Bluebond-Langner, 1978; Glaser & Strauss, 1965).

HRQoL research in the decades to follow progressively standardized and quantified HRQoL indicators, supplanting much of the psychosocial orientations that prior sociological and anthropological research typified. This empiricist turn in part gave rise to quantitative HRQoL instruments including the European Quality of Life Group-5D (European Quality of Life Group, 2009). Perhaps the widest HRQoL instrument used today is the EQ-5D domain measures of mobility, self-care, usual activities, pain/discomfort and anxiety/depression. Respondents rate the degree to which they perceive problems related to each HRQoL domain in the questionnaire on a 3- or 5-level severity scale.[d]

[d] In 2009, the EuroQol Group launched a specific instrument for youth (EQ-5D-Y) that included identical dimensions of analysis but in developmentally appropriate wording suitable to younger populations (e.g., mobility; looking after myself, doing usual activities; having pain or discomfort and feeling worried: sad or unhappy.

Although instruments have been developed to assess HRQoL facilitators, barriers and patient-reported outcomes in children (Leahy, Feudtner, & Basch, 2018; Varni & Limbers, 2009), including in global mental health contexts (Drotar, 1998; Matza, Swensen, Flood, et al., 2004; Penn et al., 2010; Solans, Pane, Estrada, et al., 2008), nearly all such instruments are modified from those developed for use in adult populations. Moreover, even pediatric-specific HRQoL instruments take on both the form and function of adult instruments, which often probe children using questionnaires that involve cognitive tasks like rating, rationing and risk-benefit assessments. While meant to be pediatric-specific, these instruments appeal to adult-oriented logics, rationalities and reasonings that children either may not have fully grasped as yet, or are wholly incapable of performing due to their neurodevelopmental or behavioral condition. The Medical Research Council report on Medical Research Involving Children confirms this:

> Standard outcome measures in adults include death and quality of life, but for many conditions different outcomes are more relevant. Measurements of these outcomes have been determined for use in adults specifically and may not be relevant for children. Quality of life measures can be used, but should be focused on the child or family and validated and tested for reliability and responsiveness to change before being used; such instruments have not always been available. It is therefore useful, and important, to consult children about outcome measures and other issues, when the research is being designed (Medical Research Council, 2004).

The methodological turn towards quantifying indicators and patient-reported outcomes in the early 1990s greatly influenced the body of HRQoL knowledge that was produced. Bjornson and McLaughlin (2001) corroborate this trend in HRQoL measures involving children with cerebral palsy: "HRQL measures may have been designed to serve one or more of three possible functions: discrimination, prediction and evaluation" (Bjornson & McLaughlin, 2001). The authors go on to define three primary purposes of HRQoL measures: a discriminative measure intended to distinguish between quality of life among children with different clinical characteristics, a predictive measure to estimate future outcome or prognosis; and an evaluative measure to indicate change in a characteristic over time (Bjornson & McLaughlin, 2001). Below, we describe a fourth, emerging category—experiential—that aims to contextualize children's HRQoL experiences not as a discreet measure, but rather as illness narratives. First, however, we call special attention to parent and health professional proxy reporting in HRQoL research with children, its effects on existing bodies of HRQoL knowledge, and how models of shared decision-making in the pediatric neuropsychiatric space inevitably takes up such knowledge.

Proxy-reporting in HRQoL research

Whereas past quantitative, qualitative and mixed methods studies have investigated various dimensions related to quality of life among childhood brain tumor patients and survivors, findings are overwhelming based on parental or clinician proxy reporting. Furthermore, many empirical studies assess late effects of pediatric brain and

CNS tumors after patients reach adulthood (Sato, Higuchi, Yanagisawa, et al., 2014). Delaying this research is a missed opportunity for preventing negative NDCS early in remission, and while patients are still young. Proxy reporting can be entirely appropriate, even necessary in some circumstances where the child is nonverbal, or perhaps suffers from severe NDCS that makes even adapted modes of communication difficult or impossible (Varni & Limbers, 2009; Varni, Limbers, & Burwinkle, 2007a). Researchers have therefore paid considerable attention to assessing interrater consistency between proxy- and patient-reports, albeit with mixed success, in effort to improve internal and external validity of HRQoL research that relies on proxy reporting (Cremeens, Eiser, & Blades, 2014; Matza et al., 2004; Meeske, Katz, Palmer, et al., 2004; Morrow, Hayen, Quine, et al., 2012; Sattoe, van Staa, & Moll, 2012; Solans et al., 2008; Theunissen, Vogels, Koopman, et al., 2014; Varni, Limbers, & Burwinkle, 2007b).

Proxy-reporting raises several key theoretical and practical limitations even under conditions of high interrater consistency. The individual HRQoL dimensions that such instruments assess—usually in the form of questionnaires—are predetermined by adults, and furthermore presented within a strictly status-based as opposed to an experiential frame. That is, patients and proxies report only discreet dimensions of HRQoL the instrument of choice outlines, e.g., mobility, pain or discomfort, feelings of worry, and without contextual appeal to what or how, if at all, such dimensions are meaningful to the child. Such instruments can delimit what is otherwise a vast expanse of HRQoL themes that may be relevant to patients and their families, including the meaning patients and proxies ascribe to these themes. Absent attention to the significance of meaning, researchers cannot expect to capture the social phenomena of HRQoL that we, and others, believe guide a child's illness experience. A combination of HRQoL data collection and analytical methods are needed therefore to produce relevant knowledge that is attuned to both the experiential and status-oriented dimensions of HRQoL to inform meaningful HRQoL interventions.

Consider for example the scenario in which patients and proxies achieve high interrater coherence on perceived feelings of fatigue, a common item on many conventional HRQoL assessment tools. It might be that child and proxy agree on the perceived status of the child's fatigue based on observable behaviors such as time and quality of sleep. But without moving beyond characterizing the status of fatigue, and towards contextualizing the global effects that fatigue may have on behaviors, practices, and abilities that can together define how children perceive their own quality of life, it is questionable whether child-proxy rater coherence provides meaningful guidance on how to mitigate fatigue in efforts to enhance HRQoL.

The decision making processes underpinning these, and other interventions, for children with NDCS, and the HRQoL knowledge used to support preferred interventions, are among the research-practice nexuses that role-playing games can feasibly create in the pediatric neuropsychiatric context. We are at times critical of the quality of children's engagement in shared decisions in this space, where HRQoL interventions for children suffering from NDCS may be based solely on information gleaned from proxy-reports, or from instrument-mediated HRQoL results. These decisional inputs alone can be problematic considering the empirical limitations explained above, to say nothing of the opportunities to facilitate children's participatory agency they inevitably miss. Such empirically limited HRQoL assessments are further problematic in LMICs, where medical paternalism may dictate child-patient-clinician behaviors and maxims of decision-making (Park & Cho, 2017). We support the position, however, that the ethos of shared decision making that can result as a positive byproduct of HRQoL research which prioritizes children's meaningful involvement is "entirely consistent with the priorities of low income settings—that is, to improve health literacy, improve patient provider communication, and empower individuals to be more involved in their healthcare (Stiggelbout, Van Der Weijden, De Wit, et al., 2012)."

Based on our above review of the unique clinical presentations among children living with NDCS, as well as the methodological features of HRQoL research involving them, NDCS post pediatric brain tumor diagnosis and treatment are diverse, frequent, and understudied from a HRQoL perspective; this is moreover a consistent research gap across low, middle and high-income countries. We elaborate in the subsequent sections twin neuroethical and empirical priorities that RPGs can fulfill in the global mental health and HRQoL research communities to enhance participatory mechanisms of knowledge production and translation.

Expanding the game-research nexus through role-playing in HRQoL

Rights to the game

Role-based research methods used to explore contextually-grounded themes of HRQoL accepts the premise that HRQoL is both interactive and relational. Researchers can capture the richness of children's HRQoL through the illness narratives that children tell during role-based interactions, as well the meaning children attribute to various dimensions of HRQoL. The research-care nexus needed to comprehensively capture the HRQoL narratives and clinical needs of this patient population thus requires an innovative research engagement approach that too adopts an interactive and relational orientation to HRQoL. Role-playing as an empirical tool is, to be sure, not novel. It has been used extensively to further the understanding, for example, of childhood development in education (Johnson, 2007; Wong, Odom, Hume, et al., 2015) and developmental psychology (Corsini, 2017; Landreth, 2012) among many others, yet fewer initiatives have combined role playing and HRQoL research, in specific (Barrera, Atenafu, Sung, et al., 2018).

RPGs, we believe, fulfill twin neuroethical and empirical priorities. They activate children's rights to participation in understanding issues that directly concern them, rights codified in international conventions such as the United Nations Declaration of Human Rights, the United Nations Convention on the Rights of the Child (UNCRC) and outlined under special conditions in national regulations governing the protection of human research participants (Box 1). As such, game-based research methods abandon categorical assumptions of children's vulnerabilities that too often mask their exclusion from research behind overly protectionist bioethical rationality.

RPGs privilege child-centeric knowledge generation by embedding HRQoL assessment into the very communicative and interactional norms unique to children, such as functional play, and thereby fulfills an empirical imperative. Put differently, RPGs fill an empirical knowledge gap by generating and translating data on HRQoL seldom derived from the child herself. The inductive approach to data collection and analysis that RPGs afford separates game-based methods of research engagement from

Box 1   Internationally relevant conventions, statutes and guidelines related to the participation of children in research

Document	Article/Statute related to participation in research
International Conventions	
UN DECLARATION OF HUMAN RIGHTS	**Article 27** *Everyone has the right **freely to participate in the cultural life** of the community, to enj[...] **share in scientific advancement and its benefits.***
UN CONVENTION ON THE RIGHTS OF THE CHILD	**Article 12** *1. States Parties shall assure to the child who is capable of forming his or her own views the **right to express those views freely in all matters affecting the child**, the views of the child being given **due weight** in accordance with the age and maturity of the child.* **Article 13** *The child shall have the **right to freedom of expression**; this right shall include freedom to **seek, receive and impart information and ideas of all kinds**, regardless of frontiers, either orally, in writing or in print, in the form of art, or through **any other media of the child's choice**.*
International Guidelines	
CIOMS— INTERNATIONAL ETHICAL GUIDELINES FOR RESEARCH INVOLVING HUMANS	**Justification of the involvement of children and adolescents in health-related research.** *The participation of children and adolescents is **indispensable** for research into diseases of childhood and conditions to which they are particularly susceptible, as well as for clinical trials of drugs that will be used for children and adolescents as well as adults* **Order of Involvement in Research** *The current Guidelines do **not** require that research **first be conducted in adults** if the research includes interventions that have a prospect for potential individual benefit for children and adolescents. This prospect is sufficient to justify the risks associated with the interventions and procedures, provided that the cumulative risk of all study interventions and procedures that do not have a prospect of potential individual benefit are no more than minimal. If research meets these conditions but the cumulative risk of all study interventions and procedures that do not have a prospect of potential individual benefit is only a minor increment above minimal risk, then research ethics committees must be convinced that the **research is of special relevance to children or adolescents** and could **not** be carried out equally well in an adult population. In such cases, older children who are **more** capable of giving assent must be selected **before** younger children or infants, unless there are sound scientific reasons for performing the research in younger children first.*
WMA DECLARATION OF OTTAWA ON CHILD HEALTH	**4. Research & monitoring for continual improvement includes:** *1. All infants will be officially registered within one month of birth.* *2. All children will be treated with **dignity and respect*** *3. Quality care is ensured through on-going monitoring of services, including collection of data, and **evaluation of outcomes*** *4. Children will **share in the benefits from scientific research** relevant to their needs*

(Continued)

Box 1   Internationally relevant conventions, statutes and guidelines related to the participation of children in research—cont'd

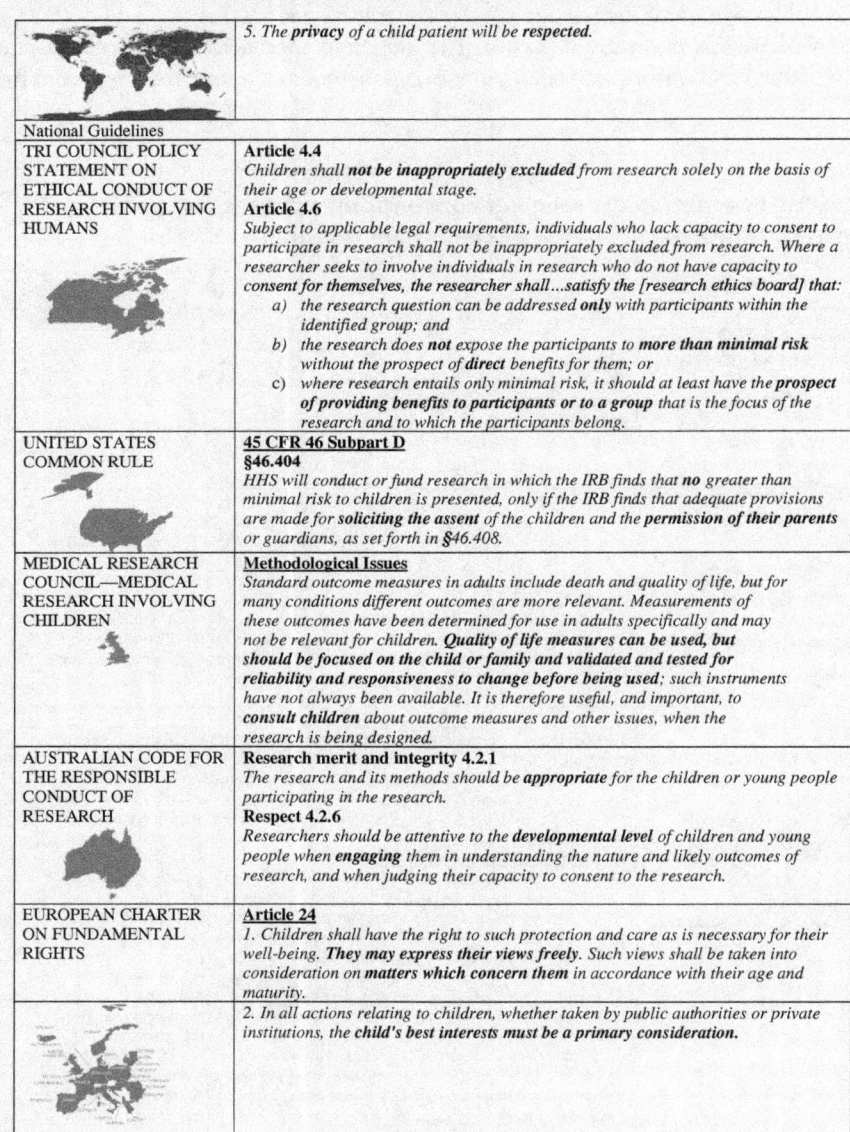

	5. The **privacy** of a child patient will be **respected**.
National Guidelines	

TRI COUNCIL POLICY STATEMENT ON ETHICAL CONDUCT OF RESEARCH INVOLVING HUMANS	**Article 4.4**
	Children shall **not be inappropriately excluded** from research solely on the basis of their age or developmental stage.
	Article 4.6
	Subject to applicable legal requirements, individuals who lack capacity to consent to participate in research shall not be inappropriately excluded from research. Where a researcher seeks to involve individuals in research who do not have capacity to consent for themselves, the researcher shall...satisfy the [research ethics board] that:
	    a) the research question can be addressed **only** with participants within the identified group; and
	    b) the research does **not** expose the participants to **more than minimal risk** without the prospect of **direct** benefits for them; or
	    c) where research entails only minimal risk, it should at least have the **prospect of providing benefits to participants or to a group** that is the focus of the research and to which the participants belong.

UNITED STATES COMMON RULE	<u>45 CFR 46 Subpart D</u> **§46.404** HHS will conduct or fund research in which the IRB finds that **no** greater than minimal risk to children is presented, only if the IRB finds that adequate provisions are made for **soliciting the assent** of the children and the **permission of their parents** or guardians, as set forth in §46.408.
MEDICAL RESEARCH COUNCIL—MEDICAL RESEARCH INVOLVING CHILDREN	<u>Methodological Issues</u> Standard outcome measures in adults include death and quality of life, but for many conditions different outcomes are more relevant. Measurements of these outcomes have been determined for use in adults specifically and may not be relevant for children. **Quality of life measures can be used, but should be focused on the child or family and validated and tested for reliability and responsiveness to change before being used**; such instruments have not always been available. It is therefore useful, and important, to **consult children** about outcome measures and other issues, when the research is being designed.
AUSTRALIAN CODE FOR THE RESPONSIBLE CONDUCT OF RESEARCH	**Research merit and integrity 4.2.1** The research and its methods should be **appropriate** for the children or young people participating in the research. **Respect 4.2.6** Researchers should be attentive to the **developmental level** of children and young people when **engaging** them in understanding the nature and likely outcomes of research, and when judging their capacity to consent to the research.
EUROPEAN CHARTER ON FUNDAMENTAL RIGHTS	<u>Article 24</u> 1. Children shall have the right to such protection and care as is necessary for their well-being. **They may express their views freely.** Such views shall be taken into consideration on **matters which concern them** in accordance with their age and maturity.
	2. In all actions relating to children, whether taken by public authorities or private institutions, the **child's best interests must be a primary consideration**.

arts based or other qualitative interviewing approaches. The latter are often criticized for their overreliance on the researchers' interpretation of qualitative data, conflating the researcher and child's voice. Grounded in these twin neuroethical and empirical imperatives, we elaborate below on the theoretical and practical foundations of RPGs to study the effects of HRQoL among children with NDCS and other neurodevelopmental/behavioral disorders.

Theory of the game

It is widely understood that children are acutely aware of social orders in which they are part. One lens through which to understand *how* and *what* children understand of their social orders is by observing them play, pretend and re-enact the archetypical roles they encounter (Bowman, 2010). RPGs harness children's methods of situational awareness and self-discovery, and are classified as *functional play with pretense* according to Barton and Wolery (2008) and Barton, Choi, and Mauldin (2019). RPGs transcend two of four taxonomic categories of functional pretend play Barton and Wolery observed in children with neurological and other developmental disabilities: substitution—assigning absent attributes—and verbalization—confirmatory vocalization. Substitution through assigning absent attributes may involve using props and other representative symbols to assume the role of another, e.g., a mother, teacher or doctor, while verbalization need not require props or motor functions to role-play (Barton & Wolery, 2008; Barton et al., 2019). Another randomized trial was able to demonstrate clinically significant improvements in social skills and quality of life among children diagnosed with brain cancer using what most closely aligns with verbalization methods of role play as the primary learning intervention (Barrera et al., 2018). Based in part on this finding, verbalization methods could be better suited for children with severe NDCS who may also have limited physical/motor abilities.

Although the ability to pretend play may not always be within the cognitive capacities of some children, one study comparing free, versus structured or functional forms of pretend play among children on the autism spectrum found significantly higher levels of engagement: "When pretend play is 'encouraged,' 'elicited,' or 'prompted,' individuals with autism benefit from these manipulations" (Jarrold & Conn, 2011) and in turn offers support for using RPGs in the pediatric population of interest to this chapter. Bergen, citing Casby (1997), corroborates that among children with language disabilities, "actual differences in symbolic play abilities appear to be quite small; they have 'a symbolic performance deficit more so than a symbolic competence deficit' (p. 477). That is, their capabilities for using symbolic ideas in play may be similar to children without language disabilities. Because of their language problems, however, they are less able to make their pretense themes and roles explicit in their play" (Bergen, 2002).

Researchers may make several modifications to the RPG system itself, game materials used to facilitate role play, e.g., cards, dice or intended players in order to meet the child's communication style, level of comprehension, modes of expression or maturity commensurate with their specific NDCS. We propose two primary ways to accommodate this neurodiversity. Researchers may adopt a more rigid role-playing structure by simplifying cognitive tasks, or by role playing with peers rather than families or clinicians to reduce power imbalances. True gamification to facilitate role play, e.g., through the use of computers, smart phones, digital graphics, and other media may also be useful modifications to traditional RPGs for children who demonstrate a preference toward technologically mediated social interactions.

We contend that RPGs in general have the ability to pique children's desire for functional forms of play, while simultaneously providing unique windows into their situational and sociocultural consciousness. Here we adopt Vygotsky's rendition of functional play as the theoretical scaffold for role-gamification of HRQoL assessment, and to better meet the therapeutic goals of children living with NDCS, neurodevelopmental and other behavioral disorders:

> ...the mistake of many accepted theories [of play] is their disregard of the child's needs – taken in the broadest sense, from inclinations to interests, as needs of an intellectual nature – or, more briefly, disregard of everything that can come under the category of incentives and motives for action. We often describe a child's development as the development of his intellectual functions, i.e., every child stands before us as a theoretical being who, according to the higher or lower level of his intellectual development, moves from one age period to another. Without a consideration of the child's needs, inclinations, incentives, and motives to act – as research has demonstrated – there will never be any advance from one stage to the next. I think that an analysis of play should start with an examination of these particular aspects. It seems that every advance from one age period to another is connected with an abrupt change in motives and incentives to act. What is of the greatest interest to the infant has almost ceased to interest the toddler. This maturing of new needs and new motives for action is, of course, the dominant factor, especially as it is impossible to ignore the fact that a child satisfies certain needs and incentives in play; and without understanding the special nature of these incentives, we cannot imagine the uniqueness of that type of activity we call play.
>
> (Vygotsky, 1967)

The potential to nuance children's incentives and motives for action that are knowable through RPGs, motivates our proposal to use play as a foray into explorations of their HRQoL. By gamifying HRQoL assessment in this way, we mean to apply gaming elements and user experience principles to redesign the terms of engagement (Deterding, Sicart, Nacke, et al., 2011). Gamification is most often discussed when transforming human-human interactions into human-computer ones. Gamification of behavior change is among the fastest growing applications of game-based techniques in the health and wellness sector. Games that aim to increase physical activity among youth have been especially popular (Johnson, Deterding, Kuhn, et al., 2016; Primack, Carroll, McNamara, et al., 2012). Johnson et al. found in a systematic review of game-based interventions that several randomized controlled trials embedded HRQoL along with other patient-reported indices in game designs (Johnson, Deterding, Kuhn, et al., 2016). No study included in the review, however, reported using games to study HRQoL as a primary, as opposed to secondary, endpoint, suggesting an untapped opportunity to explore gamification of HRQoL assessment, generally, and in a specific pediatric population with whom HRQoL research is comparatively limited (Matza, Swensen, Flood, et al., 2004).

Rules of the game

RPGs may either be person- or technologically mediated; either can be preferable depending on the cognitive abilities and resources of the players involved. For the remainder of this chapter, we focus on the design elements of a face-to-face, card-based RPG, otherwise known as a tabletop role playing game as described by Cover (2010). Tabletop role-playing games, according to Cover, unfold like a "radio drama [where] only the spoken component of a role is acted. Players may not always speak exclusively in-character but act out their role by deciding and describing what actions their characters will take within the rules of the game" (Rilstone, 1994; Tabletop Role Playing Games, 2014).[e] As is customary of other table-top role playing games from which the RPG we propose is inspired (Cover, 2010; NISE Network, 2018), we use physical character cards to assign player roles, establish the terms of the game and facilitate role-play.[f]

Table-top role-playing games typically occur in settings relative to the character profiles featured in the game. Hence, our RPG is meant for the actual clinical setting, a physician's office or hospital room, for example.[g] Players are physically present and may include children at various stages in their cancer management—from active treatment to remission—parents, friends and other family members, treating physicians and allied healthcare providers. All players receive a character card that describes a particular role in the child-parent-clinician triad. The card provides a brief description of the role, e.g., their age, gender as well as their interests, motivations and current HRQoL status. Players assume the identity and role the character card outlines during the role play, which may or may not be identical to the role they identify with in real life. Moreover, character cards are representative of the patient populations of interest. We recommend, for instance, that character cards applicable for gameplay in the global mental health context be geographically, demographically and socioeconomically consistent with empirical trends data by the World Health Organization, UNICEF and others.[h] Frameworks that enable cross-cultural adaption of HRQoL measures (Guillemin, Bombardier, & Beaton, 1993) can be especially useful in this regard to inspire the clinical situations, decision-making norms and character profiles for the RPG that is fit for purpose.

In addition to players, a physical gamemaster is present, e.g., the researcher or other game facilitator who randomly assigns and distributes the character cards, serves as

[e] This differentiates "table-top" role playing games from "live action" role playing games in which the acting is literal.

[f] Cover's volume remains the most comprehensive exploration of tabletop role playing games as a genre separate and unique unto itself in the gaming world. Her attention to the narrative and linguistic structures of tabletop role playing, and their broader implications for the construction of personal narrative is what grounds our proposal to study these narratives as they relate to experiences of HRQoL.

[g] Bolig outlines several conditions that optimize hospital settings as environments conducive to therapeutic forms of play and to our use of RPGs: The theoretical and practical implications of discerning the respective functions of play and attachment, the synergistic relationship between the two, and their respective contributions to mastery often underlies the issues of what are the *necessary* and *sufficient* conditions for play to occur in hospital settings" (Bolig, 1984).

[h] This is the approach developers of Nano Around the World adopted in designing character cards.

the arbiter of interactions between players in the game and determines when gameplay concludes. The gamemaster introduces a goal for players to achieve during the course of the RPG session based on a set of rules collectively referred to as the game system (Tabletop Role Playing Games, 2014). Once the gamemaster assigns character cards by random distribution, players share with each other the roles they are assuming in the game. Next, the gamemaster describes a clinical decision-making scenario that requires consensus from all players, a process commonly referred to as the campaign (Tabletop Role Playing Games, 2014). The scenarios provided typify actual clinical situations in which patients and families together are determining trajectories of care, in our case children living with NDCS, neurodevelopmental or other behavioral disorders. Examples of clinical scenarios in this context may involve decisions to explore treatment options that may have equivalent clinical efficacy yet different side effects with implications for quality of life; to enroll in a clinical trial that potentiates improved therapeutic benefit; or to undergo an invasive surgical procedure to hopefully improve some aspect of neurocognitive function. The game system in the RPG we propose is based on common communicative exchanges needed to reach consensus on the trajectory of care as described to us during deliberative consultations with oncologists and palliative care clinicians and where optimal HRQoL was the primary goal for terminally ill children with brain cancer.

Each player's goal is to launch a successful campaign in support of the HRQoL intervention that best meets the values, interests and priorities of their character. Players launch campaigns to optimize HRQoL in our RPG through discussion, negotiation and consensus-building in partnership with other players in the game. Over several rounds of gameplay, players advocate for their character, co-establish notions of best interests with other decision-makers, and negotiate HRQoL trade-offs between competing clinical decisions in the neurodevelopmental/behavioral context. Indeed, it is "negotiation in the [tabletop]RPG that allows for gameplay that meets a variety of interests. The TRPG as a generic form gives players agency to define the form of their game, the social interaction and the narrative that results. Whether or not the players take full advantage of this agency depends on the group. However, it is arguable that the feeling of narrative agency remains in the players' minds, even when not fully realized in action. The purpose of the TRPG is to, as a communicative act, is to foster the sense of agency over narrative" (Cover, 2010).

It is important to note that at no point in the RPG does the gamemaster cue players on how they should enact their specific roles. Likewise, player dispositions at the time of the role play necessarily direct the decisional outcomes. These game-based experiences are indeed methodological strengths because both player enactments and their HRQoL decisions should emerge inductively from the players alone absent undue influence from the gamemaster. It may therefore be relevant for the researcher to establish the child's baseline HRQoL using the instrument or approach that best aligns with the research or clinical objective the RPG is meant to supplement. A player's prior experiences and current feelings no doubt influence how they portray roles during gameplay, as well as the decisions players believe the agent they are personifying would make. It is important to note the game's outcome has no bearing on any clinical decisions facing any of the players in the immediate term. Indeed, the fictional details of the scenario and characters are what establish safe spaces for disclosure through narrative. The RPG's fictionality thereby assuages concern that a player's disposition may inappropriately skew a relevant clinical decision either positively or negatively.

In our experience piloting the game among clinicians and researchers, game sessions may last anywhere between 10 and 30 min. The session length depends foremost on the professional background of players, the familiarity of players with the clinical scenario presented, and the initial degree of consensus or conflict in opening rounds of the game. The gamemaster can analyze myriad HRQoL themes during gameplay, such as the decisional outcome—which may differ from round to round and player to player—and the content of the discussions—via transcribing game sessions with audio visual recording.

Character cards may also be more picture-based. Graphically representing potential HRQoL interventions can facilitate participation among children with whom verbal communication is difficult. The narrative content of discussions during gameplay, such as points of agreement or conflict, as well as the ways in which players interact with each other are both analytical outputs the researcher may subsequently use as sources of qualitative data. Reaching consensus on a final decision on the trajectory of care is the primary objective of the game, but need not be the most meaningful element of gameplay as we discuss further below.

Game mechanics aside, RPGs can provide children with temporal, spatial and expressive latitude to discuss HRQoL in intimate settings and with those who are directly involved in shaping it. RPGs can serve as windows into ideal HRQoL that children living with NDCS envision and indirectly communicate through advocating on behalf of their character during the course of gameplay. As one study found, role-playing was highly effective in soliciting the views of children with behavioral challenges related to learning disability on emotional wellbeing (Hill, Laybourn, & Borland, 1996). The researchers in the aforementioned study noted how RPGs forced clinical decision makers to critically engage with the HRQoL realities children constructed indirectly through their role play enactments. Such transparent disclosure of the character's preferences, values and motives—likely inspired by the child's own preferences, values and motives—results in rich, child-centric accounts of HRQoL seldom achieved in proxy-reported, or other qualitative research approaches. Transparency on otherwise sensitive topics such as death and dying, is also the cornerstone of shared-decision making that RPGs could potentially augment.

Limitations

Several practical and methodological factors can limit the use of RPGs in many pediatric neuropsychiatric settings. Integrating RPGs in global neuroethics contexts can be especially challenged where the continuity of health professionals, working equipment, health care compliance and literacy limit opportunities for meaningful engagement among patient-parent-clinician decision makers. Although card-based and other tabletop role-playing games are not resource-intensive, time may be a particularly limiting factor. This is especially true in large community hospital settings, where doctor-patient ratios make prolonged patient engagement unfeasible as needed for gameplay. One potential solution may be to incorporate short game sessions into already scheduled family meetings to discuss the child's case. These meetings can be planned around critical moments/decisions in the child's trajectory of care if they are hospitalized, or as part of routine follow up or medical rounds as an outpatient as appropriate. Meaningfulness and relevance of game-playing may also be prohibitive due to the severity of the child's condition and limited health system resources to deliver on the HRQoL interventions children may identify, if at all, during gameplay (Lipstein, Lindly, Anixt, et al., 2016). While not unique to RPGs, barriers to meaningful gameplay in global mental health environments that fulfill some or all of the data collection goals outlined earlier include poor social determinants of health. Household income, education and ethnicity are strong predictors of communication efficacy and health literacy upon which the greatest utility of RPGs for assessing HRQoL related to NDCS or other mental health conditions in LMIC depend (Smalley, Kenney, Denboba, et al., 2014; Von Rueden, Gosch, Rajmil, et al., 2006).

Critics also question the authenticity of RPG simulations based on the extent to which they reflect actual communicative events in real decision-making contexts. While we accept this critique, what warrants greater appreciation is the process by which parents and clinical teams critically engage with the alternative HRQoL realities children may conceive under the structured conditions set out in the game, rather than the decisional outcome per se. Our hope is that with consistent use of functional forms of play in clinical decision-making settings, that new normative structures, processes and skillsets for community with children on how to optimize HRQoL can then be transferable to other clinical decision contexts.

Conclusion

We elaborate in this chapter on some of the theoretical and practical underpinnings of play and their relevance to gamifying elements of HRQoL assessment in children living with NDCS. In particular, we propose role-playing as new research tool for neuroethics that can open a window into the ways children learn, self-discover and advocate for optimum HRQoL. We argue the illness narratives that unfold during gameplay affords all players—but especially children—a safe space to (i) nuance combined existential and practical features of HRQoL; (ii) better understand how stakeholders in the child-parent-clinician triad perceive their respective roles in optimizing HRQoL; and (iii) encourage collaborative problem-solving and shared decision making around HRQoL "where the disease complexity, treatment options and varying levels of evidence make [shared decision making] highly necessary" (Lipstein et al., 2016).

RPGs as a methodological tool furthermore act on rights-based protections afforded to all children as outlined in international conventions, but infrequently benefit from. As such, RPGs double as methodologically rigorous sources of empirical data on children's perceptions of HRQoL and as platforms for shared decision-making. Our application of RPGs in the pediatric neuroethics arena can achieve the latter by dismantling hierarchal decision-making coalitions most often struck between parents and clinicians, yet less so between child and clinicians. We have observed this phenomenon in pilot phases of RPG development when clinicians are asked to assume the role of the child, and when children assume a role with more formal decision- authority such as the parent or clinician.

We appreciate that neurocognitive disorders associated with brain cancer are not necessarily neuropsychiatric, although considerable overlap exists. We use brain cancer as the test case, given the stage of development of an RPG for it. We are optimistic for the translational future of RPGs to yet more layered and complex aspects of mental health disorders, and in more resource-diverse contexts globally. Our proposal to treat RPGs as new class of participatory, game-based research methods is consistent with children's rights to be included and meaningfully engaged in civic life. Optimizing HRQoL is indeed subsumed under this participatory right and codified in international human rights conventions, research ethics guidelines and philosophical notions of self/agency that underpin the field of neuroethics (Shook & Giordano, 2014). Given the diagnostic and prognostic complexities of NDCS, RPGs transfix sensitive topics into discussable rhetorical units that may include how to overcome challenges with activities of daily living, care provider burden, or pharmacological and technological choices with uncertain clinical efficacy, among others. For mental health applications in the future, and on a global scale, stigma, acceptance, culture and values can all be included and tested in line with evolving principles of international neuroethics (Shook & Giordano, 2014).

As we discuss in this chapter, RPGs can result in two mutually beneficial outcomes for players as well as the state of knowledge on HRQoL in children living with NDCS: they provide creative, adjunctive information tools for clinicians to gain insight into oft-ignored dimensions of HRQoL, and enable HRQoL researchers to study many iterations of patient/child shared decision-making in real time. The latter is useful in the future development of clinical decision aids that embed shared decision-making and prioritization of HRQoL endpoints into the tool itself.[i] Rigorous data collection and analysis of gameplay sessions from myriad contexts—involving patients with varying condition severities, and across different health systems—are needed to develop and subsequently certify a clinical decision aid based on the RPG.

The benefits as well as limitations of gamifying HRQoL assessment can be transferable across clinical settings and populations. A review by Naslund et al. on m-health interventions highlights the distinct emphasis the global mental health literature places on technological scalability, especially where technologies have shown considerable therapeutic promise in under resourced settings (Naslund, Marsch, McHugo, et al., 2015). Consistent with this literature, RPGs qualify as a "technology" in both their table-top and virtual forms. Such versatility makes scaling HRQoL assessments that use RPGs adaptable to existing resources, places and populations. Table-top RPGs can

---

[i] Based on a national study of children with special health needs, Fiks et al. recommend development of clinical decision aids to promote improved communication and parent-patient-physician partnerships in caring for children with developmental and behavioral disorders. Qualitative, quantitative and mixed methods research data derived from iterations of gameplay can serve as evidence-bases upon which such decision aids can develop.

be ideal for settings where mobile devices or internet connectivity may be ubiquitous but access limited, while virtual RPGs can be adopted in settings where such resources are both readily available and widely accessible.

We anticipate that systematic data collection and analysis from game sessions across different resource and health system contexts will identify ways of improving the game to successfully overcome time and resources limitations. The cross-specialty and, more important, cross disciplinarity inherent to game-based research design and practice make the application of RPGs as it unfolds a truly integrative approach to engagement that has potential for empirical rigor, can be clinically meaningful and ethically defensible.

References

Armstrong, D. (2009). Stabilising the construct of health related quality of life: 1970–2007. *Science Studies (St Bonaventure)*, *22*, 102–115.

Bao, P., Zheng, Y., Wang, C., et al. (2009). Time trends and characteristics of childhood cancer among children age 0–14 in Shanghai. *Pediatric Blood & Cancer*, *53*, 13–16. https://doi.org/10.1002/pbc.

Barakat, L. P., Hobbie, W., Minturn, J., et al. (2017). Survivors of childhood brain tumors and their caregivers: Transition to adulthood. *Developmental Medicine and Child Neurology*, *59*, 779–780. https://doi.org/10.1111/dmcn.13492.

Barrera, M., Atenafu, E. G., Sung, L., et al. (2018). A randomized control intervention trial to improve social skills and quality of life in pediatric brain tumor survivors. *Psychooncology*, *27*, 91–98. https://doi.org/10.1002/pon.4385.

Barton, E. E., & Wolery, M. (2008). Teaching pretend play to children: A review of the literature. *Topics in Early Childhood Special Education*, *28*, 109–125.

Barton, E. E., Choi, G., & Mauldin, E. G. (2019). Teaching sequences of pretend play to children with disabilities. *Journal of Early Intervention*, *41*(1), 13–29. https://doi.org/10.1177/1053815118799466.

Bastos, L. N. V., Silveira, J. C., Luna, C. F., et al. (2017). Childhood and adolescent cancer in the State of Pernambuco, Brazil. *Journal of Pediatric Hematology/Oncology*, *40*, 1. https://doi.org/10.1097/MPH.0000000000001017.

Bergen, D. (2002). The role of pretend play in children's cognitive development. *Early Childhood Research and Practice*, *4*, 1–13.

Bhat, S. R., Goodwin, T. L., Burwinkle, T. M., et al. (2005). Profile of daily life in children with brain tumors: An assessment of health-related quality of life. *Journal of Clinical Oncology*, *23*, 5493–5500. https://doi.org/10.1200/JCO.2005.10.190.

Bjornson, K. F., & McLaughlin, J. F. (2001). The measurement of health-related quality of life (HRQL) in children with cerebral palsy. *European Journal of Neurology*, *8*(Suppl 5), 183–193. https://doi.org/10.1046/j.1468-1331.2001.00051.x.

Bluebond-Langner, M. (1978). *The private worlds of dying children*. Princeton, NJ: Princeton University Press.

Bolig, R. (1984). Play in hospital settings. In T. D. Yawkey & A. D. Pellegrini (Eds.), *Child's play: Developmental and applied*. London: Routledge.

Bowman, S. L. (2010). *The functions of role-playing games: How participants create community, solve problems and explore identity*. Jefferson, NC: McFarland.

Buchbinder, D. K., Fortier, M. A., Osann, K., Wilford, J., Shen, V., Torno, L., et al. (2017). Quality of life among parents of adolescent and young adult brain tumor survivors. *Journal of Pediatric Hematology/Oncology, 39*, 579–584. https://doi.org/10.1097/MPH.0000000000000947.

Corsini, R. (2017). *Role playing in psychotherapy*. Routledge. https://doi.org/10.4324/9781351307208.

Cover, J. G. (2010). *The creation of narrative in tabletop role-playing games*. McFarland & Co. Publishers.

Cremeens, J., Eiser, C., & Blades, M. (2014). Factors influencing agreement between child self-report and parent proxy-reports on the pediatric quality of life inventory 4.0 (PedsQL) generic core scales. *Health and Quality of Life Outcomes, 4*, 58. https://doi.org/10.1186/1477-7525-4-58.

De Robles, P., Fiest, K. M., Frolkis, A. D., et al. (2015). The worldwide incidence and prevalence of primary brain tumors: A systematic review and meta-analysis. *Neuro-Oncology, 17*, 776–783. https://doi.org/10.1093/neuonc/nou283.

de Ruiter, M. A., Schouten-van Meeteren, A. Y. N., van Vuurden, D. G., et al. (2016). Psychosocial profile of pediatric brain tumor survivors with neurocognitive complaints. *Quality of Life Research, 25*, 435–446. https://doi.org/10.1007/s11136-015-1091-7.

Demers, C., Gélinas, I., & Carret, A. S. (2016). Activities of daily living and quality of life in survivors of childhood brain tumour. *American Journal of Occupational Therapy, 70*, 7001220040p1–7001220040p8. https://doi.org/10.5014/ajot.2016.014993.

Deterding, S., Sicart, M., Nacke, L., et al. (2011). Gamification. Using game-design elements in non-gaming contexts. In *Dl.Acm.Org.* (pp. 4–7). https://doi.org/10.1145/1979742.1979575.

Devine, K. A., Mertens, A. C., Whitton, J. A., et al. (2018). Factors associated with physical activity among adolescent and young adult survivors of early childhood cancer: A report from the childhood cancer survivor study (CCSS). *Psychooncology, 27*, 613–619. https://doi.org/10.1002/pon.4528.

Drotar, D. (1998). *Measuring health-related quality of life in children and adolescents: Implications for research and practice*. Mahwah, NJ: Lawrence Erlbaum Associates.

Dufetelle, E., 't Jong, G. W., & Kaguelidou, F. (2018). Randomized controlled trials in pediatric patients had higher completion rates than adult trials: A cross-sectional study. *Journal of Clinical Epidemiology, 100*, 53–60. https://doi.org/10.1016/j.jclinepi.2018.04.018.

Engelen, V. (2011). Monitoring quality of life in paediatric oncology practice. Doctoral Dissertation. University of Amsterdam.

European Quality of Life Group. 2009. EQ-5D, https://euroqol.org/eq-5d-instruments/.

Ezzat, S., Kamal, M., El-Khateeb, N., et al. (2016). Pediatric brain tumors in a low/middle income country: Does it differ from that in developed world? *Journal of Neuro-Oncology, 126*, 371–376. https://doi.org/10.1007/s11060-015-1979-7.

Feigin, V. L., Abajobir, A. A., Abate, K. H., et al. (2017). Global, regional, and national burden of neurological disorders during 1990–2015: A systematic analysis for the global burden of disease study 2015. *Lancet Neurology, 16*, 877–897. https://doi.org/10.1016/S1474-4422(17)30299-5.

Feinstein, J., Morrato, E. H., & Feudtner, C. (2017). Prioritizing pediatric drug research using population-level health data. *JAMA Pediatrics, 171*, 7–8. https://doi.org/10.1001/jamapediatrics.2016.3462.

Fitzmaurice, C., Allen, C., Barber, R. M., et al. (2017). Global, regional, and national cancer incidence, mortality, years of life lost, years lived with disability, and disability-adjusted life-years for 32 cancer groups, 1990 to 2015: A systematic analysis for the global burden of disease study global burden. *JAMA Oncology, 3*, 524–548. https://doi.org/10.1001/jamaoncol.2016.5688.

Forrest, C. B., Margolis, P., Seid, M., et al. (2014). PEDSnet: How a prototype pediatric learning health system is being expanded into a national network. *Health Affairs, 33*, 1171–1177. https://doi.org/10.1377/hlthaff.2014.0127.

Frazier, A. L., Piñeros, M., Fuentes, S., et al. (2017). The global burden of childhood cancer: Knowing what we do not know. *Pediatric Blood & Cancer, 64*, 64–66. https://doi.org/10.1002/pbc.26532.

Glaser, B. G., & Strauss, A. L. (1965). *Awareness of dying*. London, UK: Transaction Publishers.

Goudie, C., Coltin, H., Witkowski, L., et al. (2017). The McGill interactive pediatric OncoGenetic guidelines: An approach to identifying pediatric oncology patients most likely to benefit from a genetic evaluation. *Pediatric Blood & Cancer, 64*, 1–5. https://doi.org/10.1002/pbc.26441.

Guillemin, F., Bombardier, C., & Beaton, D. (1993). Cross-cultural adaptation of health-related quality of life measures: Literature review and proposed guidelines. *Journal of Clinical Epidemiology, 46*, 1417–14–32.

Hassan, H., Pinches, A., Picton, S. V., et al. (2017). Survival rates and prognostic predictors of high grade brain stem gliomas in childhood: A systematic review and meta-analysis. *Journal of Neuro-Oncology, 135*, 13–20. https://doi.org/10.1007/s11060-017-2546-1.

Healthy People 2020. (2019). Health-related quality of life and well-being. In *Found Heal Meas Rep 2010*. (pp. 1–6). https://doi.org/10.1016/j.soncn.2009.11.008.

Hill, M., Laybourn, A., & Borland, M. (1996). Engaging with primary school aged children about emotions and wellbeing-methodological considerations. *Children and Society, 10*, 129–144.

Hobbie, W. L., Ogle, S., Reilly, M., et al. (2016). Adolescent and young adult survivors of childhood brain tumors: Life after treatment in their own words. *Cancer Nursing, 39*, 134–143. https://doi.org/10.1097/NCC.0000000000000266.

Hocking, M. C., Hobbie, W. L., Deatrick, J. A., et al. (2011). Neurocognitive and family functioning and quality of life among young adult survivors of childhood brain tumors. *The Clinical Neuropsychologist, 25*, 942–962. https://doi.org/10.1080/13854046.2011.580284.

Howard, S. C., Davidson, A., Luna-Fineman, S., et al. (2017). A framework to develop adapted treatment regimens to manage pediatric cancer in low- and middle-income countries: The Pediatric Oncology in Developing Countries (PODC) Committee of the International Pediatric Oncology Society (SIOP). *Pediatric Blood & Cancer, 64*, 1–18. https://doi.org/10.1002/pbc.26879.

Institute of Medicine (US), Roundtable on Evidence-Based Medicine. In L. A. Olsen, D. Aisner, & J. M. McGinnis (Eds.), *The learning healthcare system: Workshop summary* (2007). Washington, DC: National Academies Press (US). Available from: https://www.ncbi.nlm.nih.gov/books/NBK53494/, https://doi.org/10.17226/11903.

Jarrold, C., & Conn, C. (2011). The development of pretend play in autism. In P. Nathan & A. D. Pellegrini (Eds.), *The oxford handbook of the development of play*. London, UK: Oxford University Press.

Johnson, D., Deterding, S., Kuhn, K. A., et al. (2016). Gamification for health and wellbeing: A systematic review of the literature. *Internet Interventions, 6*, 89–106. https://doi.org/10.1016/j.invent.2016.10.002.

Johnson, J. E. (2007). *Commentary: Play, literacy and theories of instruction*. In K. Roskos (Ed.), *Play and literacy in early childhood research from multiple perspectives*. (pp. 133–148).

Kenborg, L., Winther, J. F., Linnet, K. M., et al. (2018). Neurologic disorders in 4858 survivors of central nervous system tumors in childhood—An adult life after childhood Cancer in Scandinavia (ALiCCS) study. *Neuro-Oncology, 1*(12), https://doi.org/10.1093/neuonc/noy094.

Landreth, G. L. (2012). *Play therapy: The art f the relationship. 3rd Editio.* New York: Routledge.

Lazor, T., Tigelaar, L., Pole, J. D., et al. (2017). Instruments to measure anxiety in children, adolescents, and young adults with cancer: A systematic review. *Support Care Cancer, 25,* 2921–2931. https://doi.org/10.1007/s00520-017-3743-3.

Leahy, A. B., Feudtner, C., & Basch, E. (2018). Symptom monitoring in pediatric oncology using patient-reported outcomes: Why, how, and where next. *Patient, 11,* 147–153. https://doi.org/10.1007/s40271-017-0279-z.

Lipstein, E. A., Lindly, O. J., Anixt, J. S., et al. (2016). Shared decision making in the care of children with developmental and behavioral disorders. *Maternal and Child Health Journal, 20,* 665–673. https://doi.org/10.1016/j.bbi.2015.08.015.Chronic.

Macartney, G., Harrison, M. B., VanDenKerkhof, E., et al. (2014). Quality of life and symptoms in pediatric brain tumor survivors: A systematic review. *Journal of Pediatric Oncology Nursing, 31,* 65–77. https://doi.org/10.1177/1043454213520191.

Matza, L. S., Swensen, A. R., Flood, E. M., et al. (2004). Assessment of health-related quality of life in children: A review of conceptual, methodological, and regulatory issues. *Value Heal, 7,* 79–92. https://doi.org/10.1111/j.1524-4733.2004.71273.x.

Medical Research Council. (2004). *Medical research involving children. MRC Ethics Guide* (p. 49).

Meeske, K., Katz, E. R., Palmer, S. N., et al. (2004). Parent proxy-reported health-related quality of life and fatigue in pediatric patients diagnosed with brain tumors and acute lymphoblastic leukemia. *Cancer, 101,* 2116–2125. https://doi.org/10.1002/cncr.20609.

Morrow, A. M., Hayen, A., Quine, S., et al. (2012). A comparison of doctors', parents' and children's reports of health states and health-related quality of life in children with chronic conditions. *Child: Care, Health and Development, 38,* 186–195. https://doi.org/10.1111/j.1365-2214.2011.01240.x.

Naslund, J. A., Marsch, L. A., McHugo, G. J., et al. (2015). Emerging mHealth and eHealth interventions for serious mental illness: A review of the literature. *Journal of Mental Health, 24,* 320–331. https://doi.org/10.3109/09638237.2015.1019054.

NISE Network. (2018). *Nano Around the World card game | NISE Network.* http://www.nisenet.org/catalog/nano-around-world-card-game (Accessed July 25, 2018).

Park, E. S., & Cho, I. Y. (2017). Shared decision-making in the paediatric field: A literature review and concept analysis. *Scandinavian Journal of Caring Sciences,* 478–489. https://doi.org/10.1111/scs.12496.

Paxton, R.J.J.L.W.R.P.M.B.M.J.L.D.-W.W. (2010). Associations between leisure-time physical activity and health-related quality of life among adolescent and adult survivors of childhood cancers. *Psychooncology, 19,* 997–1003. https://doi.org/10.1002/pon.1654.

Penn, A., Shortman, R. I., Lowis, S. P., et al. (2010). Child-related determinants of health-related quality of life in children with brain tumours 1 year after diagnosis. *Pediatric Blood & Cancer, 55,* 1377–1385. https://doi.org/10.1002/pbc.

Phillips, S. M., Padgett, L. S., Leisenring, W. M., et al. (2015). Survivors of childhood cancer in the United States: Prevalence and burden of morbidity. *Cancer Epidemiology, Biomarkers & Prevention, 24,* 653–663. https://doi.org/10.1158/1055-9965.EPI-14-1418.

Primack, B. A., Carroll, M. V., McNamara, M., et al. (2012). Role of video games in improving health-related outcomes. A systematic review. *American Journal of Preventive Medicine, 42,* 630–638. https://doi.org/10.1016/j.amepre.2012.02.023.

Pui, C., Gajjar, A. J., Kane, J. R., et al. (2012). *Challenging issues in pediatric oncology. Vol. 8.* (pp. 540–549). https://doi.org/10.1038/nrclinonc.2011.95.Challenging.

Quast, L. F., Phillips, P. C., Li, Y., et al. (2018). A prospective study of family predictors of health-related quality of life in pediatric brain tumor survivors. *Pediatric Blood & Cancer,* e26976. https://doi.org/10.1002/pbc.26976.

Rilstone, A. (1994). *Role-playing games: An overview. RPGnet.* http://www.rpg.net/oracle/essays/rpgoverview.html (Accessed July 25, 2018).

Sato, I., Higuchi, A., Yanagisawa, T., et al. (2014). Impact of late effects on health-related quality of life in survivors of pediatric brain tumors. *Cancer Nursing, 37*, E1–14. https://doi.org/10.1097/NCC.0000000000000110.

Sattoe, J. N. T., van Staa, A., & Moll, H. A. (2012). The proxy problem anatomized: Child-parent disagreement in health related quality of life reports of chronically ill adolescents. *Health and Quality of Life Outcomes, 10*, 10. https://doi.org/10.1186/1477-7525-10-10.

Schulte, F., Russell, K. B., Cullen, P., et al. (2017). Systematic review and meta-analysis of health-related quality of life in pediatric CNS tumor survivors. *Pediatric Blood & Cancer, 64*, e26442. https://doi.org/10.1002/pbc.26442.

Shook, J. R., & Giordano, J. (2014). A principled and cosmopolitan neuroethics: Considerations for international relevance. *Philosophy, Ethics, and Humanities in Medicine, 9*, 1–13. https://doi.org/10.1186/1747-5341-9-1.

Simmons, B. (2014). *The PMLD ambiguity: Articulating the life-worlds of children with profound and multiple learning disabilities* (1st ed.). London: Routledge.

Smalley, L. P., Kenney, M. K., Denboba, D., et al. (2014). Family perceptions of shared decision-making with health care providers: Results of the national survey of children with special health care needs, 2009-2010. *Maternal and Child Health Journal, 18*, 1316–1327. https://doi.org/10.1007/s10995-013-1365-z.

Solans, M., Pane, S., Estrada, M. D., et al. (2008). Health-related quality of life measurement in children and adolescents: A systematic review of generic and disease-specific instruments. *Value Heal, 11*, 742–764. https://doi.org/10.1111/j.1524-4733.2007.00293.x.

Stiggelbout, A. M., Van Der Weijden, T., De Wit, M. P. T., et al. (2012). Shared decision making: Really putting patients at the centre of healthcare. *BMJ, 344*, 1–6. https://doi.org/10.1136/bmj.e256.

Stone, J., Waern, S., Khabra, K., et al. (2017). Impact of toxicities and neurocognitive impairment on the health related quality of life (HR-QoL) for survivors of medulloblastoma. *European Journal of Cancer, 72*, S171. https://doi.org/10.1016/S0959-8049(17)30631-7.

Storm, H., Engholm, G., Mägi, M., et al. (2017). Geographical variability in survival of European children with central nervous system tumours. *European Journal of Cancer, 82*, 137–148. https://doi.org/10.1016/j.ejca.2017.05.028.

Surun, A., Dujaric, M.É., Aerts, I., et al. (2018). Enrollment in early-phase clinical trials in pediatric oncology: The experience at Institut Curie. *Pediatric Blood & Cancer, 65*, 1–7. https://doi.org/10.1002/pbc.26916.

Tabletop Role Playing Games. (2014). *Wikipedia.*

Theunissen, N., Vogels, T., Koopman, H., et al. (2014). The proxy problem: Child report versus parent report in health-related quality of life research. *Quality of Life Research, 7*, 387–397.

Tock, T. I., Bhat, S., Szymonifka, J., et al. (2014). Quality of life outcomes in proton and photon treated pediatric brain tumor survivors. *Radiotherapy and Oncology, 113*, 89–94. https://doi.org/10.1016/j.radonc.2014.08.017.

Tomlinson, D., Zupanec, S., Jones, H., et al. (2016). The lived experience of fatigue in children and adolescents with cancer: A systematic review. *Support Care Cancer, 24*, 3623–3631. https://doi.org/10.1007/s00520-016-3253-8.

Vannatta, K., Gerhardt, C. A., Wells, R. J., et al. (2007). Intensity of CNS treatment for pediatric Cancer: Prediction of social outcomes in survivors. *Pediatric Blood & Cancer, 49*, 716–722. https://doi.org/10.1002/pbc.

Varni, J. W., Burwinkle, T. M., Sherman, S. A., et al. (2005). Health-related quality of life of children and adolescents with cerebral palsy: Hearing the voices of the children. *Developmental Medicine and Child Neurology, 47*, 592–597.

Varni, J. W., Limbers, C., & Burwinkle, T. M. (2007a). Literature review: Health-related quality of life measurement in pediatric oncology: Hearing the voices of the children. *Journal of Pediatric Psychology, 32*, 1151–1163. https://doi.org/10.1093/jpepsy/jsm008.

Varni, J. W., & Limbers, C. A. (2009). The pediatric quality of life inventory: Measuring pediatric health-related quality of life from the perspective of children and their parents. *Pediatric Clinics of North America, 56*, 843–863. https://doi.org/10.1016/j.pcl.2009.05.016.

Varni, J. W., Limbers, C. A., & Burwinkle, T. M. (2007b). Parent proxy-report of their children's health-related quality of life: An analysis of 13,878 parents' reliability and validity across age subgroups using the PedsQL??? 4.0 Generic Core Scales. *Health and Quality of Life Outcomes, 5*, 1–10. https://doi.org/10.1186/1477-7525-5-2.

Von Rueden, U., Gosch, A., Rajmil, L., et al. (2006). Socioeconomic determinants of health related quality of life in childhood and adolescence: Results from a European study. *Journal of Epidemiology and Community Health, 60*, 130–135. https://doi.org/10.1136/jech.2005.039792.

Vygotsky, L. S. (1967). Play and its role in the mental development of the child. *Soviet Psychology, 5*(3), 6–18. https://doi.org/10.2753/RPO1061-040505036.

Wolf, S. M., Amendola, L. M., Berg, J. S., et al. (2018). Navigating the research-clinical interface in genomic medicine: Analysis from the CSER consortium. *Genetics in Medicine, 20*, 545–553. https://doi.org/10.1038/gim.2017.137.

Wolfe, J., Orellana, L., Ullrich, C., et al. (2015). Symptoms and distress in children with advanced cancer: Prospective patient-reported outcomes from the PediQUEST study. *Journal of Clinical Oncology, 33*, 1928–1935. https://doi.org/10.1200/JCO.2014.59.1222.

Wong, C., Odom, S. L., Hume, K. A., et al. (2015). Evidence-based practices for children, youth, and young adults with autism spectrum disorder: A comprehensive review. *Journal of Autism and Developmental Disorders, 45*, 1951–1966. https://doi.org/10.1007/s10803-014-2351-z.

Neuroethics and cannabis use globally: Impact on adolescent cognition and wellbeing

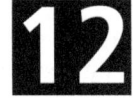

Ayla Selamoglu, Alicja Malinowska, George Savulich, Barbara J. Sahakian
Department of Psychiatry, University of Cambridge, School of Clinical Medicine and
the Behavioural and Clinical Neuroscience Institute, Cambridge, United Kingdom

Introduction

In recent years neuroethical issues surrounding neuroscience, human behavior and drug dependency have become of great social importance (Carter, Hall, & Illes, 2012). The term "neuroethics" was described as "the study of the ethical, legal and social questions that arise when scientific findings about the brain are carried into medical practice, legal interpretations and health and social policy" (Marcus, 2002) and relates to a broad range of ethical, legal and social matters due to the vast developments in neuroscience and medicine (Farah, 2012). Neuroethics also raises issues for children and adolescents as many youths are experimenting with various drugs, including substances such as cannabis which can take the form of dependency in severe cases, so warranting a need to further explore the field of neuroethics (Sahakian et al., 2015; Sahakian & Morein-Zamir, 2015). We examine the neuroethical issues associated with the use of cannabis amongst adolescents, the legalization and use of medical cannabis, and the impact cannabis has on brain development, cognition, academic achievement, wellbeing and psychiatric conditions. We will further discuss the motivations for use, socio-economic status, and the global burden of disease (GBD) associated with cannabis use.

Cannabis use disorder and free will

Cannabis use disorder (CUD) was defined as a problematic pattern of cannabis use leading to clinically significant impairment or distress with meeting at least two of the diagnostic criteria occurring within a 12-month period (American Psychiatric Association, 2013). The diagnostic criteria include: using cannabis in larger amounts and longer than initially intended, unsuccessful attempts to control cannabis use, craving to use cannabis, spending a great deal of time on activities connected to using cannabis, neglecting major areas of one's life (e.g., work, school, home responsibilities), increased tolerance, and withdrawal symptoms (American Psychiatric Association, 2013). It was estimated that 9% of cannabis users transitioned from cannabis abuse to dependence, therefore the majority of users do not develop cannabis dependency

Global Mental Health and Neuroethics. https://doi.org/10.1016/B978-0-12-815063-4.00012-5

(Florez-Salmanca et al., 2013; Lopez-Quintero & Cobos, 2011). However, some groups might be more prone to transition to dependency, for example individuals with comorbid mental illness are considered at higher risk for developing cannabis dependence (Danovitch & Gorelick, 2012). Therefore, given that cannabis is being decriminalized in certain countries, the question arises: what is the valid threshold to deem cannabis harmful for the general population and is the 9% dependence acceptable? Cannabis has long been used in medicine and its therapeutic benefits have been reported dating back to the 1890s (Reynolds, 1890). Despite this, cannabis was listed on the Schedule I of the United Nations convention in 1961 on the basis that it was deemed detrimental and having no medical use (Nutt, King, & Nichols, 2013). Since then it has remained a Schedule I drug in the United States and a Class B drug in the United Kingdom despite emerging scientific evidence of its clinical benefits (Nutt et al., 2013). Although cannabis is linked to causing harm, such as impaired cognition, overall it is less harmful than some other popular drugs and intoxicants, such as alcohol (Weissenborn & Nutt, 2012).

As cannabis use does result in dependency in some individuals, this raises questions on autonomous choice or "free will" which has long been debated in the context of addiction (Racine, Nguyen, Saigle, & Dubljevic, 2017). The fundamental argument is that dependency may compromise an individuals' ability to make good quality decisions between several courses of action, and if the behavior is considered habitual or compulsive then the individual is said to no longer exercise free will (Racine, Sattler, & Escande, 2017). For example, in cocaine-dependent individuals failure of goal-directed behavior in favor of habitual behavior has been demonstrated (Ersche et al., 2016). The results of a meta-analysis researching the link between addictive behavior and delayed reward discounting, which is a measure of impulsive decision making, suggest that addiction of various substances may be related to smaller but immediate rewards preference over larger, delayed rewards (MacKillop et al., 2011). In this context, dependency can be understood as a brain disorder, and supporters of this model suggest that substance use hijacks brain mechanisms of voluntary control and therefore individuals are unable to make rational decisions (Buchman, Skinner, & Illes, 2010). Understanding dependency as a brain disorder, rather than solely understanding it as an issue caused by an individual's lifestyle choice, impacts the views on free will, self-control and responsibility, which contribute to the stigmatization of individuals with a substance dependency (Racine, Bell, Zizzo, & Green, 2015) (see also Chapter 9). Overall, many studies report a relationship between impaired decision-making and marijuana use, however the causality is unclear and some studies suggest that impaired decision-making can be a risk factor for cannabis dependency (Gonzalez, Schuster, Mermelstein, et al., 2015; Wesley, Hanlon, & Porrino, 2011).

Prevalence and legalization of cannabis

Cannabis is one of the most widely used substances in the world, and is known to be a popular recreational drug after alcohol and tobacco (Murray, Morrison, Henquet, & Di Forti, 2007). The issue of legality changes rapidly and, as it currently stands, cannabis use is fully legalized in Canada and Uruguay and personal use has been decriminalized in Spain, Portugal, Switzerland, Solomon Islands, Norway, and The Netherlands (Robertson, 2018). For medicinal purposes cannabis use has been legalized in over 30 countries, including Australia, Denmark, Finland, Germany, Israel, Italy, The Netherlands, Sri Lanka, Turkey, and Uruguay (Robertson, 2018). The United States of America (USA) has legalized cannabis for recreational use in 10 states, including Alaska, California, Colorado, Maine, Massachusetts, Nevada, Oregon, Vermont and Washington (Robertson, 2018; Robinson & Berke, 2018). In the United Kingdom (UK) cannabis remains an illegal class B drug for both recreational and most medical use, where possession, cultivation, distribution, and sale of cannabis can result in fines or imprisonment (Harrison, 2018; UK Government, 2018). Only very recently the UK government announced its approval for a cannabis derived medicine which patients may obtain by prescription only from their GP since Autumn 2018 (Osborne, 2018). It is possible that many other countries will follow and continue to legalize cannabis use based on neuroethical arguments, such as individuals receiving a criminal record even if use only occurred once (Hall & Weier, 2015). Another important argument is the cost of implementing cannabis policies, for example one study showed that they had very little impact on overall cannabis use, and were time consuming for police officers and ultimately a burden on the judicial system (Ogrodnik, Kopp, Bongaerts, & Tecco, 2015). According to the most recent European Drug Report, expenditure and costs of drug-related complications remained mixed, with 22 countries having produced estimates of drug-related public expenditure with 0.01–0.5% of gross domestic product (GDP) reported, and about half estimated between 0.05% and 0.2% of GDP (EMCDDA, 2018).

The GBD study estimated 13.1 million cannabis dependent individuals worldwide in 2010, with a peak age between 20 and 24, and with greater prevalence in males and in high income regions (Degenhardt et al., 2013). Cannabis is currently one of the most widely used substances in the world and only alcohol is more popular amongst adolescents (Johnston, O'Malley, Miech, Bachman, & Schulenberg, 2015). The cultural context in which adolescent cannabis use occurs may be due to this mounting trend, where adolescents' perceptions of decreased harm are one of the key drivers (Johnston et al., 2015). These perceptions have likely contributed to more recreational use, with increased acceptability, and the legalization of medical cannabis in several states and countries worldwide (Cohen, 2010). A major concern might be the fact that cannabis is available in vast varieties and differs in chemical composition and potency (concentration of delta9-THC). This may pose a serious problem in evaluating cannabis' health effects and when comparing studies (Burgdoff, Kilmer, & Pacula, 2011; ElSohly et al., 2000).

Statistics from the World Health Organization (WHO) World Mental Health Survey have shown that amongst young people aged 22–29, 27% in New Zealand, 20% in the USA and only 7% in Netherlands have used this drug by the age of 15. Almost no use in this age group was reported in Asia, the Middle East and Africa (Degenhardt et al., 2008). By age 21, more than half of young adults in New Zealand (62%) and the USA (54%) had used cannabis, compared to the Netherlands (35%) (Degenhardt et al., 2008). In high schools across the USA, it has been reported that in 2014 patterns of use were common with 3.3% of students using it daily and 14.4% monthly (Johnston et al., 2015). Furthermore, results from the 2013 US National Survey on Drug Use and Health estimated that 51.9% of 18- to 25-year olds had sampled cannabis (Substance Abuse and Mental Health Services Administration, 2014).

Neuroethics of medical cannabis

Safety concerns may arise in regard to physicians providing treatment using medical cannabis. The use of cannabis for medical purposes may be relatively new for some physicians. Therefore, it is important that physicians feel they have a strong knowledge base for prescribing and for monitoring beneficial treatment effects and unwanted side effects (Sagy, Peleg-Sagy, Barski, Zeller, & Jotkowitz, 2018). There may also be issues with insurance coverage in regard to the use of medical cannabis.

There remains continued debate surrounding medical cannabis use for the purposes of treating symptoms of various diseases such as pediatric epilepsy (Elliott et al., 2018). For example, the FDA recently approved Epidiolex, essentially derived from cannabidiol, for the treatment of seizures in children with epilepsy (Devinsky et al., 2018; Wise, 2018). However, very few studies have researched the efficacy and safety of cannabinoids in pediatric disorders. A recent pilot study of 25 patients aged 1–17 with complex motor disorder examined the efficacy, safety, and tolerability of medical cannabis administered for 5 months (Libzon et al., 2018). The authors concluded significant improvements in spasticity, dystonia, sleep, mood, appetite, pain, overall motor function and quality of life, and summarized that medical cannabis was safe to administer over a 5 month period without patients experiencing severe side effects (Libzon et al., 2018). Sativex was approved in the UK in 2010 and is expected to receive Food and Drug Administration (FDA) approval; the oral mouth spray containing both cannabidiol (CBD) and tetrahydrocannabidiol (THC) is absorbed through the lining of the mouth and is administered to treat multiple sclerosis (Rubin, 2018). Sativex has been reported not to produce euphoria (Rubin, 2018). Other FDA approved drugs such as Marinol, Syndros and Cesmet are synthetic compounds and their chemical structures are very similar to THC, these are administered to cancer patients to treat nausea and vomiting whilst undergoing chemotherapy, and to patients with AIDS for lack of appetite (Rubin, 2018). Studies have also reported that cannabis can improve sleep by eliminating nightmares in patients who have experienced traumatic events (Babson, Sottile, & Morabito, 2017; Pedersen & Sandberg, 2013). Furthermore, a review of 11 articles studying cannabis use by military veterans found that many of them used cannabis to dampen posttraumatic stress disorder (PTSD) symptoms and some reported reduced anxiety, less problems with sleeping and better coping ability (Betthauser, Pilz, & Vollmer, 2015).

Experts have argued that prohibition of medical cannabis may constitute a violation of human rights preventing patients from exploring its therapeutic potential (Bone & Seddon, 2016). Largely, the message directed by public health authorities worldwide on both lawful and unlawful substances is to persuade users to abstain from or to consume certain substances in moderation in order to prevent harm to self and others, in line with the central focus of ethics on harm avoidance or reduction (Bunton & Coveney, 2011). Thus far, however, efforts made to reform legislations on prohibited substances, actively seeking to reduce punishment or administer penalties in proportion to harms caused, have been largely unsuccessful (Levine, 2003).

Influences on the developing brain

As the adolescent brain is still in its development phase, it may be that the effects of cannabis during this stage are particularly harmful. There is also a large individual variability in brain development during the adolescent phase influenced by factors such as socioeconomic status, culture and peer environment (Foulkes & Blakemore, 2018). Adolescence is a period in which the brain is exposed to profound dynamic changes, with microstructural and macrostructural transformations, primarily involving the prefrontal cortex, limbic system, white matter tracts and neurochemical alterations (Bava & Tapert, 2010; Giedd et al., 1999; Gogtay et al., 2004). During this neurodevelopmental period, increased synaptogenesis and myelination occurs, followed by considerable synaptic pruning, allowing for improved processing of higher order cognitive functions, such as complex attention, working memory, reward processing and inhibitory control (Huttenlocher & Dabholkar, 1997; Sowell, Thompson, & Tessner, 2001). Furthermore, the endocannabinoid system has an important role in the neurodevelopmental process during adolescence, including synaptic pruning and white matter development, exogenous cannabinoids may adversely affect these processes (Lubman, Cheetham, & Yücel, 2015). During adolescence, the endocannabinoid system also continues to undergo substantial changes including extensive pruning of receptor density levels in the subcortical and frontal regions, so increasing susceptibility to insults from exogenous cannabinoids (Heng, Beverley, Steiner, & Tseng, 2011; Mechoulam & Parker, 2013; Viveros et al., 2012). A neuroimaging study found that larger volumes of the vermis were correlated with poorer executive functioning in chronic adolescent cannabis users (Medina, Nagel, & Tapert, 2010). It is worth mentioning that cannabis use may have different effects on the brain depending on a user's gender. It was noted that female cannabis users demonstrated larger right amygdala volumes compared to cannabis using males and female controls, and that larger amygdala volumes were correlated with symptoms of increased depression and anxiety (Mcqueeny et al., 2011). In addition, cannabis using females acknowledged greater internalizing symptoms which are known to be related to depression, anxiety, withdrawal and loneliness (Mcqueeny et al., 2011). Total PFC volume interacted in predicting executive functioning. Among cannabis users, smaller PFC total volume was associated with better executive functioning while the opposite pattern was seen among the controls (Medina et al., 2009). While these brain changes associated with cannabis are of interest, it is unclear whether these pre-existed prior to cannabis use, since these studies were not longitudinal. This relationship between cannabis use and brain changes may be clarified further in large scale longitudinal studies of adolescents, including the IMAGEN (IMAGEN Consortium, 2018; https://imagen-europe.com/) and ABCD (ABCD Research Consortium, 2018; https://abcdstudy.org/) studies.

Effects on cognition

Early onset cannabis use in adolescent years during the crucial periods of neurodevelopment may result in lasting cognitive deficits (Castellanos-Ryan et al., 2016; Pope et al., 2003; Scott et al., 2018). A study examined 13–18 year old adolescents for the non-acute (residual effects from cannabis use) relationship between cannabis and cognitive functions with the administration of the Cambridge Neuropsychological Test Automated Battery (CANTAB) (Harvey, Sellman, Porter, & Frampton, 2007). It was concluded that there was a significant relationship between high frequency of cannabis use and impairment in executive functions and working memory, both of which are important for processing and efficiently storing information as well as utilizing strategies (Harvey et al., 2007). There is mounting evidence suggesting that adolescent cannabis use is associated with greater neurocognitive deficits in visuospatial attention (Ehrenreich et al., 1999), visual motor skills (Huestegge, Kunert, & Radach, 2010), episodic memory (Pope et al., 2003; Solowij et al., 2011), verbal fluency and inhibition (Gruber, Sagar, Dahlgren, Racine, & Lukas, 2012), and other forms of executive functioning (Fontes et al., 2011; Gruber et al., 2012), as well as lowered IQ (Meier et al., 2012). One study found that individuals with use before the age of 16 showed considerable impairment in reaction times of visual scanning, whereas those who began cannabis use after the age of 16 did not differ from controls (Ehrenreich et al., 1999). Another study demonstrated that early onset of cannabis use was associated with poorer learning, retention, and retrieval of novel verbal information even after adjusting for the frequency and dose of cannabis absorbed (Solowij et al., 2011). Moreover, chronic heavy cannabis users with an early onset age were found to perform poorly on measures of executive functions, especially in decision-making, inhibition and cognitive control, compared to late onset cannabis users (Gruber et al., 2012). Furthermore, a recent meta-analysis of 69 studies examined frequent or heavy cannabis use in adolescents and young adults and found that early cannabis use was associated with a decline in cognitive functioning (Scott et al., 2018). Moderate effect sizes were found in test of learning, delayed memory, executive functioning, speed of processing, and attention (Scott et al., 2018). These findings are important as even small changes in cognitive performance may lead to either a decline or improvement in academic achievements, for example the Academy of Medical Sciences Report (2008) stated that it is conceivable that a 10% improvement in memory score may result in better A grade scores (Horn, 2008).

Whilst the above studies have demonstrated that several cognitive domains may be affected by the use of cannabis during adolescence or early adulthood, the evidence for decline in IQ following cannabis use is mixed. A large longitudinal study of two sets of data from 789 and 2277 twin participants found that there was no significant correlation between adolescent cannabis use and IQ decline, with any deficits observed reflecting confounding factors (Jackson et al., 2016). Another longitudinal study investigated the relationship between adolescent cannabis use, IQ and academic attainment in 2235 adolescents and found that cannabis use in moderation was not causally associated to cognitive impairment, and may be due to related confounding variables, such as cigarette smoking and social adversity during adolescence (Mokrysz et al., 2016).

The authors concluded that although cannabis dependence may be associated with lowered IQ, adolescent cannabis use alone does not appear to predict lowered IQ in adulthood or the level of educational attainment (Mokrysz et al., 2016).

Research into gender differences in cognitive deficits due to adolescent cannabis use is considered an understudied area. One study reported on developmental trajectories from early adolescence to young adulthood and concluded higher levels of cannabis use by males compared to females from the ages of 11–35 (Chen & Jacobson, 2012). Another study observed when and where use occurs with males reporting use before, during, after school, and weeknights, compared to females indicating use only on weekends (Goncy & Mrug, 2013). From a cognitive perspective, reduced sequencing abilities and psychomotor speed were found to differ between male and female adolescent cannabis users where males were more affected than females even when they had similar levels of cannabis use with an average 50 days of abstinence (Lisdahl & Price, 2012).

Effects on academic performance

Although a substantial amount of research has been conducted into adolescent cannabis use and academic outcomes, it is unclear how much cannabis use impacts the risk of poor school performance and lower levels of educational attainment. A longitudinal study which followed 1601 adolescents aged 15–21 in Australia, concluded that weekly cannabis use from age 15 was associated with increased risk of early school leaving, even after being adjusted for demographics, other substance use, psychiatric morbidity and antisocial behavior (Lynskey, Coffey, Degenhardt, Carlin, & Patton, 2003). A more recent large longitudinal Australasian study with 6000 participants found that those who had not used cannabis by age 18 had a higher educational attainment than those who first used cannabis before age 15. The authors estimated that 17% of failures to complete a high school degree was connected to early cannabis use (Horwood et al., 2010). A British study investigated 1155 participants with cannabis and tobacco use by age 15 and found that weekly cannabis use was negatively associated with English and Mathematics GCSE results (Stiby et al., 2015).

A longitudinal study in a New Zealand found that cannabis users aged 16 had an elevated risk of substance use, delinquency, school dropout, and poor mental health, and 22.5% had left school before the age of 16. However, the authors state that the elevated risks can be entirely explained by social, family and individual characteristics, and only the risk of using cannabis in the future could be explained by the early onset use (Fergusson, Lynskey, & Horwood, 1996). A USA study observed adolescent cannabis users from ages 14 to 18 and concluded that persistent cannabis use during high school was associated with a lower grade point average (GPA), lower scholastic aptitude test (SAT), and greater externalizing symptoms measured by Youth Self Report. However, the effect for cannabis use became non-significant when persistent alcohol and tobacco use was controlled for (Meier, Hill, Small, & Luthar, 2015). Another study explored the relationship between early onset cannabis use and low academic attainment in 3337 twins and reported that educational attainment and school dropout in early cannabis users was likely effects of shared genetic and environmental risk factors such as social disadvantage, family dysfunction and peer affiliations (Verweij, Anja, Agrawal, Nicholas, & Lynskey, 2013). The findings from the above studies suggest that there is a link between cannabis use and lowered school performance, although there appears to be a number of additional factors contributing to this association.

Risk factor for psychiatric disorders

Several studies have demonstrated that early cannabis use is associated with transient psychotic episodes and is a risk factor for developing schizophrenia and dependency in later adulthood (Marconi, Di Forti, Lewis, Murray, & Vassos, 2016; Mathers & Ghodse, 1992; Murray & Di Forti, 2016; Negrete, Knapp, Douglas, & Smith, 1986; Thornicroft, 1990). Several longitudinal studies in the general population worldwide investigating the role of cannabis as a risk factor for schizophrenia have demonstrated that the likelihood of developing schizophrenia is double or more, with up to a sixfold risk in some cases depending on the frequency, dose, duration and age of first cannabis use (Andreasson, Engstrom, Allebeck, & Rydberg, 1987; Arseneault et al., 2002; Ferdinand et al., 2005; Fergusson, Horwood, & Swain-Campbell, 2003; Henquet et al., 2005; Stefanis et al., 2004; Van Os et al., 2002; Weiser, Knobler, Noy, & Kaplan, 2002; Wiles et al., 2003; Zammit et al., 2004). The neurobiology of cannabis induced schizophrenia might be explained by a disruption of glutamatergic transmission, where the psychoactive ingredient D9-tetrahydrocannabinol (THC) found in cannabis may result in disturbing the physiological control of the endogenous cannabinoid system over glutamate and GABA release in the developing adolescent brain (Bossong & Niesink, 2010). As such, depending on the dose, timing, and duration of use, this may cause damage to the neural circuits within the prefrontal cortex, and in the long-term may become a risk factor for psychosis (Bossong & Niesink, 2010). Cannabis use in adolescence may be a risk factor for psychotic-like symptoms given that the endocannabinoid system has a role in facilitating adolescent neurodevelopment including synaptic pruning, hence tampering with the GABAergic and dopaminergic systems (Malone, Hill, & Rubino, 2010). In 1969–1970 Swedish male military conscripts aged 18–20 (total 50,087 subjects) reported cannabis and other drug use, and after 27 years of follow up research it was concluded that early adulthood cannabis use was associated with a greater risk of developing schizophrenia, this risk further increasing with a higher frequency of use, and the correlation remained significant even whilst other drugs used were controlled for (Zammit, Allebeck, Andreasson, Lundberg, & Lewis, 2002). A more recent longitudinal study which combined data from the Canadian Saguenay Youth Study (SYS), the IMAGEN Study, and the Avon Longitudinal Study of Parents and Children (ALSPAC) analyzed a total of 1577 participants aged 12–21 years for whether adolescent cannabis use was associated with variations in neurodevelopment and whether this was mediated by polygenic risk score for schizophrenia (French et al., 2015). The authors found that adolescent cannabis use may interfere with brain maturation by accelerating cortical thinning especially in the cerebral cortices of males with high polygenic risk scores for schizophrenia (French et al., 2015). Another study explored cannabis withdrawal symptoms in young adults with psychiatric lifetime illness and found that those who used cannabis frequently, at least weekly, had more persistent cannabis withdrawal symptoms, this was also in line with previous findings indicating that psychiatric diagnosis was related with several indicators of greater severity of cannabis use (Schuster et al., 2017).

Other psychiatric conditions that may be precipitated by cannabis use in adolescents or young adults include depression and anxiety. A meta-analysis examined 76,058 participants, mostly adolescents and young adults from 14 longitudinal studies to establish whether cannabis use was associated with the development of depression, and found that cannabis use was correlated with a modest increased risk for developing depressive disorders and that heavy cannabis use was associated with a stronger, yet still moderate risk for developing depression (Lev-Ran et al., 2014). Another study which included four Australasian cohorts comprised of 6900 adolescents and young adults, found a significant correlation between frequency of cannabis use and severity of depression which was similar across all cohorts, was age dependent, and suggested that stronger associations were evident in mid-adolescence and that this effect weakened towards mature adulthood (Horwood et al., 2012). However, contradictory findings have also been reported by other studies where no significant relation was found between cannabis use and depression (Fergusson & Horwood, 1997; Manrique-Garcia, Zammit, Dalman, Hemmingsson, & Allebeck, 2012; Windle & Wiesner, 2004). Research on cannabis use and anxiety is more mixed with a systematic review study suggesting that cannabis use and anxiety symptoms or disorders often co-occur (Crippa et al., 2009). The majority of the literature especially longitudinal studies often combine depressive and anxiety disorders when investigating cannabis use, and so are unable to distinguish the unique relations between these conditions (McGee, Williams, Poulton, & Moffitt, 2000). A meta-analysis of 31 longitudinal and cross-sectional studies with 112,000 cases derived from 10 countries (Australia, Canada, Columbia, France, Germany, The Netherlands, New Zealand, Switzerland, UK, and USA) assessed the relationship between cannabis and anxiety, and found that cohorts with anxiety or concurrent anxiety and depression were more likely to use cannabis, and prospective analyses revealed that cannabis use at baseline was positively correlated with anxiety at follow-up (Kedzior & Laeber, 2014). In contrast, a longitudinal study which assessed for cannabis use based on a self-report questionnaire with a 7 point Likert scale of 'never used' to 'used every day' was completed by 15- to 17-year olds and concluded that there was no clear evidence to suggest that chronic users would develop anxiety disorders during their early to mid-20s (Windle & Wiesner, 2004). Nonetheless, a majority of studies confirm findings indicating a relationship between cannabis use promoting the development of depressive symptoms and anxiety (Bovasso, 2001; Brook, Brook, Zhang, Cohen, & Whiteman, 2002; Fergusson, Horwood, & Swain-Campbell, 2002; Hayatbakhsh et al., 2007; Patton et al., 2002; Rey, Sawyer, Raphael, Patton, & Lynskey, 2002; Van Laar, Van Dorsselaer, Monshouwer, & De Graaf, 2007).

Reasons for use and socioeconomic status (SES)

The motives for substance and cannabis use by adolescents suggest that this behavior is driven by a range of reasons. A study investigating the role of motivation of recently graduated high-school students who provided open-ended reasons for cannabis use, resulting in 19 distinct motive categories (Lee, Neighbors, & Woods, 2007). The authors concluded that amongst these categories, enjoyment/fun motives were the most prevalent reasons, followed by conformity, experimentation, social enhancement, boredom and relaxation (Lee et al., 2007). A study which included young adults in its sample of 105 male cannabis users requested participants to respond to 29 author complied potential reasons for cannabis use, and results indicated that "to have fun/to enjoy the feeling," "to see things differently/expand awareness/to be more creative," "to fit in with peers/to help socialize," and "to help when feeling down/to forget about problems/as an escape" were the most common responses (Hecimovic, Barrett, Darredeau, & Stewart, 2014). Next to the motives for cannabis use, it is also worth mentioning that a co-occurrence of other substances used can be observed. A systematic review examining 31 studies on co-occurring cannabis and tobacco users found that simultaneous use of cannabis and tobacco was associated with a higher likelihood of cannabis use disorders, as well as greater psychosocial problems resulting in poorer cannabis cessation outcomes and therefore continued cannabis use (Peters, Budney, & Carroll, 2012). Another study assessed the use of e-cigarettes in a sample of 621 (308 females) high-school students across 35 schools and its association with current tobacco and cannabis smokers as well as alcohol users, and found that e-cigarette users were more likely to be current tobacco and cannabis smokers and to have misused alcohol in the past month (Surís, Berchtold, & Akre, 2015). Understanding the motives and risks specific to cannabis may improve the predications of use as well as help establish which communities under what social circumstances may require tailored interventions.

The socioeconomic status (SES) of adolescents and their families is another factor that may have an impact on cannabis use amongst teenagers (Table 1). A systematic review analyzing the associations between SES and cannabis use amongst adolescents evaluated 25 studies and found that the majority of the studies (60%) had not reported a significant relationship between SES and cannabis use (Hanson & Chen, 2007). Of the 25 studies, six reported positive correlations where adolescents from high SES backgrounds used more cannabis than adolescents from low SES families and four of the studies resulted in a negative correlation, with low SES associated with more cannabis use than high SES adolescents. Those opposite results may be explained by different studies using different measures of SES. The researchers found that SES measured via family social status was negatively associated with marijuana use, while positive association was observed when family financial resources was the measure of SES (Hanson & Chen, 2007). One study used two measures of SES (parents' education and income) and reported a non-linear correlation between SES and adolescent cannabis use, where those who came from both low and high SES backgrounds reported greater use compared to adolescents from middle class SES backgrounds.

Table 1 Motives for cannabis use amongst adolescents and young adults

Motive	Description
Enjoyment	For fun, to be happy, get high, or enjoy the feeling
Conformity	Influence of peer pressure, because friends do it, to fit in with peers
Experimentation	Considered a novelty and new experience, or genuinely curious
Social enhancement	Allows to bond with friends and hang out with them, easier to socialize
Boredom	Gives them something to do, or they have nothing better to do
Relaxation	Helps to relax, or helps with sleep
Coping	Allows to better manage self in a depressed state of mind, allows to relieve stress
Availability	Was easy to acquire cannabis, or was offered cannabis, was easier to get than other drugs
Relative low risk	Perceptions of low health risk, no result of experiencing a hangover, or it was safer to use compared to other drugs
Altered or enhanced perception	To enhance experiences, makes things more fun, heighten senses (any of the five senses)
Activity enhancement	Music sounds better, everyday activates seem more interesting, to become more open to experiences
Rebellion	Rebelling against parents, the thrill of doing something illegal
Alcohol intoxication	Was under the influence of alcohol
Food	To enjoy good food, food tastes better, to reduce appetite, or manage weight
Anxiety reduction	To become more extrovert, be less shy, to feel less insecure, or to feel more confident
Image enhancement	To be cool, too look or feel cool
Celebration	Use on special occasions, to celebrate
Medical use	To alleviate physical pain, or to treat a headache
Habit	The feeling was addictive, it became a habit
Co-occurring use	Already a current smoker (tobacco/e-cigarette), or already using with other substances such as alcohol and or/other drugs, to increase/decrease the effects of another drug
Creative	To be more creative
Escape	To forget about ones' problems, to use as a way to escape and free the mind
Study	To help study or concentrate
Sexual	For sexual reasons
Withdrawal	To avoid withdrawal from cannabis, or to help withdrawal from another drug
Energy	To give one more energy
Alert	To stay awake or alert

This table gathered information from: Hecimovic et al. (2014), Lee et al. (2007), Peters et al. (2012), and Surís et al. (2015).

However this effect was only observed when SES was measured by education not income (Goodman & Huang, 2002). A French study investigated the relationship between cannabis use in adolescence and SES measured using parents' occupational status. Additionally, the researchers focussed on the intensity and frequency of cannabis use, which may be another reason for the variation across different studies. The main finding was that adolescents from higher SES backgrounds were more likely to experiment with cannabis, however they were less prone to engage in more dangerous and intensive use than their peers from lower SES backgrounds (Legleye, Beck, Khlat, Peretti-Watel, & Chau, 2012).

Burden of disease

It is important in neuroethical discussions of cannabis use to consider its risks, therefore it is crucial to understand how cannabis dependence contributes to the global burden of disease. Disability adjusted life years (DALY) is a measure of disease burden and can be used to comprehend the overall impact of a given disease. DALY consist of years of life lost due to premature mortality (YLLs) and the years lived with disability (YLDs) (Degenhardt et al., 2013). In a systematic analysis for the GBD conducted in 84 risk categories, the authors reported statistically significant increase of 3.68% in DALY associated with cannabis use disorders (CUD) between 2006 and 2016. However, the increase for disorders connected to opioids, cocaine and other drugs was double or more. It is also worth mentioning that no deaths were reported in connection to CUD, unlike other drug disorders (Gakidou et al., 2017). Similarly, Degenhardt et al. (2013) reported in their 2010 study that cannabis dependence had not increased mortality as dependence on other drugs had.

Conclusion

Overall, this chapter summarized adolescent cannabis use and the impact it has on mental health and wellbeing. Cannabis Use Disorder may result in raising discussion around free will. This places the individual in a position where they may not be able to conceptualize, plan and execute sound decisions in their daily lives. Neuroethical issues surrounding cannabis use also have important implications for physicians and other treating professionals who under legal obligations must attend to patients by providing care at acknowledged standards. Gradually medical cannabis is becoming present in the pharmaceutical industry, with this doctors face the dilemma of whether to prescribe medical cannabis or to advise alternative treatments.

We further discussed the extensive developments in neuroscience and medicine by reviewing adolescent cannabis use in a neuroethical context. The use of cannabis by adolescents globally has led to debates on legalization and many countries around the world have authorized cannabis use in some form, either for recreational or medical purposes. At the same time concerns have been raised by experts given the data on the adverse effects that adolescent cannabis use may have for the developing brain, and associated cognitive impairments. Another important factor is the effect adolescent cannabis use may have on school performance and how this may impact overall academic achievements and the level of qualifications. It was shown that there was a relationship between cannabis use in adolescents and educational attainment, however a number of additional factors seemed to contribute to this association. The link between SES and cannabis use is unclear as there are many factors, like frequency and intensity of cannabis use, and different measures of SES, to be considered. The level of burden produced by CUD was also discussed, the burden of disease associated with CUD has been shown to increase over a decade, however CUD is still less harmful than other drug-related disorders, and unlike other drugs, for example opioids or cocaine, it is not accountable for an increase in mortality.

Governments worldwide need to consider the legal status of cannabis use in detail, including the potential adverse effects on domains, including alterations in brain function and structure, cognitive and intellectual functioning, academic and occupational performance, motor vehicle accidents, antisocial and delinquent behavior, and psychiatric disorders. To ensure healthy brain function, effective cognition, mental wellbeing, and success in school and society, it is important to identify those adolescents at risk of chronic cannabis use. Additional research is required on the drivers of cannabis use disorder and on programs for prevention and effective treatments. Only by undertaking comprehensive analyses of these factors, will it be possible to ensure that adolescents can realize their potential and flourish in society.

Acknowledgments

Barbara J. Sahakian received funding from the NIHR Cambridge Biomedical Research Centre (Mental Health Theme) and from Eton College and the Wallitt Foundation. George Savulich is funded by Eton College and the Wallitt Foundation and is supported by the NIHR Cambridge Biomedical Research Centre (Mental Health Theme).

References

ABCD Research Consortium. (2018). *Adolescent brain cognitive development study.* https://abcdstudy.org/index.html (Accessed July 25, 2018).

American Psychiatric Association. (2013). *Diagnostic and statistical manual of mental disorders* (5th ed.). Arlington, VA: American Psychiatric Publishing.

Andreasson, S., Engstrom, A. N. N., Allebeck, P., & Rydberg, U. L. F. (1987). Cannabis and schizophrenia: A longitudinal study of Swedish conscripts. *Lancet*, 1483–1486.

Arseneault, L., Cannon, M., Poulton, R., Murray, R., Caspi, A., & Moffitt, T. E. (2002). Cannabis use in adolescence and risk for adult psychosis: Longitudinal prospective study. *British Medical Journal*, *325*, 1212–1213. https://doi.org/10.1136/bmj.325.7374.1212.

Babson, K. A., Sottile, J., & Morabito, D. (2017). Cannabis, cannabinoids, and sleep: A review of the literature. *Current Psychiatry Reports*, *19*. https://doi.org/10.1007/s11920-017-0775-9.

Bava, S., & Tapert, S. F. (2010). Adolescent brain development and the risk for alcohol and other drug problems. *Neuropsychology Review*, *20*, 398–413. https://doi.org/10.1007/s11065-010-9146-6.

Betthauser, K., Pilz, J., & Vollmer, L. E. (2015). Use and effects of cannabinoids in military veterans with posttraumatic stress disorder. *American Journal of Health-System Pharmacy*, *72*, 1279–1284. https://doi.org/10.2146/ajhp140523.

Bone, M., & Seddon, T. (2016). Human rights, public health and medicinal cannabis use. *Critical Public Health*, *26*, 51–61. https://doi.org/10.1080/09581596.2015.1038218.

Bossong, M. G., & Niesink, R. J. M. (2010). Adolescent brain maturation, the endogenous cannabinoid system and the neurobiology of cannabis-induced schizophrenia. *Progress in Neurobiology*, *92*, 370–385. https://doi.org/10.1016/j.pneurobio.2010.06.010.

Bovasso, G. B. (2001). Cannabis abuse as a risk factor for depressive symptoms. *The American Journal of Psychiatry*, *158*, 2033–2037. https://doi.org/10.1176/appi.ajp.158.12.2033.

Brook, D. W., Brook, J. S., Zhang, C., Cohen, P., & Whiteman, M. (2002). Drug use and the risk of major depressive disorder, alcohol dependence, and substance use disorders. *Archives of General Psychiatry*, *59*, 1039. https://doi.org/10.1001/archpsyc.59.11.1039.

Buchman, D. Z., Skinner, W., & Illes, J. (2010). Negotiating the relationship between addiction, ethics, and brain science. *AJOB Neuroscience*, *1*, 36–45. https://doi.org/10.1080/21507740903508609.

Bunton, R., & Coveney, J. (2011). Drugs' pleasures. *Critical Public Health*, *21*, 9–23. https://doi.org/10.1080/09581596.2010.530644.

Burgdoff, J., Kilmer, B., & Pacula, R. (2011). Heterogeneity in the composition of marijuana seized in California. *Drug and Alcohol Dependence*, *117*, 59–61. https://doi.org/10.1016/j.drugalcdep.2010.11.031.

Carter, A. N., Hall, W. D., & Illes, J. (2012). Introduction: What is addiction neuroethics and why does it matter? In A. Carter, W. Hall, & J. Illes (Eds.), *Addiction neuroethics: The ethics of addiction neuroscience research and treatment* (1st ed., pp. xvii–xxv). London, UK: Elsevier. https://doi.org/10.1016/B978-0-12-385973-0.00019-3.

Castellanos-Ryan, N., Pingault, J.-B., Parent, S., Vitaro, F., Tremblay, R. E., & Séguin, J. R. (2016). Adolescent cannabis use, change in neurocognitive function, and high-school graduation: A longitudinal study from early adolescence to young adulthood. *Development and Psychopathology*, *29*, 1–14. https://doi.org/10.1017/S0954579416001280.

Chen, P., & Jacobson, K. C. (2012). Developmental trajectories of substance use from early adolescence to young adulthood: Gender and racial/ethnic differences. *Journal of Adolescent Health*, *50*, 154–163. https://doi.org/10.1016/j.jadohealth.2011.05.013.

Cohen, P. J. (2010). Medical Marijuana 2010: It's time to fix the regulatory vacuum. *The Journal of Law Medicine and Ethics*, *38*(3), 654–666.

Crippa, J. A., Zuardi, A. W., Martin-Santos, R., Bhattacharya, S., Atakan, Z., McGuire, P., et al. (2009). Cannabis and anxiety: A critical review of evidence. *Human Psychopharmacology*, *24*, 515–523. https://doi.org/10.1002/hup.

Danovitch, I., & Gorelick, D. (2012). State of the art treatments for cannabis dependence. *The Psychiatric Clinics of North America*, *35*, 309–326. https://doi.org/10.1016/j.psc.2012.03.003.State.

Degenhardt, L., Chiu, W. T., Sampson, N., Kessler, R. C., Anthony, J. C., Angermeyer, M., et al. (2008). Toward a global view of alcohol, tobacco, cannabis, and cocaine use: Findings from the WHO world mental health surveys. *PLoS Medicine*, *5*, 1053–1067. https://doi.org/10.1371/journal.pmed.0050141.

Degenhardt, L., Ferrari, A. J., Calabria, B., Hall, W. D., Norman, R. E., McGrath, J., et al. (2013). The global epidemiology and contribution of Cannabis use and dependence to the global burden of disease: Results from the GBD 2010 study. *PLoS One*, *8*, 1–13. https://doi.org/10.1371/journal.pone.0076635.

Devinsky, O., Patel, A. D., Cross, J. H., Villanueva, V., Wirrell, E. C., Privitera, M., et al. (2018). Effect of cannabidiol on drop seizures in the Lennox-Gastaut syndrome. *The New England Journal of Medicine*, *378*, 1888–1897. https://doi.org/10.1056/NEJMoa1714631.

Ehrenreich, H., Rinn, T., Kunert, H. J., Moeller, M. R., Poser, W., Schilling, L., et al. (1999). Specific attentional dysfunction in adults following early start of cannabis use. *Psychopharmacology*, *142*(3), 295–301. https://doi.org/10.1007/S002130050892.

Elliott, J., DeJean, D., Clifford, T., Coyle, D., Potter, B., Skidmore, B., et al. (2018). Cannabis for pediatric epilepsy: Protocol for a living systematic review. *Systematic Review*, *7*, 95. https://doi.org/10.1186/s13643-018-0761-2.

ElSohly, M. A., Ross, S. A., Mehmedic, Z., Arafat, R., Yi, B., Banahan, B. F., 3rd. (2000). Potency trends of delta9-THC and other cannabinoids in confiscated marijuana from 1980–1997. *Journal of Forensic Sciences*, *45*, 24–30. https://doi.org/10.1111/j.1556-4029.2010.01441.x.

EMCDDA. (2018). *European Drug Report*.

Ersche, K. D., Gillan, C. M., Jones, P. S., Williams, G. B., Laetitia, H. E., Luijten, M., et al. (2016). Europe PMC Funders Group: Carrots and sticks fail to change behavior in cocaine addiction. *Science*, *352*, 1468–1471. https://doi.org/10.1126/science.aaf3700.Carrots.

Farah, M. J. (2012). Neuroethics: The ethical, legal, and societal impact of neuroscience. *Annual Review of Psychology*, *63*, 571–591. https://doi.org/10.1146/annurev.psych.093008.100438.

Ferdinand, R. F., Sondeijker, F., Van Der Ende, J., Selten, J., Huizink, A., Verhulst, F. C., et al. (2005). Cannabis use predicts future psychotic symptoms, and vice versa. *Addiction*, *100*(5), 612–618. https://doi.org/10.1111/j.1360-0443.2005.01070.x.

Fergusson, D., Horwood, L., & Swain-Campbell, N. (2003). Cannabis dependence and psychotic symptoms in young people. *Psychological Medicine*, *33*(1), 15–21.

Fergusson, D. M., & Horwood, L. J. (1997). Early onset cannabis use and psychosocial adjustment in young adults. *Addiction*, *92*, 279–296. https://doi.org/10.1111/j.1360-0443.1997.tb03198.x.

Fergusson, D. M., Horwood, L. J., & Swain-Campbell, N. (2002). Cannabis use and psychosocial adjustment in adolescence and young adulthood. *Addiction*, *97*, 1123–1135. https://doi.org/10.1046/j.1360-0443.2002.00103.x.

Fergusson, D. M., Lynskey, M. T., & Horwood, L. J. (1996). The short-term consequences of early onset cannabis use. *Journal of Abnormal Child Psychology*, *24*, 499–512. https://doi.org/10.1007/BF01441571.

Florez-Salmanca, L., Secedes-Villa, R., Hasin, D. S., Cottler, L., Wang, S., Grant, B. F., et al. (2013). Probability and predictors of transition from abuse to dependence on alcohol, cannabis, and cocaine: Results from the National Epidemiologic Survey on alcohol and related conditions. *American Journal of Drug and Alcohol Abuse*, *39*, 168–179. https://doi.org/10.3109/00952990.2013.772618.Probability.

Fontes, M. A., Bolla, K. I., Cunha, P. J., Almeida, P. P., Jungerman, F., Laranjeira, R. R., et al. (2011). Cannabis use before age 15 and subsequent executive functioning. *The British Journal of Psychiatry*, *198*, 442–447. https://doi.org/10.1192/bjp.bp.110.077479.

Foulkes, L., & Blakemore, S. J. (2018). Studying individual differences in human adolescent brain development. *Nature Neuroscience*, *21*, 315–323. https://doi.org/10.1038/s41593-018-0078-4.

French, L., Gray, C., Leonard, G., Perron, M., Pike, G. B., Richer, L., et al. (2015). Early cannabis use, polygenic risk score for schizophrenia, and brain maturation in adolescence. *JAMA Psychiatry*, *72*, 1002–1011. https://doi.org/10.1001/jamapsychiatry.2015.1131.

Gakidou, E., Afshin, A., Abajobir, A. A., Abate, K. H., Abbafati, C., Abbas, K. M., et al. (2017). Global, regional, and national comparative risk assessment of 84 behavioural, environmental and occupational, and metabolic risks or clusters of risks, 1990–2016: A systematic analysis for the global burden of disease study 2016. *Lancet*, *390*, 1345–1422. https://doi.org/10.1016/S0140-6736(17)32366-8.

Giedd, J. N., Blumenthal, J., Jeffries, N. O., Castellanos, F. X., Liu, H., Zijdenbos, A., et al. (1999). Brain development during childhood and adolescence: A longitudinal MRI study. *Nature Neuroscience, 2,* 861–863. https://doi.org/10.1038/13158.

Gogtay, N., Giedd, J. N., Lusk, L., Hayashi, K. M., Greenstein, D., Vaituzis, A. C., et al. (2004). Dynamic mapping of human cortical development during childhood through early adulthood. *Proceedings of the National Academy of Sciences of the United States of America, 101,* 8174–8179. https://doi.org/10.1073/pnas.0402680101.

Goncy, E. A., & Mrug, S. (2013). Where and when adolescents use tobacco, alcohol, and marijuana: comparisons by age, gender, and race. *Journal of Studies on Alcohol and Drugs, 74,* 288–300. https://doi.org/10.15288/jsad.2013.74.288.

Gonzalez, R., Schuster, R. M., Mermelstein, R. M., et al. (2015). The role of decision-making in cannabis-related problems among young adults. *Drug and Alcohol Dependence, 154,* 214–221.

Goodman, E., & Huang, B. (2002). Socioeconomic status, depressive symptoms, and adolescent substance use. *Archives of Pediatrics & Adolescent Medicine, 156,* 448–453.

Gruber, S. A., Sagar, K. A., Dahlgren, M. K., Racine, M., & Lukas, S. E. (2012). Age of onset of marijuana use and executive function. *Psychology of Addictive Behaviors, 26,* 496–506. https://doi.org/10.1037/a0026269.Age.

Hall, W., & Weier, M. (2015). Assessing the public health impacts of legalizing recreational Cannabis use in the USA. *Clinical Pharmacology and Therapeutics, 97,* 607–615. https://doi.org/10.1002/cpt.110.

Hanson, M. D., & Chen, E. (2007). Socioeconomic status and health behaviors in adolescence: A review of the literature. *Journal of Behavioral Medicine, 30,* 263–285. https://doi.org/10.1007/s10865-007-9098-3.

Harrison, G. (2018). *Put it bluntly. Is weed illegal in the UK, where is cannabis legal ad what are the laws on buying or smoking marijuana?* https://www.thesun.co.uk/news/4094039/is-weed-legal-uk-law-cannabis-marijuana/. (Accessed July 25, 2018).

Harvey, M. A., Sellman, J. D., Porter, R. J., & Frampton, C. M. (2007). The relationship between non-acute adolescent cannabis use and cognition. *Drug and Alcohol Review, 26*(3), 309–319. https://doi.org/10.1080/09595230701247772.

Hayatbakhsh, M. R., Najman, J. M., Jamrozik, K., Mamun, A. A., Alati, R., & Bor, W. (2007). Cannabis and anxiety and depression in young adults: A large prospective study. *Journal of the American Academy of Child and Adolescent Psychiatry, 46,* 408–417. https://doi.org/10.1097/chi.0b013e31802dc54d.

Hecimovic, K., Barrett, S. P., Darredeau, C., & Stewart, S. H. (2014). Cannabis use motives and personality risk factors. *Addictive Behaviors, 39,* 729–732. https://doi.org/10.1016/j.addbeh.2013.11.025.

Heng, L., Beverley, J. A., Steiner, H., & Tseng, K. Y. (2011). Differential developmental trajectories for CB1 cannabinoid receptor expression in limbic/associative and sensorimotor cortical areas. *Synapse, 65,* 278–286. https://doi.org/10.1002/syn.20844.

Henquet, C., Krabbendam, L., Spauwen, J., Kaplan, C., Lieb, R., & Wittchen, H. (2005). Prospective cohort study of cannabis use, predisposition for psychosis, and psychotic symptoms in young people. *British Medical Journal,* 1–5.

Horn, G. (2008). *Brain science, addiction and drugs. An Academy of Medical Sciences working group report.*

Horwood, L. J., Fergusson, D. M., Coffey, C., Patton, G. C., Tait, R., Smart, D., et al. (2012). Cannabis and depression: An integrative data analysis of four Australasian cohorts. *Drug and Alcohol Dependence, 126,* 369–378. https://doi.org/10.1016/j.drugalcdep.2012.06.002.

Horwood, L. J., Fergusson, D. M., Hayatbakhsh, M. R., Najman, J. M., Coffey, C., Patton, G. C., et al. (2010). Cannabis use and educational achievement: Findings from three Australasian cohort studies. *Drug and Alcohol Dependence, 110,* 247–253. https://doi.org/10.1016/j. drugalcdep.2010.03.008.

Huestegge, L., Kunert, H. J., & Radach, R. (2010). Long-term effects of cannabis on eye movement control in reading. *Psychopharmacology, 209,* 77–84. https://doi.org/10.1007/s00213-009-1769-z.

Huttenlocher, P.R., Dabholkar, A.S., 1997. Regional differences in synaptogenesis in human cerebral cortex. The Journal of Comparative Neurology 387, 167–178. https://doi.org/10.1002/(SICI)1096-9861(19971020)387:2<167::AID-CNE1>3.0.CO;2-Z.

IMAGEN Consortium. (2018). *IMAGEN study.* https://imagen-europe.com/. (Accessed July 25, 2018).

Jackson, N. J., Isen, J. D., Khoddam, R., Irons, D., Tuvblad, C., Iacono, W. G., et al. (2016). Impact of adolescent marijuana use on intelligence: Results from two longitudinal twin studies. *Proceedings of the National Academy of Sciences, 113,* E500–E508. https://doi.org/10.1073/pnas.1516648113.

Johnston, L., O'Malley, P., Miech, R., Bachman, J., & Schulenberg, J. (2015). *Monitoring the future: National survey results on drug use: 1975–2014. Overview, key findings on adolescent drug use,* (pp. 1–98). https://doi.org/10.1017/CBO9781107415324.004.

Kedzior, K. K., & Laeber, L. T. (2014). A positive association between anxiety disorders and cannabis use or cannabis use disorders in the general population—A meta-analysis of 31 studies. *BMC Psychiatry, 14,* 136. https://doi.org/10.1186/1471-244X-14-136.

Lee, C. M., Neighbors, C., & Woods, B. A. (2007). Marijuana motives: Young adults' reasons for using marijuana. *Addictive Behaviors, 32,* 1384–1394. https://doi.org/10.1016/j. addbeh.2006.09.010.

Legleye, S., Beck, F., Khlat, M., Peretti-Watel, P., & Chau, N. (2012). The influence of socioeconomic status on cannabis use among French adolescents. *Journal of Adolescent Health, 50,* 395–402. https://doi.org/10.1016/j.jadohealth.2011.08.004.

Lev-Ran, S., Roerecke, M., Le Foll, B., George, T. P., McKenzie, K., & Rehm, J. (2014). The association between cannabis use and depression: A systematic review and meta-analysis of longitudinal studies. *Psychological Medicine, 44,* 797–810. https://doi.org/10.1017/S0033291713001438.

Levine, H. G. (2003). Global drug prohibition: Its uses and crises. *International Journal of Drug Policy, 14,* 145–153. https://doi.org/10.1016/S0955-3959(03)00003-3.

Libzon, S., Schleider, L.B.-L., Saban, N., Levit, L., Tamari, Y., Linder, I., et al. (2018). Medical Cannabis for pediatric moderate to severe complex motor disorders. *Journal of Child Neurology, 33,* 565–571. https://doi.org/10.1177/0883073818773028.

Lisdahl, K. M., & Price, J. S. (2012). Increased marijuana use and gender predict poorer cognitive functioning in adolescents and emerging adults. *Journal of the International Neuropsychological Society, 18,* 678–688. https://doi.org/10.1017/S1355617712000276.

Lopez-Quintero, C., & Cobos, J. (2011). From first use to dependence on nicotine, alcohol, cannabis, and cocaine: Results of the National Epidemiologic Survey on alcohol and related conditions (NESARC). *Drug Alcohol Depend, 115,* 120–130. https://doi.org/10.1016/j. drugalcdep.2010.11.004.Probability.

Lubman, D. I., Cheetham, A., & Yücel, M. (2015). Pharmacology & therapeutics cannabis and adolescent brain development. *Pharmacology & Therapeutics, 148,* 1–16. https://doi.org/10.1016/j.pharmthera.2014.11.009.

Lynskey, M. T., Coffey, C., Degenhardt, L., Carlin, J. B., & Patton, G. (2003). A longitudinal study of the effects of adolescent cannabis use on high school completion. *Addiction, 98,* 685–692. https://doi.org/356.

MacKillop, J., Amlung, M. T., Few, L. R., Ray, L. A., Sweet, L. H., & Munafò, M. R. (2011). Delayed reward discounting and addictive behavior: A meta-analysis. *Psychopharmacology, 216,* 305–321. https://doi.org/10.1007/s00213-011-2229-0.

Malone, D. T., Hill, M. N., & Rubino, T. (2010). Adolescent cannabis use and psychosis: Epidemiology and neurodevelopmental models. *British Journal of Pharmacology, 160,* 511–522. https://doi.org/10.1111/j.1476-5381.2010.00721.x.

Manrique-Garcia, E., Zammit, S., Dalman, C., Hemmingsson, T., & Allebeck, P. (2012). Cannabis use and depression: A longitudinal study of a national cohort of Swedish conscripts. *BMC Psychiatry, 12,* 112. https://doi.org/10.1186/1471-244X-12-112.

Marconi, A., Di Forti, M., Lewis, C. M., Murray, R. M., & Vassos, E. (2016). Meta-analysis of the association between the level of cannabis use and risk of psychosis. *Schizophrenia Bulletin, 42,* 1262–1269. https://doi.org/10.1093/schbul/sbw003.

Marcus, S. (2002). *Neuroethics: Mapping the field.* In *Proceedings of the landmark conference 2002, Stanford University and the University of California. Dana Foundation.*

Mathers, D. C., & Ghodse, A. H. (1992). Cannabis and psychotic illness. *The British Journal of Psychiatry,* 648–653.

McGee, R., Williams, S., Poulton, R., & Moffitt, T. (2000). A longitudinal study of cannabis use and mental health from adolescence to early adulthood. *Addiction, 95,* 491–503. https://doi.org/10.1046/j.1360-0443.2000.9544912.x.

Mcqueeny, T., Padula, C. B., Price, J., Lisdahl, K., Logan, P., & Tapert, S. F. (2011). Gender effects on amygdala morphometry in adolescent marijuana users. *Behavioural Brain Research, 224,* 128–134. https://doi.org/10.1016/j.bbr.2011.05.031.

Mechoulam, R., & Parker, L. A. (2013). The Endocannabinoid system and the brain. *Annual Review of Psychology, 64,* 21–47. https://doi.org/10.1146/annurev-psych-113011-143739.

Medina, K. L., Nagel, B. J., & Tapert, S. F. (2010). Abnormal cerebellar morphometry in abstinent adolescent marijuana users. *Psychiatry Research, 182,* 152–159. https://doi.org/10.1016/j.pscychresns.2009.12.004.Abnormal.

Medina, K. L., Ph, D., Mcqueeny, T., Nagel, B. J., Hanson, K. L., Yang, T. T., et al. (2009). Prefrontal cortex morphometry in abstinent adolescent marijuana users: Subtle gender effects. *Addiction Biology, 14,* 457–468. https://doi.org/10.1111/j.1369-1600.2009.00166.x .Prefrontal.

Meier, M. H., Caspi, A., Ambler, A., Harrington, H., Houts, R., Keefe, R. S. E., et al. (2012). Persistent cannabis users show neuropsychological decline from childhood to midlife. *Proceedings of the National Academy of Sciences, 109,* E2657–E2664. https://doi.org/10.1073/pnas.1206820109.

Meier, M. H., Hill, M. L., Small, P. J., & Luthar, S. S. (2015). Associations of adolescent cannabis use with academic performance and mental health: A longitudinal study of upper middle class youth. *Drug and Alcohol Dependence, 156,* 207–212. https://doi.org/10.1016/j.drugalcdep.2015.09.010.

Mokrysz, C., Landy, R., Gage, S. H., Munafò, M. R., Roiser, J. P., & Curran, H. V. (2016). Are IQ and educational outcomes in teenagers related to their cannabis use? A prospective cohort study. *Journal of Psychopharmacology, 30,* 159–168. https://doi.org/10.1177/0269881115622241.

Murray, R. M., & Di Forti, M. (2016). Cannabis and psychosis: What degree of proof do we require? Biol. *Psychiatry, 79,* 514–515. https://doi.org/10.1016/j.biopsych.2016.02.005.

Murray, R. M., Morrison, P. D., Henquet, C., & Di Forti, M. (2007). Cannabis, the mind and society: The hash realities. *Nature Reviews. Neuroscience, 8,* 885–895. https://doi.org/10.1038/nrn2253.

Negrete, J. C., Knapp, W. P., Douglas, D. E., & Smith, W. B. (1986). Cannabis affects the severity of schizophrenic symptoms: Results of a clinical survey. *Psychological Medicine, 16,* 515–520.

Nutt, D. J., King, L. A., & Nichols, D. E. (2013). Effects of schedule I drug laws on neuroscience research and treatment innovation. *Nature Reviews. Neuroscience, 14,* 577–585. https://doi.org/10.1038/nrn3530.

Ogrodnik, M., Kopp, P., Bongaerts, X., & Tecco, J. M. (2015). An economic analysis of different cannabis decriminalization scenarios. *Psychiatria Danubina, 27,* 309–314.

Osborne, S. (2018). *Medical cannabis to be available on prescription in UK after being approved for use by government.* https://www.independent.co.uk/news/health/medical-cannabis-uk-prescription-legal-epilepsy-pain-relief-home-office-moj-nhs-a8464766.html. (Accessed July 27, 2018).

Patton, G. C., Coffey, C., Carlin, J. B., Degenhardt, L., Lynskey, M., & Hall, W. (2002). Cannabis use and mental health in young people: Cohort study. *British Medical Journal, 325,* 1195–1198. https://doi.org/10.1136/bmj.325.7374.1195.

Pedersen, W., & Sandberg, S. (2013). The medicalisation of revolt: A sociological analysis of medical cannabis users. *Sociology of Health and Illness, 35,* 17–32. https://doi.org/10.1111/j.1467-9566.2012.01476.x.

Peters, E. N., Budney, A. J., & Carroll, K. M. (2012). Clinical correlates of co-occurring cannabis and tobacco use: A systematic review. *Addiction, 107,* 1404–1417. https://doi.org/10.1111/j.1360-0443.2012.03843.x.

Pope, H. G., Gruber, A. J., Hudson, J. I., Cohane, G., Huestis, M. A., & Yurgelun-Todd, D. (2003). Early-onset cannabis use and cognitive deficits: What is the nature of the association? *Drug and Alcohol Dependence, 69,* 303–310. https://doi.org/10.1016/S0376-8716(02)00334-4.

Racine, E., Bell, E., Zizzo, N., & Green, C. (2015). Public discourse on the biology of alcohol addiction: Implications for stigma, self-control, essentialism, and coercive policies in pregnancy. *Neuroethics, 8,* 177–186. https://doi.org/10.1007/s12152-014-9228-x.

Racine, E., Nguyen, V., Saigle, V., & Dubljevic, V. (2017). Media portrayal of a landmark neuroscience experiment on free will. *Science and Engineering Ethics, 23,* 989–1007. https://doi.org/10.1007/s11948-016-9845-3.

Racine, E., Sattler, S., & Escande, A. (2017). Free will and the brain disease model of addiction: The not so seductive allure of neuroscience and its modest impact on the attribution of free will to people with an addiction. *Frontiers in Psychology, 8,* 1–17. https://doi.org/10.3389/fpsyg.2017.01850.

Rey, J. M., Sawyer, M. G., Raphael, B., Patton, G. C., & Lynskey, M. (2002). Mental health of teenagers who use cannabis. *The British Journal of Psychiatry, 180,* 216–221. https://doi.org/10.1192/bjp.180.3.216.

Reynolds, J. R. (1890). Therapeutical uses and toxic effects of cannabis indica. *Lancet, 637*–638.

Robertson, S. (2018). *Where is cannabis legal around the world and where can you only use it for medicinal purposes?* https://metro.co.uk/2018/06/20/where-is-cannabis-legal-7645777/. (Accessed July 25, 2018).

Robinson, M., & Berke, J. (2018). *Here's where you can legally consume marijuana in the US in 2018.* UK: Bus. Insid. http://uk.businessinsider.com/where-can-you-can-legally-smoke-weed-2018-1/#alaska-1. (Accessed July 25, 2018).

Rubin, R. (2018). The path to the first FDA-approved Cannabis-derived treatment and what comes next. *JAMA, 320,* 1227–1229. https://doi.org/10.1001/JAMA.2018.11914.

Sagy, I., Peleg-Sagy, T., Barski, L., Zeller, L., & Jotkowitz, A. (2018). Ethical issues in medical cannabis use. *European Journal of Internal Medicine*, *49*, 20–22. https://doi.org/10.1016/j. ejim.2018.01.016.

Sahakian, B. J., Bruhl, A. B., Cook, J., Killikelly, C., Savulich, G., Piercy, T., et al. (2015). The impact of neuroscience on society: Cognitive enhancement in neuropsychiatric disorders and in healthy people. *Philosophical Tranactions of the Royal Society B*, 1–13. https://doi. org/10.1098/rstb.2014.0214.

Sahakian, B. J., & Morein-Zamir, S. (2015). Pharmacological cognitive enhancement: Treatment of neuropsychiatric disorders and lifestyle use by healthy people. *The Lancet Psychiatry*, *2*, 357–362. https://doi.org/10.1016/S2215-0366(15)00004-8.

Schuster, R. M., Fontaine, M., Nip, E., Zhang, H., Hanly, A., & Eden Evins, A. (2017). Prolonged cannabis withdrawal in young adults with lifetime psychiatric illness. *Preventive Medicine (Baltimore)*, *104*, 40–45. https://doi.org/10.1016/j.ypmed.2017.02.019.

Scott, J. C., Slomiak, S. T., Jones, J. D., Rosen, A. F. G., Moore, T. M., & Gur, R. C. (2018). Association of cannabis with cognitive functioning in adolescents and young adults. *JAMA Psychiatry*, *19104*, 585–595. https://doi.org/10.1001/jamapsychiatry.2018.0335.

Solowij, N., Jones, K. A., Rozman, M. E., Davis, S. M., Ciarrochi, J., Heaven, P. C. L., et al. (2011). Verbal learning and memory in adolescent cannabis users, alcohol users and non-users. *Psychopharmacology*, *216*, 131–144. https://doi.org/10.1007/s00213-011-2203-x.

Sowell, E. R., Thompson, P. M., Tessner, K. D., & Toga, A. W. (2001). Mapping continued brain growth and gray matter density reduction in dorsal frontal cortex: Inverse relationships during postadolescent brain maturation. *The Journal of Neuroscience*, *21*, 8819–8829. https://doi.org/21/22/8819.

Stefanis, N. C., Delespaul, P., Henquet, C., Bakoula, C., Stefanis, C. N., & Van Os, J. (2004). Early adolescent cannabis exposure and positive and negative dimensions of psychosis. *Addiction*, *99*, 1333–1341. https://doi.org/10.1111/j.1360-0443.2004.00806.x.

Stiby, A. I., Hickman, M., Munaf, M. R., Heron, J., Yip, V. L., & Macleod, J. (2015). Adolescent cannabis and tobacco use and educational outcomes at age 16: Birth cohort study. *Addiction*, *110*, 658–668. https://doi.org/10.1111/add.12827.

Substance Abuse and Mental Health Services Administration, 2014. Results from the 2013 National Survey on Drug Use and Health: Summary of National Findings. NSDUH Ser. H-48, HHS Publ. No. 14-4863. Rockville, MD Subst. Abus. Ment. Heal. Serv. Adm., 1–143, https://doi.org/NSDUHSeriesH-41, HHS Publication No. (SMA) 11-4658.

Surís, J. C., Berchtold, A., & Akre, C. (2015). Reasons to use e-cigarettes and associations with other substances among adolescents in Switzerland. *Drug and Alcohol Dependence*, *153*, 140–144. https://doi.org/10.1016/j.drugalcdep.2015.05.034.

Thornicroft, G. (1990). Cannabis and psychosis is there epidemiological evidence for an association? *British Journal of Psychiatry*, *157*, 25–33.

UK Government. (2018). *Drug penalties*. GOV.UK. https://www.gov.uk/penalties-drug-possession-dealing. (Accessed July 25, 2018).

Van Laar, M., Van Dorsselaer, S., Monshouwer, K., & De Graaf, R. (2007). Does cannabis use predict the first incidence of mood and anxiety disorders in the adult population? *Addiction*, *102*, 1251–1260. https://doi.org/10.1111/j.1360-0443.2007.01875.x.

Van Os, J., Bak, M., Hanssen, M., Bijl, R. V., De Graaf, R., & Verdoux, H. (2002). Cannabis use and psychosis: A longitudinal population-based study. *American Journal of Epidemiology*, *156*, 319–327. https://doi.org/10.1093/aje/kwf043.

Verweij, J. H. K., Anja, H. C., Agrawal, A., Nicholas, M. G., & Lynskey, T. M. (2013). Is the relationship between early-onset cannabis use and educational attainment causal or due to common liability? *Drug and Alcohol Dependence*, *31*, 1713–1723. https://doi.org/10.1109/ TMI.2012.2196707.Separate.

Viveros, M. P., Llorente, R., Suarez, J., Llorente-Berzal, A., López-Gallardo, M., & Rodriguez De Fonseca, F. (2012). The endocannabinoid system in critical neurodevelopmental periods: Sex differences and neuropsychiatric implications. *Journal of Psychopharmacology*, *26*, 164–176. https://doi.org/10.1177/0269881111408956.

Weiser, M., Knobler, H. Y., Noy, S., & Kaplan, Z. (2002). Invited Paper: Clinical characteristics of adolescents later hospitalized for schizophrenia. *American Journal of Medical Genetics*, *955*, 949–955. https://doi.org/10.1002/ajmg.10647.

Weissenborn, R., & Nutt, D. J. (2012). Popular intoxicants: What lessons can be learned from the last 40 years of alcohol and cannabis regulation? *Journal of Psychopharmacology*, *26*, 213–220. https://doi.org/10.1177/0269881111414751.

Wesley, M. J., Hanlon, C. A., & Porrino, L. J. (2011). Poor decision-making by chronic marijuana users is associated with decreased functional responsiveness to negative consequences. *Psychiatry Research*, *191*, 51–59.

Wiles, N. J., Zammit, S., Bebbington, P., Singleton, N., Meltzer, H., & Lewis, G. (2003). Self-reported psychotic symptoms in the general population results from the longitudinal study of the British National Psychiatric Morbidity Survey. *British Journal of Psychiatry*, *188*, 519–526.

Windle, M., & Wiesner, M. (2004). Trajectories of marijuana use from adolescence to young adulthood: Predictors and outcomes. *Development and Psychopathology*, *16*, 1007–1027. https://doi.org/10.1017/S0954579404040118.

Wise, J. (2018). FDA approves its first cannabis based medicine. *British Medical Journal*, https://doi.org/10.1136/bmj.k2827.

Zammit, S., Allebeck, P., Andreasson, S., Lundberg, I., & Lewis, G. (2002). Self reported cannabis use as a risk factor for historical cohort study. *British Medical Journal*, *325*, 1–5.

Zammit, S., Spurlock, G., Williams, H.Y.W.E.L., Norton, N., Williams, N., Donovan, M. C. O., et al. (2004). Genotype effects of CHRNA7, CNR1 and COMT in schizophrenia: interactions with tobacco and cannabis use. *British Journal of Psychiatry*, *191*, 402–427.

Further reading

Badiani, A., Belin, D., Epstein, D., Calu, D., & Shaham, Y. (2013). NIH public access. *Nature Reviews Neuroscience*, *12*, 685–700. https://doi.org/10.1021/nl061786n.Core-Shell.

Becker, J. B., & Chartoff, E. (2018). Sex differences in neural mechanisms mediating reward and addiction. *Neuropsychopharmacology*, https://doi.org/10.1038/s41386-018-0125-6.

Fernández-Serrano, M. J., Pérez-García, M., & Verdejo-García, A. (2011). What are the specific vs. generalized effects of drugs of abuse on neuropsychological performance? *Neuroscience and Biobehavioral Reviews*, *35*, 377–406. https://doi.org/10.1016/j.neubiorev.2010.04.008.

Hyman, S. E. (2005). A disease of learning and memory. *The American Journal of Psychiatry*, *162*, 1414–1422. https://doi.org/10.1176/appi.ajp.162.8.1414.

Hyman, S. E., Malenka, R. C., & Nestler, E. J. (2006). Neural mechanisms of addiction: The role of reward-related learning and memory. *Annual Review of Neuroscience*, *29*, 565–598. https://doi.org/10.1146/annurev.neuro.29.051605.113009.

Disease, wellness, and addiction: A global perspective

13

Anthony Barnett[a], Wayne Hall[b,c], Adrian Carter[a,d]
[a]School of Psychological Sciences and Turner Institute for Brain and Mental Health, Monash University, Melbourne, VIC, Australia, [b]Centre for Youth Substance Abuse Research, The University of Queensland, Brisbane, QLD, Australia, [c]National Addiction Centre, Institute of Psychiatry, Psychology and Neuroscience, Kings College London, London, United Kingdom, [d]University of Queensland Centre of Clinical Research, University of Queensland, Brisbane, QLD, Australia

Introduction

The global mental health movement (Becker & Kleinman, 2013; Patel, 2012; Stein & Giordano, 2015) has a critical role to play in addressing the burden of disease resulting from substance use disorders (SUDs). Global mental health is an emergent field that advocates for culturally appropriate forms of mental health care that can be scaled up to reduce the population impact of mental disorders across all nations and peoples, particularly lower income countries and socially marginalized populations. The global mental health movement assumes that access to healthcare is a human right and that there should be "no health without mental health" (Prince et al., 2007). It recognizes a global 90:10 research gap in which the vast majority of mental health research (90%) has been done in high-income countries (HICs) to the benefit of 10% of the world's population who live in those countries. The movement emphasizes that mental disorders remain underdiagnosed and undertreated across the world, with the widest treatment gap in low- and middle-income countries (LMICs) (Saxena, Paraje, Sharan, Karam, & Sadana, 2006). It advocates for evidence-based clinical practice while recognizing that mental disorders need to be understood within their sociocultural context (Stein & Giordano, 2015).

Within this consensus, however, there are varying philosophical approaches about how best to reduce the global burden of mental illness and drug addiction. In this chapter we review two prominent approaches that produce different priorities for global mental health. We contrast a more clinical, technology driven approach against one that emphasizes a population level approach to global mental health, and examine the effectiveness of each of these prioritization exercises in the area of drug addiction. In particular we look at the impact that drug addiction has globally, and critically analyze the effectiveness of the National Institute on Drug Abuse (NIDA) brain disease approach (Leshner, 1997; Volkow, Koob, & Mclellan, 2016) in reducing the global burden of drug addiction. We make some provisional recommendations about the most appropriate and effective approaches to global mental health in drug addiction, and reflect on the role of addiction neuroethics in guiding decisions about research investment.

Global Mental Health and Neuroethics. https://doi.org/10.1016/B978-0-12-815063-4.00013-7

Competing approaches to prioritizing global mental health

The US National Institute for Mental Health's (NIMH) *Grand Challenges in Global Mental Health* initiative identified priorities for research over the coming decade in order to improve the lives of people living with mental, neurological and substance-use (MNS) disorders (Collins et al., 2011). The key tenets of this initiative were that it: (1) had a global scope; (2) used the Delphi method; (3) covered the full range of MNS disorders; and (4) hoped to build a wide ranging community of research funders to help implement the research.

The prioritization exercise brought together the largest Delphi panel to consider global mental health research. It was guided by a scientific advisory board consisting of over 400 researchers, clinicians and program implementers working in more than 60 countries (Collins et al., 2011). Over a number of rounds, panelists were asked: "What are the grand challenges in global mental health?" that if successfully implemented, would aid in solving an important health problem.

The exercise identified 25 grand challenges for global mental health. These included research on the etiology and treatment of MNS disorders and the implementation of interventions targeting individuals experiencing drug addiction that may be scaled up to have a population impact. Importantly, NIMH's approach emphasized the role of neuroscientific and pharmacological research in delivering more effective treatments for MNS disorders. It argued that "…breakthroughs are likely to depend on discoveries in genomics and neuroscience, in tandem with exploration of the role of sociocultural and environmental contexts" (Collins et al., 2011, p. 3).

Another influential research prioritization exercise for global mental health emphasized a different vision of priorities. The *Lancet Mental Health Group* (Tomlinson et al., 2009) assessed priorities for a more efficient use of funds for global mental health research. Their assessment involved a systematic evaluation of research investment options for four broad classes of disorders, one of which was alcohol and other SUDs. Members of the group adopted a priority-setting approach that listed research questions and scored them using criteria such as answerability, effectiveness, deliverability, equity and potential impact on persisting burden of mental health disorders.

The *Lancet Mental Health Group* (Tomlinson et al., 2009) gave the highest priority to research on health policy and systems. These included research on how to deliver cost-effective interventions in low-resource settings, and epidemiological research on child and adolescent mental disorders including alcohol and other drugs of abuse. They gave the lowest priority to developing new interventions and new drugs or pharmacological interventions, vaccines or other technologies. The Lancet exercise concluded that critical knowledge gaps were best filled by research on health policy and systems, the epidemiology of disorders and better ways to deliver cost-effective interventions.

Priorities for the treatment of addiction

The NIMH prioritization of genomic and neuroscience research for global mental health research is reflected in the priorities for drug research led by NIDA

(Leshner, 1997; Volkow et al., 2016). In 1997, Alan Leshner, then director of NIDA, claimed that addiction was best understood as a chronic, relapsing brain disease and that advances in neuroscience research would substantially reduce the scale of the problem (Leshner, 1997). Researchers from NIDA argued that chronic drug use hijacks the brain's reward systems, making it difficult for people to stop using drugs and resulting in high rates of relapse (Dackis & O'Brien, 2005).

NIDA has invested heavily in neuroscience research in the strong belief that it will produce novel breakthrough treatments for addiction (Hall, Carter, & Forlini, 2015). Advocates of the BDMA claimed that it would deliver novel and more effective pharmacological treatments with fewer side effects to prevent drug addiction in vulnerable individuals (Kosten & Owens, 2005; Veilleux, Colvin, Anderson, York, & Heinz, 2010). Other promises include the use of direct brain interventions, such as deep brain stimulation (Luigjes et al., 2012), and neuroimaging technologies to better diagnose and treat people with addictions (Franken & van de Wetering, 2015; Lubman, 2007). Advocates of the NIDA approach have also claimed that it will benefit people with addictions by reducing moral judgment, stigma and discrimination, improving their access to quality health care and reducing the use of punitive approaches to addiction, such as imprisonment (Leshner, 1997; Volkow et al., 2016).

However, critics have argued that the BDMA may increase (rather than decrease) stigma for those with addictions and bias policies toward medical solutions to social problems (Hall, Carter, & Barnett, 2017; Hall, Carter, & Forlini, 2015; Hammer et al., 2013; Trujols, 2015). Opinions differ on the impact of the BDMA on treatment: some treatment providers see the BDMA as having potentially positive impacts for clients (e.g., increased insight into their condition, reduced self-blame), whereas others view the BDMA as having potential negative impacts (e.g., making people feel helpless about their recovery, reducing self-efficacy and treatment-seeking) (Barnett, Hall, Fry, Dilkes-Frayne, & Carter, 2018).

NIDA's focus on addiction neuroscience research and medical treatments of the individual (Hall, Carter, & Forlini, 2015) can be contrasted with support for more public health and health services research suggested by the *Lancet Mental Health Group's* prioritization exercise. In the remainder of the chapter we attempt to evaluate these differing visions, while paying particular attention to how they might reduce the scale of global addiction problems.

Substance use across the globe

Both NIMH and The Lancet group's global mental health exercises focussed on alcohol and SUDs, without discussing tobacco use. Given the health burden that tobacco represents across the globe and the co-morbidity of tobacco use with other drugs, we include it in our analysis of substance use. Tobacco policy and treatment also provides an instructive case for understanding the relative impacts of the NIMH and The Lancet group's approaches to research tackling addiction globally.

Tobacco

Cigarettes and other forms of tobacco smoking remain a significant and increasing burden on global public health (Jha et al., 2006; Jha, Ranson, Nguyen, & Yach, 2002; Ng et al., 2014). A systematic review of studies in 139 countries estimating worldwide smoking prevalence in 1995 (Jha et al., 2002), found that globally 29% of people aged 15 years or over were regular smokers. Of the world's 1.1 billion smokers in 1995, four-fifths lived in LMICs. Countries in East Asia accounted for a disproportionately high percentage (38%) of the world's smokers and four-fifths of all smokers were male. There were, however, large reductions in the prevalence of daily smoking from 1980 to 2012 (Institute for Health Metrics and Evaluation, 2018; Ng et al., 2014) at the global level, but due to population growth the number of daily smokers increased significantly over this period. From 1980 to 2012, it was estimated that the number of cigarettes consumed globally increased by approximately 26%.

In 2000, it was estimated that approximately 4.8 million (Ezzati & Lopez, 2003) premature deaths were attributable to smoking worldwide; a figure that has increased to 5.7 million in 2010 (Ng et al., 2014). In 2000, approximately half of these deaths occurred in LMICs (Ezzati & Lopez, 2003). The leading causes of death were cardiovascular diseases, chronic obstructive pulmonary disease, and lung cancer. Furthermore, a higher prevalence of smoking has been found in individuals experiencing mental illness (Lê Cook et al., 2014). In 2010, smoking remained among the top risk factors for global disease burden, with tobacco smoking, including second hand smoke, representing approximately 6% of global disability adjusted life years (DALYs) (Lim et al., 2012).

Alcohol

Generally, HICs have the highest levels of per capita alcohol consumption and prevalence of heavy episodic drinking. The highest alcohol consumption continues to be found in Europe and the Americas, with intermediate levels in the Western Pacific and African regions, and the lowest in South-East Asia and the Eastern Mediterranean (Griswold et al., 2018; World Health Organization, 2014). Worldwide between 2006 and 2010, there was an increase in per capita alcohol consumption. This was mainly driven by increased per capita alcohol consumption in China and India. Globally women drink less alcohol than men and have a lower prevalence of alcohol use disorders (World Health Organization, 2014).

DALYs attributable to alcohol use disorder varied by more than ten times between regions such as North Africa or the Middle East and Eastern Europe. The largest burden of disease for alcohol use disorders was found in the 25–50 age group, followed by a gradual decline with age (Whiteford et al., 2013). Globally, the age-standardized DALY rate (per 100,000) decreased for alcohol use disorders in both men and women between 1990 and 2010 (Whiteford, Ferrari, Degenhardt, Feigin, & Vos, 2015). In 2010, the global proportion of total DALYs for alcohol use disorder (including alcohol dependence and fetal alcohol syndrome) was 0.7% (Whiteford et al., 2015). Alcohol remains an important risk factor for premature mortality that disproportionally affects

LMICs, with more than 85% of global deaths attributable to alcohol in these nations (Medina-Mora et al., 2015).

Illicit drugs

Cannabis products (e.g., marijuana, hashish) remain the most widely used illicit drugs, followed by amphetamine-type stimulants (e.g., cocaine, methamphetamine) and illicit opioids (e.g., heroin, diverted pharmaceutical opioids) (UNODC, 2013). In 2010, the rates of opioid and cannabis dependence were higher in HICs than in LMICs; cocaine use and dependence rates were highest in North America and Latin America (Degenhardt et al., 2011); and rates of amphetamine dependence were be highest in Southeast Asia and Australasia (Degenhardt et al., 2014).

The proportion of DALYs attributed to illicit drug dependence was 20 times higher in some regions than others. The countries with the highest burden included the United States, United Kingdom, Russia, and Australia (Degenhardt et al., 2013). Illicit drug dependence (with opioid dependence the largest contributor) accounted for 20 million DALYs in 2010 and represented approximately 0.8% of all global DALYs (Degenhardt et al., 2013). Across the globe, the age-standardized DALY rate (per 100,000) increased for opioid dependence in both men and women, and remained stable for cocaine, amphetamine and cannabis dependence between 1990 and 2010 (Whiteford et al., 2015).

Comparing NIMH and the Lancet's approach to reducing the burden of SUDs

In this section we summarize evidence on the effectiveness of interventions and treatment for SUDs, paying particular attention to LMICs. We then assess how the NIMH and The Lancet group's research priorities fit with the existing evidence on interventions to reduce the harms of drug use and SUDs.

Tobacco

A growing body of studies in HICs has examined the efficacy of interventions in reducing demand for tobacco products (Jha & Chaloupka, 2000; Jha et al., 2006). Fewer studies have compared differences in the effectiveness of these interventions between HICs and LMICs. There is robust evidence from HICs and LMICs that increasing taxes on cigarettes and other tobacco products significantly reduces tobacco smoking (Chaloupka, Yurekli, & Fong, 2012; Farrelly, Pechacek, Thomas, & Nelson, 2008; Jha et al., 2006; US Department of Health Human Services, 2014; Wakefield et al., 2008). So does legislation restricting smoking in public and private places (e.g., smoking bans in workplaces) (Fichtenberg & Glantz, 2002), bans on cigarette advertising (World Health Organization, 2013), and counter-advertising campaigns (Friend & Levy, 2002) in HICs. However, most smokers in LMICs remain unaware of the risks of smoking because their governments have made little effort to inform them (Steptoe et al., 2002; Yang, Hammond, Driezen, Fong, & Jiang, 2010).

A number of pharmacological treatments are available to help smokers quit. These include nicotine replacement therapy (NRT), bupropion (Cahill, Stevens, Perera, & Lancaster, 2013) and varenicline. These treatments only modestly increase the success of quit attempts when given with psychological support and counseling. Policies that decrease the cost of pharmacological treatments and increase their availability may lead to significant increases in smoking cessation (Jha et al., 2006).

The substantial interest among smokers in new forms of nicotine delivery, such as e-cigarettes and nicotine vaporisers, has taken the tobacco control field by surprise and produced strongly polarized policy responses. Proponents see these as disruptive technologies that will accelerate the end of tobacco smoking by increasing quitting and providing a safer long-term alternative to combustible cigarettes (Gartner & Hall, 2016; McNeil et al., 2015). Their opponents see them as a threat to tobacco control that will allow the cigarette industry to subvert tobacco control policies, renormalize smoking and recruit new smokers (Grana, Benowitz, & Glantz, 2014; Kalkhoran & Glantz, 2016).

It has been very difficult to assess the plausibility of these radically different scenarios in the absence of good evidence on who uses these devices and how they are used. Most evidence to date has been limited to cross-sectional studies. Prospective studies are needed to clarify how many smokers are using them to quit and with what success.

Nations have adopted very different approaches to regulating e-cigarettes. Some have treated non-combustibles as a medical device/medicine for cessation use only, others as a tobacco product, and some as a general consumer good. Restricting smokers' access to nicotine vaporisers only when they are approved for use as medicines (as has occurred in Australia) may have the unintended effect of conferring a monopoly on products owned by the tobacco industry. Over-regulation of vaping products can also have the perverse effect of denying smokers access to a less harmful option, while allowing much more dangerous cigarettes to remain freely available (Hall, Gartner, & Forlini, 2015).

Under-regulation may also prevent smokers who could benefit from switching if consumers lack confidence in the safety of the devices and liquids. Finding the optimal regulatory sweet spot between prohibition and regulatory anarchy is a difficult task given the lack of consensus in the tobacco control community about how much regulation is necessary and what aspects of these products should be regulated and how. A similar challenge exists in finding the optimal regulatory framework for cannabis products in countries that have decriminalized it (Caulkins, Kilmer, & Kleiman, 2016).

Alcohol and illicit drugs

There are a range of interventions at the population, community and health care levels that have been identified as effective in reducing the harms of alcohol and illicit drug dependence. These are summarized in Table 1. Although this framework focuses

Table 1 Summary of interventions for alcohol and illicit drug dependence.

	Alcohol use and dependence[a]	Illicit drug use and dependence[b]
Population platform interventions	Prohibition, rationing, and partial bans Taxation Minimum Prices Restrictions on sales and advertising	Regulation (e.g., law enforcement) Awareness campaigns Inter-sector collaboration (e.g., court mandated treatment)
Community platform interventions	Family-based interventions Mass media campaigns	Workplace drug testing Drug education (incl. children and adolescents) Self-help groups (e.g., SMART Recovery)
Health care platform interventions	Screening and brief interventions Medical and social detoxification, counseling, follow up, and referral Self-help and support groups (e.g., AA)	Community based care (e.g., emergency naloxone provision) Specialist healthcare (e.g., detoxification and withdrawal) Brief psychological interventions Medications (e.g., MMT, sustained release naltrexone, medications for cannabis dependence)

[a] Medina-Mora et al. (2015).
[b] Degenhardt, Stockings, Strang, Marsden, and Hall (2015).
Table information adapted from Disease Control Priorities (3rd edition).

on alcohol and illicit drug dependence, similar approaches have been applied to interventions for behavioral addictions including gambling (cf. Gainsbury, Blankers, Wilkinson, Schelleman-Offermans, & Cousijn, 2014).

An evidence-based approach to global treatment of SUDs

A number of broad statements can be made about how the evidence on the effectiveness of polices to reduce tobacco and alcohol and illicit drug harm fits with the global mental health research priorities of NIMH's *Grand Challenges in Global Mental Health* initiative and the *Lancet Mental Health Group*. Firstly, there is strong evidence in HICs, and to a lesser degree in LMICs, supporting the efficacy of increased tobacco taxes, legislation restricting smoking in public places, bans of advertising, and public health campaigns on the risks of smoking in reducing tobacco smoking. In Asia, which has a disproportionately high proportion of the world's smokers there will be major benefits from research on how to implement these policies. The *Lancet Mental Health Group's* prioritization of health policy and systems research is supported by robust evidence about the effectiveness of population level demand reduction initiatives.

There is also evidence that pharmacological treatments (e.g., NRT, bupropion, varenicline) are only modestly effective in increasing the success of quit attempts when combined with psychosocial interventions. In this regard, NIMH's prioritization in global mental health funding for research exploring the etiology and treatment of SUDs and addiction may have benefits for tobacco use reduction in the future. This may occur after population level approaches have reduced the prevalence of smoking to a low level, as has happened in some HICs. However, these pharmacological treatments are rarely provided with the sorts of psychosocial interventions that trials show are required for their efficacy. Effectiveness and cost-effectiveness studies would need to take this into consideration when examining the role of pharmacological treatments, particularly in LMICs with limited resources and infrastructure to provide ongoing counseling and psychosocial support.

Our synthesis of strategies to address alcohol and illicit drug dependence drawn from the Disease Control Priorities report (Degenhardt et al., 2015; Medina-Mora et al., 2015) describes interventions on three levels (see Table 1): population platform; community platform; and health care platform interventions. The *Lancet Mental Health Group's* priorities for global mental health funding aligns with the two higher level platforms. For example, future research in LMICs exploring taxation and restriction of sales for alcohol, and the regulation of illicit drugs at the population platform level, fit better with The Lancet group's global mental health research prioritization strategy than that of NIMH.

There is an important role for the assessment and treatment of individuals who are dependent on alcohol and illicit drugs. Health care interventions (see Table 1) include screening and brief interventions and medical detoxification that may reduce the burden of alcohol dependence. Naloxone provision, specialist detoxification and withdrawal services, and pharmacotherapies (e.g., opioid replacements therapies) have scope to reduce harm related to illicit drug use and dependence in HIC and LMICs. NIMH's research priorities to examine the etiology and treatment of substance use and the effectiveness of policies to scale up access to interventions align with evidence supporting these health care interventions. So too does the *Lancet Mental Health Group's* prioritization of research on health systems and research on improved delivery of cost-effective interventions.

In LMICs epidemiological research and better surveillance systems are critical to understand the prevalence, patterns and harms of SUDs in these countries. Both the *Lancet Mental Health Group's* and NIMH's prioritization exercises include epidemiological research as a focus area in order to better capture the prevalence of SUDs in LMICs.

However, in contrast to the *Lancet Mental Health Group's* approach, one of the defining features of NIMH's global health research priorities is the importance attached to curiosity driven research in genomics and neuroscience. NIMH's approach runs the risk of being overly optimistic about how soon neuroscience research might produce breakthrough treatments. Critically, lessons can be learnt from the translational failures that have characterized NIDA's focus on neuroscience research to deliver new treatments. Although there continues to be a debate about whether or not addiction is a brain disease, there is more agreement that the promises made by Leshner that addiction neuroscience would lead to improved treatment (such as novel pharmacotherapies) remain unfulfilled. Leshner predicted over 20 years ago that the BDMA would deliver more effective drug vaccines and long-acting, implantable drugs to reduce relapse; pharmacogenomic tests to match patients to the most effective treatment; drugs to modulate the stress response or the salience of drug-related cues; and most recently, drugs to reverse epigenetic changes produced by chronic drug use (Hall, Carter, & Forlini, 2015).

Despite NIDA investing over US$1 billion a year on addiction research, the vast majority on neurobiological or clinical research (Hall, Carter, & Forlini, 2015), the most widely used treatments for addiction remain those that were discovered over three decades ago before the exponential increase in addiction neuroscience research (e.g., methadone, NRT). Despite almost three decades of neuroscience research, very few of the clinical promises espoused by the BDMA have been realized (Hall, Carter, & Forlini, 2015; Kalant, 2010). During this time, population-based policy approaches have reduced smoking rates from around 50% to under 15% in some countries. This failure would suggest that a population-based, public health approach as described by The Lancet group would yield more effective and cost-effective results in reducing disease burden sooner in LMICs.

Is there a role for neuroethics in setting funding priorities?

Two expert led prioritization exercises have reached conclusions that emphasize differing priorities about where research funds should be allocated in global mental health research. Does *addiction neuroethics* (Carter & Hall, 2011) as a discipline have a useful role to play in deciding between these competing views?

There have already been a number of suggestions made about how neuroethics might assist the global mental health movement. Stein and Giordano (2015) noted that historically the two fields have had little interaction and outlined some important differences between the fields that may explain why. They argued that: (1) global mental health has focused on reducing problems in LMICs, while neuroethics has focussed more on ethical issues most relevant to Western HICs; (2) global mental health has focussed on implementation science while neuroethics has more often focussed on ethical issues raised by new neurotechnologies and novel interventions being developed in HICs; and (3) global mental health has emphasized the value of employing community health workers for mental health interventions, whereas neuroethics has explored technological procedures such as neuroimaging and deep brain stimulation that require significant costs and infrastructure and highly trained medical and other staff to implement them. These differences reflect the historical development of neuroethics as a field, rather than any inherent priorities in a neuroethical approach.

Nonetheless, Stein and Giordano (2015) argued that global mental health and neuroethics have a number of converging perspectives that may enable collaboration. They specifically suggested that neuroethics might explore issues that arise at the intersection between global mental health and clinical neuroscience, such as, what constitutes disease and wellness, human rights issues in neuropsychiatric care, and the value of inclusion and patient empowerment in service delivery.

We agree with Stein and Giordano's (2015) view. The field of neuroethics and its engagement with global mental health research needs to broaden its focus to engage with wider debates in bioethics about the rationing of scarce resources to addiction research to reduce the global burden caused by these disorders. Such approaches, commonly considered within healthcare research funding allocation, are informed by cost-benefit analyses and economic evaluations with the aim of maximizing health outcomes by use of the most cost effective interventions with the largest public health impacts. In doing so, neuroethics may overcome the criticism that it is overly focused on neurotechnologies in HICs. In the context of global mental health, neuroethics has an important contribution to make in influencing decisions on where funding for addiction neuroscience research might best be invested. Furthermore, it is vital for neuroethics research to explore the social impact of neuroscientific discourses by ex-amining how clinicians, policy makers and service users view the role of the brain in addiction in LMICs.

One of the difficulties with deciding how to allocate resources to maximize health benefits is uncertainty about what future benefits may accrue from curiosity driven research (Sassi, Archard, & Le Grand, 2001). This issue is particularly salient for genomics and neuroscience research on SUDs and addiction. As we and others have argued, despite a sustained financial investment in addiction neuroscience, the brain disease paradigm has not yet fulfilled the promises of delivering more effective ther-apies for addiction problems promised by Alan Leshner in 1997 (Hall, Carter, & Forlini, 2015; Heather et al., 2017; Kalant, 2010; Lewis, 2015). In view of this, the current level of investment in genomics and neuroscience assumed by NIMH's *Grand Challenges in Global Mental Health* initiative may not be justified.

We support some funding of speculative curiosity driven research. Science and medicine as a profession has a duty to advance scientific knowledge and pursue novel therapies by investing in research with more speculative longer term benefits. Investment in scientific and medical research also provides economic benefits in terms of increased employment and industrial development. However, these are seldom the goals used to justify investment in medical research and innovation which stress the short term benefits of the research. It is a question of balance in which more weight should be given to funding health services research than blue sky research than has been the case at NIDA over the past three decades.

Conclusion

Two prioritization exercises for global mental health research on SUDs have produced different recommendations on where research funding should be allocated to improve global mental health. On the one hand, NIMH has prioritized research on the etiology and treatment of MNS disorders, with an emphasis on the role of genomic, neuro-scientific and pharmacological research to deliver more effective treatments. On the other, The Lancet group's prioritization exercise recommended that critical knowledge gaps were best filled by research on health policy and systems, epidemiology and the improved delivery of cost-effective interventions.

NIMH's prioritization of research on the etiology of SUDs may have limited benefits for health care interventions in the future, for example, in medical detoxification and pharmacotherapies. However, The Lancet group's commitment to a population-based, public health approach to treating SUDs across the globe is likely to yield more cost-effective and timely results, especially in LMICs. NIMH's commitment to speculative neuroscience research is likely to face the same translational difficulties as NIDA has with its focus on addiction neuroscience research at the expense of public health interventions and health services research. In the future, a greater participation by addiction neuroethics may improve debates on how funding and other resources are allocated toward addiction research globally.

References

Barnett, A. I., Hall, W., Fry, C. L., Dilkes-Frayne, E., & Carter, A. (2018). Drug and alcohol treatment providers' views about the disease model of addiction and its impact on clinical practice: A systematic review. *Drug and Alcohol Review*, *37*(6), 697–720.

Becker, A. E., & Kleinman, A. (2013). Mental health and the global agenda. *New England Journal of Medicine*, *369*(1), 66–73.

Cahill, K., Stevens, S., Perera, R., & Lancaster, T. (2013). Pharmacological interventions for smoking cessation: An overview and network meta-analysis. *Cochrane Database of Systematic Reviews*, (5), https://doi.org/10.1002/14651858.CD009329.pub2.

Carter, A., & Hall, W. (2011). *Addiction neuroethics: The promises and perils of neuroscience research on addiction*. Cambridge University Press.

Caulkins, J. P., Kilmer, B., & Kleiman, M. A. (2016). *Marijuana legalization: What everyone needs to know*. Oxford University Press.

Chaloupka, F. J., Yurekli, A., & Fong, G. T. (2012). Tobacco taxes as a tobacco control strategy. *Tobacco Control*, *21*(2), 172–180.

Collins, P. Y., Patel, V., Joestl, S. S., March, D., Insel, T. R., Daar, A. S., et al. (2011). Grand challenges in global mental health. *Nature*, *475*(7354), 27.

Dackis, C., & O'Brien, C. (2005). Neurobiology of addiction: Treatment and public policy ramifications. *Nature Neuroscience*, *8*(11), 1431.

Degenhardt, L., Baxter, A. J., Lee, Y. Y., Hall, W., Sara, G. E., Johns, N., et al. (2014). The global epidemiology and burden of psychostimulant dependence: Findings from the Global Burden of Disease Study 2010. *Drug & Alcohol Dependence*, *137*, 36–47.

Degenhardt, L., Bucello, C., Calabria, B., Nelson, P., Roberts, A., Hall, W., et al. (2011). What data are available on the extent of illicit drug use and dependence globally? Results of four systematic reviews. *Drug & Alcohol Dependence*, *117*(2), 85–101.

Degenhardt, L., Stockings, E., Strang, J., Marsden, J., & Hall, W. (2015). Illicit drug dependence. In V. Patel, D. Chisholm, T. Dua, R. Laxminarayan, & M. E. Medina-Mora (Eds.), *Disease control priorities third edition: Mental, neurological, and substance use disorders*. Washington: International Bank for Reconstruction and Development/The World Bank.

Degenhardt, L., Whiteford, H. A., Ferrari, A. J., Baxter, A. J., Charlson, F. J., Hall, W. D., et al. (2013). Global burden of disease attributable to illicit drug use and dependence: Findings from the Global Burden of Disease Study 2010. *The Lancet*, *382*(9904), 1564–1574.

Ezzati, M., & Lopez, A. D. (2003). Estimates of global mortality attributable to smoking in 2000. *The Lancet*, *362*(9387), 847–852.

Farrelly, M. C., Pechacek, T. F., Thomas, K. Y., & Nelson, D. (2008). The impact of tobacco control programs on adult smoking. *American Journal of Public Health*, *98*(2), 304–309.

Fichtenberg, C. M., & Glantz, S. A. (2002). Effect of smoke-free workplaces on smoking behaviour: Systematic review. *BMJ*, *325*(7357), 188.

Franken, I. H. A., & van de Wetering, B. J. M. (2015). Bridging the gap between the neurocognitive lab and the addiction clinic. *Addictive Behaviors*, *44*, 108–114.

Friend, K., & Levy, D. T. (2002). Reductions in smoking prevalence and cigarette consumption associated with mass-media campaigns. *Health Education Research*, *17*(1), 85–98.

Gainsbury, S. M., Blankers, M., Wilkinson, C., Schelleman-Offermans, K., & Cousijn, J. (2014). Recommendations for international gambling harm-minimisation guidelines: Comparison with effective public health policy. *Journal of Gambling Studies*, *30*(4), 771–788.

Gartner, C., & Hall, W. (2016). *Assessing the place of nicotine vaporisers in tobacco control.* BMJ Publishing Group Ltd.

Grana, R., Benowitz, N., & Glantz, S. A. (2014). E-cigarettes: A scientific review. *Circulation*, *129*(19), 1972–1986.

Griswold, M. G., Fullman, N., Hawley, C., Arian, N., Zimsen, S. R., Tymeson, H. D., et al. (2018). Alcohol use and burden for 195 countries and territories, 1990–2016: A systematic analysis for the Global Burden of Disease Study 2016. *The Lancet*, *392*(10152), 1015–1035.

Hall, W., Carter, A., & Barnett, A. (2017). Disease or developmental disorder: Competing perspectives on the neuroscience of addiction. *Neuroethics*, *10*(1), 103–110.

Hall, W., Carter, A., & Forlini, C. (2015). The brain disease model of addiction: Is it supported by the evidence and has it delivered on its promises? *The Lancet Psychiatry*, *2*(1), 105–110.

Hall, W., Gartner, C., & Forlini, C. (2015). Ethical issues raised by a ban on the sale of electronic nicotine devices. *Addiction*, *110*(7), 1061–1067.

Hammer, R., Dingel, M., Ostergren, J., Partridge, B., Mccormick, J., & Koenig, B. A. (2013). Addiction: Current criticism of the brain disease paradigm. *AJOB Neuroscience*, *4*(3), 27–32.

Heather, N., Best, D., Kawalek, A., Field, M., Lewis, M., Rotgers, F., et al. (2017). *Challenging the brain disease model of addiction: European launch of the addiction theory network.* Taylor & Francis.

Institute for Health Metrics and Evaluation. (2018). *Smoking and tobacco.* Seattle, WA: University of Washington. Available from: http://www.healthdata.org/smoking-tobacco (Accessed July 25, 2018).

Jha, P., & Chaloupka, F. J. (2000). *Tobacco control in developing countries.* Oxford University Press.

Jha, P., Chaloupka, F. J., Moore, J., Gajalakshmi, V., Gupta, P. C., Peck, R., et al. (2006). *Tobacco addiction.*

Jha, P., Ranson, M. K., Nguyen, S. N., & Yach, D. (2002). Estimates of global and regional smoking prevalence in 1995, by age and sex. *American Journal of Public Health*, *92*(6), 1002–1006.

Kalant, H. (2010). What neurobiology cannot tell us about addiction. *Addiction*, *105*(5), 780–789.

Kalkhoran, S., & Glantz, S. A. (2016). E-cigarettes and smoking cessation in real-world and clinical settings: A systematic review and meta-analysis. *The Lancet Respiratory Medicine*, *4*(2), 116–128.

Kosten, T., & Owens, S. M. (2005). Immunotherapy for the treatment of drug abuse. *Pharmacology & Therapeutics*, *108*(1), 76–85.

Lê Cook, B., Wayne, G. F., Kafali, E. N., Liu, Z., Shu, C., & Flores, M. (2014). Trends in smoking among adults with mental illness and association between mental health treatment and smoking cessation. *JAMA*, *311*(2), 172–182.

Leshner, A. I. (1997). Addiction is a brain disease, and it matters. [Cover story]. *Science*, *278*(5335), 45–47.

Lewis, M. (2015). *The biology of desire: Why addiction is not a disease*. Public Affairs.

Lim, S. S., Vos, T., Flaxman, A. D., Danaei, G., Shibuya, K., Adair-Rohani, H., et al. (2012). A comparative risk assessment of burden of disease and injury attributable to 67 risk factors and risk factor clusters in 21 regions, 1990–2010: A systematic analysis for the Global Burden of Disease Study 2010. *The Lancet*, *380*(9859), 2224–2260.

Lubman, D. I. (2007). Addiction neuroscience and its relevance to clinical practice. *Drug and Alcohol Review*, *26*(1), 1–2.

Luigjes, J., Van Den Brink, W., Feenstra, M., Van Den Munckhof, P., Schuurman, P., Schippers, R., et al. (2012). Deep brain stimulation in addiction: A review of potential brain targets. *Molecular Psychiatry*, *17*(6), 572–583.

McNeil, A., Brose, L., Calder, R., Hitchman, S., Hajek, P., & Mcrobbie, H. (2015). *E-cigarettes: An evidence update. A report commissioned by Public Health England*. Public Health England.111.

Medina-Mora, M. E., Monteiro, M., Room, R., Rehm, J. R., Jernigan, D., Sánchez-Moreno, D., et al. (2015). Alcohol use and alcohol use disorders. In V. Patel, D. Chisholm, T. Dua, R. Laxminarayan, & M. E. Medina-Mora (Eds.), *Disease control priorities third edition: Mental, neurological, and substance use disorders*. Washington, DC: International Bank for Reconstruction and Development/The World Bank.

Ng, M., Freeman, M. K., Fleming, T. D., Robinson, M., Dwyer-Lindgren, L., Thomson, B., et al. (2014). Smoking prevalence and cigarette consumption in 187 countries, 1980–2012. *JAMA*, *311*(2), 183–192.

Patel, V. (2012). Global mental health: From science to action. *Harvard Review of Psychiatry*, *20*(1), 6–12.

Prince, M., Patel, V., Saxena, S., Maj, M., Maselko, J., Phillips, M. R., et al. (2007). No health without mental health. *The Lancet*, *370*(9590), 859–877.

Sassi, F., Archard, L., & Le Grand, J. (2001). Equity and the economic evaluation of healthcare. *Health Technology Assessment (Winchester, England)*, *5*(3), 1.

Saxena, S., Paraje, G., Sharan, P., Karam, G., & Sadana, R. (2006). The 10/90 divide in mental health research: Trends over a 10-year period. *The British Journal of Psychiatry*, *188*(1), 81–82.

Stein, D. J., & Giordano, J. (2015). Global mental health and neuroethics. *BMC Medicine*, *13*(1), 44.

Steptoe, A., Wardle, J., Cui, W., Baban, A., Glass, K., Tsuda, A., et al. (2002). An international comparison of tobacco smoking, beliefs and risk awareness in university students from 23 countries. *Addiction*, *97*(12), 1561–1571.

Tomlinson, M., Rudan, I., Saxena, S., Swartz, L., Tsai, A. C., & Patel, V. (2009). Setting priorities for global mental health research. *Bulletin of the World Health Organization*, *87*(6), 438–446.

Trujols, J. (2015). The brain disease model of addiction: Challenging or reinforcing stigma? *The Lancet Psychiatry*, *2*(4), 292.

UNODC. (2013). *World drug report 2013*.

US Department of Health Human Services. (2014). *The health consequences of smoking—50 years of progress: A report of the surgeon general*. Atlanta, GA: US Department of

Health and Human Services, Centers for Disease Control and Prevention, National Center for Chronic Disease Prevention and Health Promotion, Office on Smoking and Health.17.

Veilleux, J. C., Colvin, P. J., Anderson, J., York, C., & Heinz, A. J. (2010). A review of opioid dependence treatment: Pharmacological and psychosocial interventions to treat opioid addiction. *Clinical Psychology Review*, *30*(2), 155–166.

Volkow, N. D., Koob, G. F., & Mclellan, A. T. (2016). Neurobiologic advances from the brain disease model of addiction. *New England Journal of Medicine*, *374*(4), 363–371.

Wakefield, M. A., Durkin, S., Spittal, M. J., Siahpush, M., Scollo, M., Simpson, J. A., et al. (2008). Impact of tobacco control policies and mass media campaigns on monthly adult smoking prevalence. *American Journal of Public Health*, *98*(8), 1443–1450.

Whiteford, H. A., Degenhardt, L., Rehm, J., Baxter, A. J., Ferrari, A. J., Erskine, H. E., et al. (2013). Global burden of disease attributable to mental and substance use disorders: Findings from the Global Burden of Disease Study 2010. *The Lancet*, *382*(9904), 1575–1586.

Whiteford, H. A., Ferrari, A. J., Degenhardt, L., Feigin, V., & Vos, T. (2015). The global burden of mental, neurological and substance use disorders: An analysis from the Global Burden of Disease Study 2010. In V. Patel, D. Chisholm, T. Dua, R. Laxminarayan, & M. E. Medina-Mora (Eds.), *Mental, neurological, and substance use disorders*. (3rd ed.).

World Health Organization. (2013). *WHO report on the global tobacco epidemic, 2013: Enforcing bans on tobacco advertising, promotion and sponsorship*. World Health Organization.

World Health Organization. (2014). *Global status report on alcohol and health, 2014*. World Health Organization.

Yang, J., Hammond, D., Driezen, P., Fong, G. T., & Jiang, Y. (2010). Health knowledge and perception of risks among Chinese smokers and non-smokers: Findings from the Wave 1 ITC China Survey. *Tobacco Control*, *19*(Suppl 2), i18–i23.

Further reading

American Society of Addiction Medicine. (2011). *Public policy statement: Definition of addiction* Available from: http://www.asam.org/for-the-public/definition-of-addiction.

Office of National Drug Control Policy. (2014). *National drug control strategy*.

Disease and wellness across the lifespan: A global perspective on the mental health burden of dementia

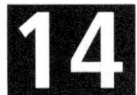

Veljko Dubljević
Science Technology and Society Program, Department of Philosophy and Religious Studies, North Carolina State University, Raleigh, NC, United States

Introduction

Dementia, and especially behavioral variant frontotemporal dementia (bvFTD), which I will focus on in this chapter, reverses the hard won freedoms and rights that are enjoyed by most adult human beings. We take for granted that we have the right to drive, control our finances and property, vote and drink (Dubljević, 2013). Yet, with the onset of dementia, there is widespread recognition that deficits in cognitive and decisional faculties are sufficiently pronounced that such rights—and indeed, autonomy in general—need to be curbed.

However, it is the specific nature of the behavioral variant frontotemporal dementia that impedes this recognition until it is too late.[a] BvFTD cases are the most common type of frontotemporal dementia (Chare et al., 2014), and are characterized by the absence of obvious cognitive impairment (Lanata & Miller, 2016). BvFTD is recognized by presence of symptoms such as disinhibition, social inappropriateness, personality changes, hyper-sexuality and hyper-orality (Rascovsky et al., 2011) along with markedly impaired socio-moral judgments (Manes et al., 2011). Individuals in early stages of bvFTD—that is, before the family intervenes and curbs their autonomy—usually commit immoral and illegal acts that have lasting repercussions (Mendez, Anderson, & Shapira, 2005). The disease starts with disinhibition and leads to frontotemporal lobar degeneration, also known as "Pick's disease" (Birkhoff, Garberi, & Re, 2016). The prognosis is poor, and, as in other types of dementia, bvFTD ultimately ends in death, in most cases approximately 5 years after the diagnosis has been made (Chare et al., 2014). In the early stages of the disease progression, the affected person starts making decisions and actions that are increasingly disinhibited and socially inappropriate while at the same time manifesting a lack of concern. This lack of concern is evident in behaviors and responses regarding social standing and expectations as well as financial decisions (Rascovsky et al., 2011).

Based on clinical and statistical data alone, it is very hard to imagine what it is like to interact with bvFTD patients. The lack of "qualitative" experience of interacting

---

[a] In this paragraph, I draw on Dubljević (2019).

Global Mental Health and Neuroethics. https://doi.org/10.1016/B978-0-12-815063-4.00014-9

with these individuals as human beings is easily populated with social stereotypes, misinformation and outright prejudice. I have had the opportunity to meet, observe and talk with two bvFTD patients and their families as part of my research visit to a prestigious medical center.[b] In what follows, I will describe my encounters with persons that were part of a comprehensive research program on bvFTD and reflect on what is known about the social and ethical impacts of dementia, most notably in terms of mental health burdens and stigma. I will end with a message of hope: the people I talked to won me over, and I feel the need to speak on their behalf—to advocate for and praise efforts of de-stigmatization, prevention of discrimination, and inclusion of the perspective of individuals living with dementia in social debates on their future and well-being. Not knowing what to expect, I assumed that bvFTD patients would be callous and immoral individuals, interested only in themselves and their short-term pleasure. I was very wrong about that.

Conversations with Jake and Barbara

I first had the opportunity to interact with Jake. While I was sitting in the medical center's waiting room for the chance to observe a cognitive testing procedure with an early stage bvFTD patient, an energetic 60-year-old engaged me in a conversation by noting the quality of my leather satchel and asking me where I bought it. He seemed very friendly and eager to share advice on the best places to find good seafood with someone who was obviously a newcomer to his birthplace. He soon found out that he and I had much in common: I live in North Carolina, and his son recently graduated from a prestigious university there. If I was surprised by his straightforward and direct manner, this was counterbalanced by the obvious goodwill and trustworthiness he seemed to radiate. When he asked me if I thought that there are many racists in North Carolina, I had to concede that indeed there are some. Just as he told me that his wife died 8 years ago, our conversation was interrupted by the clinical research assistant: it was time to observe the cognitive testing and it turned out that my waiting room acquaintance was Jake, the patient being tested today. He noted that, of course, he wouldn't object to me being there. His daughter, Barbara, told me afterwards that she had qualms about outside observers, but she is still coming to terms with his illness and doesn't want to contradict Jake unless she has to.

I found in observing Jake that his cognitive skills are fairly good: he is good with numbers and words, and if he can't remember who wrote Hamlet, it could be explained by his lack of formal education. As he jokingly noted, he prefers reading magazines to "those Russian bores," and that's why he chose to be self-employed in his butcher shop and not seek higher education and work as an architect or an engineer. It appeared that his quick wit had served him well: he said that his butcher shop supplied

---

[b] Due to the need to protect the privacy of patients and family members, their names have been changed and details about the place where the encounters took place are omitted.

catering to the hotel I stayed in, and he boasted about the size of his yacht, the speed of his new truck, and how big his house and garden are ("I've never felt better in my life"). After a prompting from the clinical research assistant, he conceded that he had to retire 2 years ago due to the onset of his illness ("it was time to leave work to others and enjoy life"), but it seems his past financial success could provide him with many comforts, including a gardener. This information was later confirmed by Barbara, who had also warmed up to me after her initial distrust. She maintained a wary expression at all times and explained that people had taken advantage of Jake in the past ("he is too trusting of strangers – I worry about him a lot"). As Jake's main family contact, Barbara is torn between work and looking after her father: he lives alone, with paid help, but she worries what he may do.

Indeed, Jake's cognitive deficits are very subtle, yet his disinhibition is what makes him at the same time very happy and a danger for his own future. I will say more about Jake's and Barbara's prospects after I have introduced another patient I interacted with: Dan.

Conversations with Dan and Jane

Unlike Jake, Dan was examined together with Jane, his wife. The need for that became obvious immediately: while Dan happily related that there were no problems ("I am happy, I have a good wife"), his wife Jane added crucial pieces of information. When asked about his financial situation, Dan, who used to be a professional driver, shrugged and said: "I feel like the same guy, but then they take my driver's license." Jane added that this is with good reason and happened after he was involved in a "hit and run" incident in March of 2015. Dan shrugged again and told us that it was "no big deal," that now he is used to not driving and that he actually prefers to be driven around. After the examining neurologist asked him if he was always ok with that, Dan told us that he might have been a bit upset before. Jane informed us that Dan used to have crying episodes: he was actually very upset about not having a job and not being able to drive. After a prompting from the neurologist, Dan said: "I've accepted it, I feel lucky." Jane, on the contrary, confided that the crying episodes lasted for a year and a half and that they got so bad that Dan tried to take all of his medication at once and die. After that time, Jane realized she had to retire from her job and take over managing most aspects of Dan's life.

Gradually, the neurologist and I were informed, Dan lost all of his usual freedoms. After engaging in shopping sprees (he spent $2500 on materials to build a sauna), Jane canceled all his credit cards. After an incident where Dan cut off a tip of his finger while woodworking, she locked up his tools. After a period of 6 months in which he was obsessively watching pornographic content, Jane disconnected his Internet access. After Dan started rapidly gaining weight due to cravings for unhealthy food, she limited the size of his portions. When Dan wanted to engage me in a side conversation about his many hobbies, Jane squeezed his hand and told him: "let's not bore other people with this." Dan seemed to take all this in stride: "You learn to accept it, otherwise you're gonna go crazy."

The problem

Here lies the crux of the matter I am exploring in this chapter. As the population around the world ages and prevalence of dementias such as those affecting Jake and Dan increases, more and more mental health issues will arise, either as co-morbidities or due to considerable strain on care-givers and family. In the spirit of using qualitative methods in empirical neuroethics, I have chosen to showcase the global mental health burden of dementia by putting human faces and names (Jake, Barbara, Dan and Jane as well as others) to a mounting problem that is usually treated as a mere statistic.

So, let's start with some facts and follow up by putting a face, name and subjective experience to them. The world is aging rapidly and transitioning to an "aging society," where the number of people over people in later life stages outweighs the number being born. This transition has taken decades in the developed nations in the West, such as United States (U.S. Congress, Office of Technology Assessment [OTA], 1987), but it is much more pronounced in developing countries such as Vietnam, where the change is so rapid that it occurred in one generation (Cheng, Chou, & Zarit, 2013). The rising burden of aging and accompanying complications cause immense human suffering and pose unprecedented challenges for society, most notably for families, healthcare, and even the justice system. For example, dementia not only progressively destroys essential mental functions such as memory and socio-moral decision making, but it is also an incredibly costly chronic disease (Ramos & Koroshetz, 2017). It was reported that there were 36 million people living with dementia worldwide in 2010, and it is estimated that this number will increase to 66 million by 2030 and 115 million by 2050 (Batsch & Mittelman, 2012). The global cost of dementia in 2010 was reported at $604 billion (Family Caregiver Alliance, 2016). In addition, the World Health Organization estimated that there were 7.7 million new cases of dementia in the year 2010, or one new case every 4 seconds (World Health Organization [WHO], 2012).

The number of adults (such as Jane and Barbara) that provide care to relatives with dementia (such as Jake and Dan) is also growing. In the United States, it is estimated that 15.7 million adult family caregivers look after a person with dementia (Family Caregiver Alliance, 2016). It is estimated that 75% of the care for persons with dementia is provided directly by family, while 25% represents services purchased by family members (Schulz & Martire, 2004). At $470 billion in 2013, the value of unpaid caregiving exceeded the value of paid home care and total Medicaid spending in the same year, and it nearly matched the value of the sales of the world's largest company (Family Caregiver Alliance, 2016). Upwards of 75% of all caregivers are female, and they may spend as much as 50% more time providing care than males.

Family members provide care at substantial personal cost and risk to their own psychological and physical wellbeing (Sorensen, Duberstein, Gill, & Pinquart, 2006). A few examples might help put things into perspective. Even innocuous sounding deficits that dementia patients experience, such as "having trouble organizing time" can have an enormous burden on family members. In case of Dan, his wife Jane relates that he often wakes up in the middle of the night and dresses to go to work. Apart from losing sleep, family caregivers like Jane have to deal with managing behavior of their loved ones and dealing with an emotional burden of lack of understanding and social support (more on that below). The key problem is that at times, interactions with a person suffering from dementia can be severely mentally taxing. Jane tells that "[In the] first three hours he doesn't comprehend anything. Dan is always confused in the morning. He hears me but [he is] not comprehending."

The difficulties in communication lead to other hardships, and this is not limited to bvFTD, as all forms of dementia share three dominant groups of symptoms: impairment in memory and language retention; altered mood and depression; and aggression and agitation (Spiro, 2010). The crucial thing to understand is that mental health issues associated with dementia are on the rise, and that the bulk of the care for dementia patients is provided by family members. Even though the medical community and the media sometimes speak about the global impact of dementia in catastrophic terms, such as the "dementia tsunami" which is "worse than death" for the affected individual and their family (Peel, 2014), I will try to abstain from "scaremongering" as much as possible. Instead, listening to the voices of people living with dementia and their caregivers gives an insight into how the "panic-blame" framework (Hillman & Latimer, 2017; Peel, 2014) is driving the social representation of dementia, contributing to social isolation, stigmatization and ultimately denying of legitimate claims for adequate healthcare and support.

Mental health issues associated with dementia

Dementia ranks among the most feared conditions by older adults (Robillard & Wight, 2017). In fact, according to some reports, people fear dementia more than cancer and even more than death (Brooks, 2011; Peel, 2014). This fear contributes to mental health issues and social stigma surrounding dementia (see below). Analysis of qualitative data, such as what I'm providing with careful reading of quotes from Jake, Barbara, Dan and Jane, is an important window into the perspectives of dementia patients and caregivers—the fears and hopes they might have for themselves and their loved ones. However, it is equally important to understand what preconceived notions older adults, the population most likely to be affected by dementia, have about affected individuals and the value of their life. The greatest factor for developing dementia is age itself, as prevalence increases in stark increments, doubling every 5–7 years after living for 65 years, making the thoughts of aging populations of prime importance.

A study of British older adults revealed a range of fears and anxieties, so much so that these emotions affect treatment of others and self care (Corner & Bond, 2004). Namely, older adults predominantly feel uncomfortable with friends or relatives with dementia and are at the same time reluctant to contact health professionals about memory problems. This behavior seems to be reinforced by popular media articles, which present dementia in a kind of "despair and loss" panic discourse (Hillman & Latimer, 2017), which fuels stereotypes that dementia is "social death" and that any "dementia sufferer" is a "liminal or non-person making a transition from life to death"

(Peel, 2014). Newspaper headlines speak of dementia as a "demographic time-bomb," constructing or defining it as a threat or imminent catastrophe.

Such messages are clearly increasing anxiety among caregivers, especially children of persons living with dementia, as revealed by a qualitative study of caregiver perspectives (Peel, 2014). Sue, a daughter of a person living with vascular dementia echoes the "time-bomb" metaphor:

> It's the time bomb, isn't it, you know, we're all going to get it because we're going to live – if we live long enough we're all going to get it because simple biology, you're going to get dementia. So it's 'Oh my God'. It's like something to be frightened of that's coming down the path ... I think it's talked about in quite a negative way, as if it's a terrifying – I mean it is frightening in a way when you've got it – it must be terrifying, because my mum says, 'I'm losing my mind'
>
> *(Peel, 2014, p. 892).*

Words and phrases such as "merciless assault," "dreaded," "cruel," "horror," "terrible affliction," "harrowing descent" and "crippling brain-wasting disease" in popular media (Peel, 2014) convey the message that those associated with dementia in any way are somehow on the dark side, beyond reason, and dangerous. The cultural representation of dementia contributes to the growing fear, which in turn produces social and mental health problems for people living with dementia, those that are at risk for developing dementia, and especially for caregivers.

Derek, a male caregiver from a qualitative study in England, echoes this social representation almost in terms of "evil" or "sinful" characteristics of dementia:

> [D]ementia, [...] it's an absolutely wicked illness. Wicked. Wicked for the person that's suffering, and wicked for the carer that's looking after that person. Terrible, terrible thing, it is
>
> *(Peel, 2014, p. 891).*

The fear and anxiety about dementia dovetails with the already present reduction in the sense of social value. The feelings about the lack of respect afforded to elderly individuals in society are summarized in this quote by an anonymous participant in a study of social perspectives on dementia among older adults in the United Kingdom:

> [W]hen you're old, you're on the scrap-heap, or at least you feel as if you are, that is people make you feel as if you are. I suppose I think that people who have Alzheimer's and dementia are at the bottom of the scrap-heap and ... most people would just think they should die
>
> *(Corner & Bond, 2004, p. 148).*

Such preconceived notions are clearly influencing behavior of affected individuals, as we can see with Dan. Before he found his peace and, more or less, came to terms with his condition, Dan attempted suicide by taking all of his medication at once. However, social perspectives on dementia are not limited to a perception that a life of a "demented individual" is not worth living—they are providing value judgments of healthcare expenses and allocation of medical resources, as neatly (if bluntly) summarized by another anonymous study participant:

> *I don't think it's right that money is taken away from children and the like … to treat the elderly and the demented*
>
> *(Corner & Bond, 2004, p. 148).*

Indeed, both Dan and Jake experience barriers in receiving proper care. Namely, there just aren't sufficient healthcare resources for treatment of dementia, and when they are present, they come with substantial financial costs and major reductions in rights and dignity. Jake (still) appears to have sufficient funds to live a comfortable life—if the finances are prudently managed—but he is a fiercely independent person that does not want to be treated like a child. It remains to be seen if he will struggle with depression as Dan did. Also, appearances can be deceiving: similar to Jake who likes to boast about the size of his yacht and his new truck, Dan was enthusiastic about new purchases and costly projects. Until Jane put a stop to them, Dan had carefree shopping sprees. In January of 2016, after driving Jane to the hospital to have surgery, Dan went off to spend $2500 for materials for "building a sauna" ("I've always wanted one, I'm gonna have one"). This careless disregard for the prudent and feasible forced Jane to retire and significantly strained their financial resources, so Dan, Jane, and their family are now struggling to cope. Since he is a US army veteran, they tried to get the Veterans Administration to help, but to receive aid, Dan would have to be in lock-down and in Memory care, which is geared toward Alzheimer's and not Frontotemporal dementia. As is the case in many instances, the family chose to sacrifice almost everything for their loved one in need.

Dementia is also seen as a "dirty secret." Dan, for instance, is very touchy about other people knowing he has dementia, and this impedes his access to social and healthcare support. But Dan's attitude seems to be a reflection of a general attitude shared by many. As succinctly formulated by one study participant, this is generally viewed to be a sort of a secret personal failing:

> *Never heard about it when I was young … of course anybody was mental, you never thought, you didn't talk about it. It was kept under cover, they didn't get any sympathy for it…*
>
> *(Corner & Bond, 2004, p. 151).*

All in all, dementias seem to personify all that is feared in growing old—and this has attracted considerable media attention. The proliferation of stories that seek to represent dementia in mainstream press and television news as well as works of fiction tends to evoke frightening images of "living death," freakish stories of extremes that happen to "them," as opposed to "us" (Hillman & Latimer, 2017). This leads to social alienation of persons and families struggling with dementia and serious mental health issues. Caring for people with dementia is associated with well-documented increases in burden, distress and detrimental effects of mental health and well-being (Sorensen et al., 2006). The important questions to ask are the following: how much of the burden is due to the difficulties in interaction, communication and behavior of people living with dementia, and how much is due to social stereotypes and stigma or due to lack of resources (extended families or frail care facilities)?

Stigma and dementia

Dementia is a condition associated with significant prejudice and stigma. Three kinds of stigma (Structural stigma, Social stigma and Self-stigma) can lead to a range of negative outcomes (Carter & Hall, 2017). Structural stigma can lead to institutional discrimination that deprives individuals with dementia of effective healthcare. For instance, if they are labeled as "demented," their preferences may no longer be taken into account. Social stigma involves interpersonal victimization or discrimination that may discourage the affected individual from seeking treatment. Finally, self-stigma is a collection of negative attitudes toward oneself that can lead to loss of self esteem, depression and poorer health behaviors, such as substance misuse.

We appear to have seen very little to suggest self-stigma with Jake (although appearances may be misleading). However, he is still very early in the progression of dementia, and in the position to do serious damage to himself. For instance, his family persuaded him to retire after he became rude to customers in 2016, but he is still very much involved in financial decisions and fiercely guards his independence. Indeed, as I argue at length elsewhere (Dubljević, 2019), dementia (and especially bvFTD) presents a unique challenge for our ethical value system, most notably in terms of respect for autonomy. The effects of stigma are more observable with Barbara: she seems to be deeply ashamed of Jake's behavior, and appears to be dreading every interaction he might have with strangers. The structural stigma of dementia will make it virtually impossible for Jake to enjoy a degree of independence and respect for his (still considerable) cognitive faculties in his retirement without endangering his future. Namely, even when taken over by a family member (as opposed to a "professional guardian"), guardianship is a massive intrusion into personal life and all aspects of decision making adults take for granted. What's more, it is haphazardly regulated, and people labeled as "demented" and "legally incapacitated" have fewer rights than even incarcerated individuals (Reed, 2018).

With Dan, we see how all three types, the structural, social and self-stigma, are at play. Dan hides his diagnosis as much as he can. In fact, he has been referred to the Frontotemporal dementia research study even though he is currently not officially diagnosed—the chief neurologist suggested diagnosing him with "mild cognitive decline" so that Dan can get support from the healthcare system. Dan doesn't want others to look at him differently ("I feel like the same guy, but then they take my driver's license") and treat him as a child. He coped with the new reality by engaging in substance use—heavy drinking, pain medication, marijuana. Dan goes to such lengths to hide his condition that he would rather end up in trouble with the law than disclose his condition: in one incident, he was apprehended by the police after placing items on and repeatedly trying to unlock what he thought was his truck. To Dan, this was unfair treatment for an honest mistake ("no malice in that"), and he resented the way the officers looked at him after the family intervened by disclosing his condition to release him from custody.

The way forward

Dementia will perhaps never be seen without some measure of fear: it may be safe to assert that there is no way to completely eliminate the sense of obliteration, or gradual chipping away of humanity that is associated with the condition. However, stories of people like Jake, Barbara, Dan, and Jane provide us with another image: they are very much human as actors and acted upon in socio-moral and legal contexts, as beings who laugh and cry, as people who try to remain connected to the world. The obstacles are many. For Dan, even though he has found a measure of peace, he has still not fully come to terms with his condition. For Jane—and other caregivers like her who are exposed to the severe and chronic stress of dealing with problem behaviors and navigating the healthcare system—their physical and mental well-being are at serious risk. One study found that 10% of caregivers of dementia patients with mood disorder co-morbidities met criteria for major depressive disorder, while 62% met criteria for minor depression (Schulz & Martire, 2004). For Jake in particular (considering he is in the early stages of disease progression, at the start of the journey, and since his wife passed away), he is likely to continue living alone. Even with the best effort, his daughter, Barbara thinks that his prospects are grim.

There is hope, however. Worldwide efforts to de-stigmatize dementia are underway, as well as new dementia-friendly communities across Europe, Japan and United States (Batsch & Mittelman, 2012). These efforts should be followed up by changes in healthcare policy that fully recognize the role of caregivers as healthcare resources. Healthcare, financial and workplace policies, such as reimbursement, tax credits, retirement plans, caregiving leaves, etc. may need to be implemented (Sorensen et al., 2006). Global differences in the way healthcare systems are set up will most likely come to the forefront; a comprehensive strategy in countries such as the United States is less likely than in countries with a "single payer" health system. Nevertheless, the global neuroethics and mental health community should compare experiences and solutions, such as the UK comprehensive strategy for dementia (Department of Health [DoH], 2009). This is all the more urgent as the public, and even health care professionals seem to equate all forms of dementia with Alzheimer's and have limited knowledge of different types of dementia (and associated distinct challenges). High income countries (such as United Kingdom, France, Norway, United States and South Korea) provide some resources, such as memory clinics and specific dementia strategies, whereas in low and middle income countries resources and even know-how are limited (Cheng et al., 2013; Parra et al., 2018). For instance, even basic recommendations and guidelines for dementia diagnosis are available in only a subset of countries in Latin America (e.g., in Chile, Argentina, Mexico and Brazil), while most low income countries in Latin America have minimal mental health facilities and do not have mental health policies or budgets specific to dementia (Parra et al., 2018). This situation is mirrored in East Asia: there are relatively few programs in low and middle income countries for elderly care, and those that are available tend to offer generic programs, rather than specific resources for dementia (Cheng et al., 2013).

The mental health burden of dementia is a global problem which can only be solved after innovative policies across the world are assessed for enabling healthcare delivery and empowering patients to lead as dignified lives as possible. On the one hand, funds and resources are limiting the amount of care that societies can reasonably be expected to provide. On the other hand, knowledge about and due respect toward persons living with dementia are not necessarily limited by wealth, and the global neuroethics and mental health community can provide a great service by promoting them.

References

Batsch, N. L., & Mittelman, M. S. (2012). *World Alzheimer report 2012: Overcoming the stigma of dementia*. London: Alzheimer's Disease International.

Birkhoff, J. M., Garberi, C., & Re, L. (2016). The behavioral variant frontotemporal dementia: An analysis of the literature and a case report. *International Journal of Law and Psychiatry, 47*, 157–163.

Brooks, L. (2011). Comment: Alzheimer's is compelling in fiction because it's so cruel in life. *The Guardian*, (30 September).

Carter, A., & Hall, W. (2017). Looking to the future: Clinical and policy implications of the brain disease model of addiction. In J. Illes (Ed.), *Neuroethics: Anticipating the future* (pp. 497–514). Oxford: Oxford University Press.

Chare, L., Hodges, J. R., Leyton, C. E., McGinley, C., Tan, R. H., Krill, J. J., et al. (2014). New criteria for frontotemporal dementia syndromes: Clinical and pathological diagnostic implications. *Cognitive Neurology, 85*, 866–871.

Cheng, S. T., Chou, K. L., & Zarit, S. H. (2013). Dementia in Asia: Introduction to a special section. *Aging & Mental Health, 17*(8), 911–914.

Corner, L., & Bond, J. (2004). Being at risk of dementia: Fears and anxieties of older adults. *Journal of Aging Studies, 18*, 143–155.

Department of Health [DoH]. (2009). *Living well with dementia: A national dementia strategy*. London: The Stationery Office.

Dubljević, V. (2013). Autonomy in neuroethics: Political and not metaphysical. *American Journal of Bioethics Neuroscience, 4*(4), 44–51.

Dubljević, V. (2019). *The principle of autonomy and behavioral variant frontotemporal dementia*. [Under Review].

Family Caregiver Alliance. (2016). https://www.caregiver.org/caregiver-statistics-demographics.

Hillman, A., & Latimer, J. (2017). Cultural representations of dementia. *PLoS Medicine, 14*(3), e1002274.

Lanata, S. C., & Miller, B. C. (2016). The behavioral variant frontotemporal dementia (bvFTD) syndrome in psychiatry. *Journal of Neurology, Neurosurgery, and Psychiatry, 87*, 501–511.

Manes, F., Torralva, T., Ibáñez, A., Roca, M., Bekinschtein, T., & Gleichgerrcht, E. (2011). Decision-making in frontotemporal dementia: Clinical, theoretical and legal implications. *Dementia and Geriatric Cognitive Disorders, 32*, 11–17.

Mendez, M. F., Anderson, E., & Shapira, J. S. (2005). An investigation of moral judgments in frontotemporal dementia. *Cognitive and Behavioral Neurology, 18*, 193–197.

Parra, M. A., Baez, S., Allegri, R., Nitrini, R., Lopera, F., Slachevsky, A., et al. (2018). Dementia in Latin America: Assessing the present and envisioning the future. *Neurology, 90,* 222–231.

Peel, E. (2014). 'The living death of Alzheimer's' versus 'Take a walk to keep dementia at bay': Representations of dementia in print media and carer discourse. *Sociology of Health & Illness, 36*(6), 885–901.

Ramos, K. M., & Koroshetz, W. J. (2017). Integrating ethics into neurotechnology research and development: The US National Institutes of Health BRAIN Initiative. In J. Illes (Ed.), *Neuroethics: Anticipating the future* (pp. 144–156). Oxford: Oxford University Press.

Rascovsky, K., Hodges, J. R., KNopman, D., Mendez, M. F., Kramer, J. H., Neuhaus, J., et al. (2011). Sensitivity of revised diagnostic criteria for the behavioural variant of frontotemporal dementia. *Brain, 134,* 2456–2477.

Reed, R. (2018). John Oliver explains how legal guardians abuse their power. *The Rolling Stone,* (June 4, 2018). Available from: https://www.rollingstone.com/tv/tv-news/john-oliver-explains-how-legal-guardians-abuse-their-power-629697/.

Robillard, J. M., & Wight, E. (2017). Communicating about the brain in the digital era. In J. Illes (Ed.), *Neuroethics: Anticipating the future* (pp. 554–569). Oxford: Oxford University Press.

Schulz, R., & Martire, L. M. (2004). Family caregiving of persons with dementia: Prevalence, health effects, and support strategies. *The American Journal of Geriatric Psychiatry, 12*(3), 240–249.

Sorensen, S., Duberstein, P., Gill, D., & Pinquart, M. (2006). Dementia care: Mental health effects, intervention strategies, and clinical implications. *Lancet Neurology, 5,* 961–973.

Spiro, N. (2010). Music and dementia: Observing effects and searching for underlying theories. *Aging & Mental Health, 14*(8), 891–899.

U.S. Congress, Office of Technology Assessment [OTA]. (1987). *Losing a million minds: Confronting the tragedy of Alzheimer's disease and other dementias, OTA-BA-323.* Washington, DC: U.S. Government Printing Office.

World Health Organization [WHO]. (2012). *Dementia: A public health priority.* Geneva: World Health Organization. ISBN: 978-92-4-156445-8.

Further reading

Diehl-Schmid, J. K., Perneczky, R., Koch, J., Nedopil, N., & Kurz, A. (2013). Guilty by suspicion? Criminal behavior in frontotemporal lobar degeneration. *Cognitive and Behavioral Neurology, 26*(2), 73–77. https://doi.org/10.1097/WNN.0b013e31829cff11.

McDermot, O., Charlesworth, G., Hogervorst, E., Stoner, C., Moniz-Cook, E., Spector, A., et al. (2018). Psychosocial interventions for people with dementia: A synthesis of systematic reviews. *Aging and Mental Health,* https://doi.org/10.1080/13607863.2017.1423031.

Addressing disability in global mental health and neuroethics: Challenges and hopes

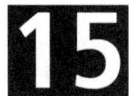

Kevin Chien-Chang Wu
Graduate Institute of Medical Education and Bioethics, National Taiwan University College of Medicine, Taipei, Taiwan, Department of Psychiatry, National Taiwan University Hospital, Taipei, Taiwan

Introduction

In recent decades, using measures of disability adjusted life years (DALYs), global health studies have repeatedly found that neuropsychiatric conditions are major contributors to the global burden of disease (GBD). More than a quarter of years lived with disability have been attributed to these conditions (Mathers & Loncar, 2006; Murray & Lopez, 1994). Depression was the fourth leading contributor to DALYs in 1990, the third in 2000 and the second in 2010, and is projected to be the leading contributor in 2020 and 2030 (Ferrari et al., 2013; Mathers & Loncar, 2006; Murray & Lopez, 1996). Such findings have given impetus to synchronized efforts to prioritize mental health as a key component of global health (Prince et al., 2007). Emphasizing the slogan of "no health without mental health," global mental health has matured into a discipline that aims to reduce the treatment gap of mental health conditions and the human rights inequality in mental health care and outcome (Patel, 2012; Prince et al., 2007). Furthermore, a continuous exchange with critiques of global mental health has arguably led the field to give greater consideration to socio-cultural contexts and developmental issues (Cherepanov, 2018; Patel et al., 2018).

As neuroscience advances with improved molecular and imaging techniques, it may facilitate our understanding of the pathogenesis of mental disorders, the construction of more reliable diagnostic criteria of mental disorders, and more targeted and effective treatment and prevention of mental disorders (Stein et al., 2015). As an interdisciplinary field that investigates "neuroscience of ethics" and "ethics of neuroscience," neuroethics could examine ethical issues in synergy with global mental health and neuroscience (Illes & Hossain, 2017). Scholars have argued for a mutually beneficial relationship between global mental health and neuroethics, warning against a neuro-reductionistic style of thinking and disregard of cultural contexts (Stein & Giordano, 2015).

First, since neuroethics emphasizes naturalistic empirical approach to philosophy of mind and bioethical issues, it could expand and reinforce the ethical vantage points of global mental health in conducting neuropsychiatric studies in low- and middle-income countries (Stein & Giordano, 2015). Second, as neuroethics addresses both treatment and enhancement of mental conditions using neuroscience-technology, it might contribute to ethical discourses on how global mental health could achieve the WHO definition of health as "complete physical, mental and social wellbeing" (Stein & Giordano, 2015). Third, as neuroethics explores implication of neuroscience-technology in social institution and distributive justice, the nature of human rights and other moralities, it could help clarify and solidify the discourse of global mental health on human rights and parity for mental health (Stein & Giordano, 2015). Finally, as neuroethics probes the concept and construction of the subjective and objective aspects of self and related ethical concepts such as responsibility, free will and autonomy, it could help deepen the efforts of global mental health in responding to the claim of "nothing about us without us" by including community and patient groups for designing schemes of promoting mental health (Stein & Giordano, 2015).

Consistent with a view that mental health conditions are quite closely related to disability issues, Stein and Giordano (2015) have incorporated work from disability studies insofar as they address human rights, social inclusion and consumer participation. However, whether disability models, global mental health and neuroethics make good bedfellows is still an open question. Therefore, this chapter will undertake a preliminary analysis of the opportunities and challenges for addressing disability issues in global mental health and neuroethics. The next section delineates major models of disability and their relevance to mental or psychosocial disability. The "Challenges to global mental health and neuroethics" section covers major challenges of disability research to the intersection of global mental health and neuroethics. Many critiques of global mental health and neuroethics have themes that resonate with work in disability studies. The "Opportunities for addressing disability in GMH and neuroethics: A proposal" section covers opportunities for addressing disability in global mental health and neuroethics and proposes an integrated model of disability as a comprehensive framework for future analysis.

Models of disability

In a very broad sense, almost everyone will become or have to care a person with disability. According to the 2011 World Report on Disability, 15% of the world's population have disability, among which 88% live in the world's poor countries (World Health Organization, 2011). Thus, global mental health and neuroethics definitely have to address those with mental or psychosocial disabilities and mental health distress related to disability. The way we represent and construe disability is closely linked with how we intervene to address suffering and problems experienced by people with disability (Hacking, 1983). Therefore, it is important to first explore what disability is before addressing it in global mental health and neuroethics.

In this chapter, a number of models of disability will be used because it is almost impossible to adhere to one universal definition of disability for the complex issues in global mental health and neuroethics. Different definitions of disability have been proposed for different clinical, administrative, research or political purposes (Altman, 2001; An interview with Tina Minkowitz, 2015; Wasserman, Asch, Blustein,

& Putnam, 2016). For administrative reasons, disability definitions may differ in different regions or countries. For example, regarding social welfare coverage, substance addiction is excluded from the definition of disability in the United States, but not in Canada (Flacks, 2012). In the same country, the United States, the definition of disability in the Americans with Disability Act is different from that in the social security system (Altman, 2001). Article 1 of the UN Convention on the Rights of Persons with Disabilities (CRPD) uses the wording "[p]ersons with disabilities include..." instead of "persons with disabilities are..." (*United Nations Convention on the Rights of Persons with Disabilities*, 2006), in order to maintain a leeway for the signatories of the convention to make adjustments for their jurisdiction.

The large variety (physical, mental, intellectual, sensory, etc.) of impairment characteristics, compounds the difficulty of constructing a definition of disability that satisfies all stakeholders (An interview with Tina Minkowitz, 2015). Thus, for the purpose of this chapter, major models of disability are addressed to pave the way for further discussions on their potential impacts on disability conceptualization and management in global mental health and neuroethics. Three caveats need, however, to be emphasized. First, the boundaries between the models are not always rigid. Second, the models might not be universally applicable for persons with disabilities everywhere (Goodley, 2017). Third, this review is for the purpose of creating a preliminary framework for addressing disability in global mental health and neuroethics.

Traditionally, disability is viewed as impaired human function caused by a medical condition, the severity of which is above a certain threshold and warrants specific government welfare compensation (Davis, 2017). Alongside the civil rights movement, there have been advocates for protecting and promoting the rights or identities of people with disabilities or disabled people (Wasserman et al., 2016). In general, major models of disability have emphasized long-term impairments and limitations in social lives, although the terms used and their meanings might differ (Altman, 2001).

Thus, for example, a person is deemed to be impaired according to a standard set by statistics, biological prototype, evolutionary construct, normative criteria, or a combination of these (Altman, 2001; Wakefield, 1992; Wasserman et al., 2016). Such a person with impairment will be deemed to have disability when having limitations in different kinds of activities or social participation. Generally speaking, impairment is a necessary factor for the making of disability, but whether it is a sufficient one depends on the models of disability (Wasserman et al., 2016). Historically, governments have restricted freedom and rights of people in certain races and genders, but we tend not to view them as having disability given the above perspective (Shakespeare, 2014; Wasserman et al., 2016). Furthermore, short-term flu might impair our health, but we tend not recognize a person with it as having disability, because it is not a chronic trait or attribute of the person (*United Nations Convention on the Rights of Persons with Disabilities*, 2006; Wasserman et al., 2016).

Before modern times, disabilities (e.g., disfigurement) were often construed as evidence of religious sin or moral failure. People with disability and their families were often socially excluded and ostracized (Goodley, 2017). Stigmatization was unavoidable. In this moral or religious model of disability, potentially harsh moral or religious treatment focused on the individual person with disability. The purpose of the treatment was unfortunately not necessarily of any benefit to the person. Even though this kind of approach still prevails in many places around the world, it is not a model of disability worthy of adoption given its strongly unethical consequences.

Based on construal of the relationship between impairment and the social environment, there are three basic models of disability. The first is the medical (or individualist) model, according to which we can measure disability mainly by assessing how severely the impairment interferes with activities and social participation. Thus, the source of disability is located in the body and the person, and is caused by physical or mental impairment (Altman, 2001; Goodley, 2017; Shakespeare, 2014; Wasserman et al., 2016). In its extreme form, a diagnosis of disease or disorder means the existence of disability. People with disability may become the object of professional gaze, with diminished agency (Linton, 1998; Sherry, 2006). Laws and policies based on the medical model usually stress medical treatment and rehabilitation. If disability remains, care and remedy provided by the social welfare system or charity is typically offered (Altman, 2001). Since both the medical model and the moral model focus on individuals' intrinsic characteristics, they are also called individualist models (Goodley, 2017).

A second model is the social model, in which the major concern is how the social environment (interpersonal interaction, social structure and institution, etc.) exerts a negative influence and makes the person with impairment unable to perform activities or participate in social affairs. The influence might be straightforwardly restricting or just failing to accommodate or support (e.g., in an awkward physical environment) such that a person becomes disabled. Thus proponents of this model prefer to use "disabled person" instead of "person with disability" to stress that persons are disabled by society (Russo & Shulkes, 2015; Sapey, Spandler, & Anderson, 2015). This chapter will use these terms interchangeably unless specified otherwise.

In the original British social model proposed by the Union of Physically Impaired Against Segregation (UPIAS), disability is defined as "the disadvantage or restriction of activity caused by a contemporary social organization which takes little or no account of people who have physical impairments and thus excludes them from participation in the mainstream of social activities." (UPIAS, 1976, pp. 3–4). On the face of things, this model almost neglects the causal role of impairment in disability; it instead emphasizes the inadequacy in material resources in society for changing the situations of persons with impairment, so it is also called British materialist model (Shakespeare, 2014). To some observers, its law and policy recommendations seem aggressive and anti-intellectual (Vehmas, 2008), but it is possible that despite the advocacy rhetoric of the social model, supporters of the British materialist model do consider the impact of impairment on the formation of disability (Beaudry, 2016).

There are several subtypes of the social model approach. According to the minority group model, persons with disabilities are disabled through social exclusion and stigmatization. Thus the appropriate response to diminish disability is through laws and policies focused on anti-discrimination and civil/human rights protection. For example, the policy goal of the Americans with Disability Act is to protect "a discrete and insular minority," as in the case of racial minorities (Goodley, 2017; Wasserman et al., 2016). Based on the disablism model, social oppression and barriers, including those maintained through interpersonal relations, not only restrict the activities and participation of persons with impairment, but also have negative impact on their psychosocial wellbeing (Reeve, 2012). The symbolic systems (e.g., texts and practices) might evolve with the advancement of science and humanity, but they still restrain persons with disabilities from full participation in society (Garland-Thomson, 2002).

The human variation model takes disability as a mismatch between a person's attributes and the physical and social environment; or put it in another way, "an extension of the variability in physical and mental attributes beyond the present – but not the potential – ability of social institutions to routinely respond" (Scotch & Schriner, 1997). Disability may be a universal human condition (Zola, 1989) or shared human identity (Davis, 2002) that disabled persons can affirm or be proud of (Curtis, Dellar, Leslie, & Watson, 2000), since every human variation may be a disability in some physical and social settings (Wasserman et al., 2016). For proponents of this model, impairment and disability are not abnormality. Even so-called "impairment" may be viewed as part of human diversity, which is constructed as pathology by society. On its farthest end of this approach, the social is the culprit for both the impairment and the disability, either in a real or constructive sense (Goodley, 2017).

In the cultural model of disability, body and impairment are deemed socio-cultural entities full of meanings. It is important to examine and deconstruct how cultural practices in science, professions, media, etc. represent impairment and disabilities, in order to do its cultural work (Goodley, 2017). In laws and policies based on these social model subtypes, the major theme is how society and culture should be modified to accommodate the disabled persons and discontinue the disablement discourses as soon as possible if not immediately. One of the major problems is what costs we are willing and justified to afford and allocate (Stein, 2008); pragmatic and feasible solutions must be found.

The third basic disability model that emphasizes the interactions between impairment and social environment is often called the interaction model of disability (Goodley, 2017; Shakespeare, 2014). The interaction model emphasizes both the non-negligible roles of impairment (including individual pain and suffering) and the social (including interpersonal attitudes, social structures and institutions) in rendering disability. One example is the definition given by Article 1 of the CRPD: "Persons with disabilities include those who have long-term physical, mental, intellectual or sensory impairments which in interaction with various barriers may hinder their full and effective participation in society on an equal basis with others." In another, adopting a biopsychosocial approach, the International Classification of Functioning, Disability and Health (ICF) views disability as the "outcomes of interactions between health conditions (diseases, disorders and injuries) and contextual factors" (World Health Organization, 2002). Because in the CRPD disability is construed as a human rights issue that stresses physical and social barriers and discrimination, this interaction model may be called the human rights model, in which human rights discourse is the foundation of law and policy making.

One of its variations is called the Nordic relational model of disability, which does not take challenging society as a major goal. In a "good enough" welfare context, the theme is on promoting community participation of persons with disabilities (especially intellectual disability). As impairment and disability are not so separable and disability is deemed relative to environment, the model aims to create a social environment that allows those with disabilities to lead ordinary lives (Goodley, 2017; Shakespeare, 2014; World Health Organization, 2011). In the eyes of some advocates of social models, the interaction model is overly biomedical discourses and so may minimize the impact of social oppression on disability (Shakespeare, 2014). At present, however, interaction model is predominant in UN and WHO documents addressing disability.

Within the disability models that take the social environment into consideration, the British social model (or the materialist model) has been criticized for how it construes impairment. On the one hand, it downplays the importance of impairment, such as pain and suffering, either as an objective basis (Bickenbach, 1993) or as a source of disability (Shakespeare, 2014). On the other hand, it is hard to tease apart the mutual embeddedness of the biological and the social in rendering disability (Anastasiou & Kauffman, 2013; Martiny, 2015). Moreover, impairment could be a social construction by medical sciences (e.g., homosexuality) or a creation of the changing social environment (e.g., dyslexia) (Amundson, 2000; Cole, 2007; Tremain, 2001). Thus, both the social model and the interaction model have to consider how to adapt policy making to the view that impairment is itself a result of social value judgments.

Psychosocial disability and mental impairment

It is important for global mental health and neuroethics to consider how best to accommodate different models of disability. Since psychosocial disability is the term preferred by the CRPD committee, this chapter will use the terms mental impairment and psychosocial disability. Individuals with mental impairment and psychosocial disabilities have been the most discriminated against and stigmatized (Wasserman, 2018). Compared to people with physical disabilities, such individuals are more likely to be viewed as lacking autonomy or competence in decision making. Even now, treatment against their will and preferences is accepted in countries that have ratified the CRPD (An interview with Tina Minkowitz, 2015).

In the anti-psychiatry movement of the 1960s, Szasz argued that mental illness is a myth, since beliefs and emotions could not be manifestations of brain diseases (Szasz, 1960). Although the persuasiveness of his arguments has been challenged by both philosophical reasoning and neuropsychiatric research, arguments against biomedical models of mental impairment continue to be articulated, and with more vigor than in the case of physical impairment. Although people who embrace deaf culture do not view deafness as a physical impairment, it is difficult to extrapolate this kind of approach to other typical kinds of physical impairment (Scully, 2012; Shakespeare, 2014). However, at an individual level, the boundaries between "healthy" and "impaired" mental functions are blurry and debatable. Furthermore, social forces impact on mental impairment and psychosocial disability in multiple ways (Amundson, 2000; Tremain, 2001).

According to the social model of disability, the social environment engenders disability by setting barriers for those with mental impairment. However, for scholars adopting a critical disability approach, "the 'problem' of disability does not lie with the person with disabilities but rather in the way that normalcy is constructed." (Davis, 2017, p. 1). It is the power of the norm that constructs impairment and disability. Thus, in the discourse of "mad pride," madness as a mental difference is affirmed without negative connotations (Curtis et al., 2000). Just like other minority groups, people with madness are disabled by social oppression. Even if neuroscientific explanations for mental conditions are adopted, the human variation model emphasizes the term neuro-diversity, to indicate that these mental conditions do not represent mental impairment, but are natural differences needing social accommodation (Graby, 2015).

On the other hand, in the medical model of mental disability, gene-environment interactions or social determinants of mental health (e.g., poverty, inequality, etc.) (Allen, Balfour, Bell, & Marmot, 2014) can still be used to explain how the social modifies the effects of the neuropsychiatric mechanisms underlying mental impairment. Therefore, embracing the biopsychosocial interaction model of the ICF, the World Report on Disability views disability as brought about by the interaction between contextual factors and health conditions that results in impaired body functions and structure, activity limitation or participation restrictions (World Health Organization, 2011).

However, the ICF has been criticized for using the stigmatizing labels of mental disorders and not focusing on subjective experiences of autonomy and meaning that are closely related to life satisfaction and happiness (Hemmingsson & Jonsson, 2005). Therefore, some have advocated for adopting Amartya Sen's capabilities approach to disabilities; this emphasizes the type of life people are capable of having. Capability refers to practical opportunity, and functioning refers to actual achievement. Compatible with this approach and emphasizing resource provision and environment adjustment, the human development model aims to enhance a person's capability set, and the functioning components, that a person has freedom to choose. A person is disabled when deprived of capability and/or functioning (Mitra, 2018). Thus, it is important for societies to examine whether persons with mental impairment lower their expectations for development due to entrenched restrictive social practices (Wallcraft & Hopper, 2015).

In Article 3, the CRPD promotes the general principles of respect for inherent dignity and individual autonomy, respect for differences, non-discrimination, equality of opportunity, full and effective participation and inclusion in society, accessibility, gender equality, and respect for children's evolving capacities and right to preserve their identities. These principles not only protect the human rights of people with psychosocial disabilities, but also may lessen the risk of mental impairment and lower social barriers against this population. In its general comment on Article 12 (Committee on the Rights of Persons with Disabilities, 2014), the CRPD Committee demands signatories to abolish disabling practices such as the deprivation of legal capacity in guardianship and compulsory psychiatric admission. It adopts a model of relational autonomy, in which all of us make decisions more or less with the support from others, but the decisions are still ours (Series, 2015). Mental incapacity, as a lack of decisional skill determined through professional assessment, is not an acceptable condition for disregard of the rights, will and preference of a person with disability (Committee on the Rights of Persons with Disabilities, 2014). If a person with disability cannot communicate his/her will and preference through the best available support, the best interpretation of the person's will and preference is the recommended way of decision making.

According to the committee's guideline to Article 14, no matter what extra conditions (e.g., danger to self or others) are added to justify practices of compulsory psychiatric admission of persons with disabilities, these practices still fail to comply with the requirements of Article 14 that "the existence of a disability shall in no case justify a deprivation of liberty" (Committee on the Rights of Persons with Disabilities, 2015). It has been argued that these interpretations of Article 12 and Article 14 may hinder the realization of other important human rights, such as the right to health and life (Freeman et al., 2015). How to deal with self-impairing or self-disabling behavior of persons with disabilities indeed remains a challenge under the current framework of the CRPD. For the time being, no country has abolished all practices of substitutive decision making.

Arguably, the optimal way forwards is to aim to achieve the goal of incremental human rights protection through procedures that are transparent, fully informed, fully participatory and respecting differences, avoiding both absolute human rights and cultural relativism (Bickenbach, 2009). Addressing disabilities, the intersection between global mental health and neuroethics needs to find ways to negotiate with various models of disability. It is fair to say that many critiques of the disciplines of both global mental health and neuroethics resonate with the views of advocates of social models of disability. In the next sections, the chapter will first review briefly the challenges faced by global mental health and neuroethics, and then propose an integrated model of disability that might create a platform for addressing disability in a pragmatic and dynamic way.

Challenges to global mental health and neuroethics

The basic components of models of disability include impairment, physical/social barriers, and social oppression. To address disability in the global mental health framework we must delineate how this discipline can best respond to social models of disability (Mitra, 2018). Addressing disability in neuroethics requires a parallel response. Such a discussion is certainly not intended to indicate that global mental health and neuroethics cannot address disability issues. Rather it aims to create a space for global mental health and neuroethics to evolve in a way that meets the needs of different stakeholders. As will be argued, both global mental health and neuroethics do incorporate wider transdisciplinary frameworks and multilevel domains that can be used to address disability issues.

Challenges to global mental health

Global mental health gained momentum due to findings that neuropsychiatric disorders contribute a prominent proportion to DALYs globally (Wildeman, 2013). However, the term "disability" used in this measure does not have the same meaning as those used in models of disability, especially social models of disability. In calculating the DALY, a severity weight for each health condition for discounting the value of a lived year was given by health professionals in the program's early years; 1 for death, 0 for perfect health and in between for others. In its revised form, in which severity weight values were assigned by health professionals through person tradeoff games, the DALY is a pure medical model of disability which carries a strong utilitarian flavor and an emphasis on the productivity of individuals (Grosse, Lollar, Campbell, & Chamie, 2009; Laurie, 2015; Wildeman, 2013). Although a version of DALYs has incorporated the valuation of health conditions by the general public (Salomon et al., 2015), the usefulness of DALY in addressing disabilities is potentially limited by the failure to consider the subjective preference or experience of the general public, or of persons with impairment, as well as the objective social context (Grosse et al., 2009; Laurie, 2015). DALY may therefore be misleading in understanding disabilities and relevant policy making.

The second issue that presents a challenge for global mental health is its emphasis on Western style mental health assessments and services. Critics argue that the expansion of mental disorders by pathologizing and biomedicalizing our daily experiences is unlikely to be beneficial to people all around the world (Frances, 2013). A shift to biological explanations may worsen stigmatization (Summerfield, 2012). People in different cultures may have their own ways of approaching and managing mental distress/impairment, which provide better outcomes. Evidence based mental health practices should not exclude local communities' epistemic authority in their cultural contexts (Kirmayer, 2012). Reckless or unintended promotion of pharmaceutical treatments that lack effectiveness data in low and middle income countries may disconnect people from community experiences and adversely change the ways they perceive mental impairment and disability (Summerfield, 2012; Wildeman, 2013).

Global mental health therefore needs to conduct additional research on what services are acceptable and effective, and so worthy of scaling up in different sociocultural contexts (Jain & Orr, 2016). Local and population measures that modify disabling social oppression/barriers to enable people need to be addressed (Ingleby, 2014; Whitley, 2015). Advocates for social and interaction models of disability may have important points about impairment that global mental health needs to be cognizant of. For example, people with mental impairments in different cultures may be able to construe their own identities/selves, and figure out ways of living good lives in their peculiar sociocultural contexts. To meet the extreme accusation of global mental health as a postcolonial medical imperialism, global mental health needs strategies to integrate the local with the global and to connect closely with communities in the form of real mutual partnerships (Miller, 2014; Whitley, 2015).

To facilitate the operations of global mental health in different countries, extensive collection of data is necessary. Indeed, a third challenge for global mental health is the concern that this discipline represents a Foucauldian regime of government control, which closely impacts on people's selves and lives (Fullagar, 2017; Wildeman, 2013). The previous Director-General of the WHO Dr. Margaret Chan often reminded people attending her speech that "what gets measured gets done" (https://www.who.int/dg/speeches/2015/health-measurement-summit/en/). Global mental health has to heed the negative impacts of collecting and producing metrics for measuring mental impairment and psychosocial disability, in ways that do not meet the information requirement for distributive justice (Anand & Hanson, 1997; Laurie, 2015). For global mental health to succeed, it also has to strengthen its outcome measures to include not only symptoms and signs of mental disorders, but also the reality of subjective well-being. The CRPD may be useful for global mental health in addressing inequalities that restrict and suppress people with mental impairments and disabilities. However, global mental health needs to further develop a theoretical framework for justice, such as the capabilities approach, in order to optimize its impact (White, Imperiale, & Perera, 2016).

Challenges to neuroethics

The field of neuroethics was given impetus by the potential power of neuroscience-technology. It is important to address the ethical, legal and social implications of these science and technology developments. In the long run, neuroscientific understanding of constructs central to humanity (e.g., self, will, responsibility, competence, etc.) may in turn influence how we conduct ourselves (Greene & Cohen, 2004; Hacking, 1983). Indeed, neuroscience-technology may be viewed as part of the regime of biopower that governs people's lives, and neuroethics may be seen as also saturated with biopolitics (Jotterand & Ienca, 2017).

Based on medical models of disability, advancement of neuroscience-technology, such as pharmaceuticals and neural devices, are the best way to treat and rehabilitate people with mental impairment and disabilities. As a discipline scrutinizing and facilitating the ethics of researching and utilizing brain science and technology (Conrad & De Vries, 2011), neuroethics promotes their importance and power in individual interventions (Amadio et al., 2018; Evers, 2017; Illes, 2010). Along with the globalization of brain research initiatives, the role of neuroethics in consolidating the perceived pathology of people with mental impairment and disability will be vigorously opposed to by those who advocate for social and interaction models of psychosocial disabilities (Whitehouse, 2011).

Neuroethics relies on neuroscience, molecular biology and other mind sciences research, and may discount lay expert knowledge. Thus, the controversy about epistemological issues encountered in global mental health recurs in neuroethics. The issues involve not only how to use neuroscience knowledge to improve mental health and wellbeing of people in non-Western culture countries, but also how to conduct neuroscience research especially when local people hold worldviews and moralities that differ from individualist neoliberal ones (Brief & Illes, 2010). One example is the question of how to integrate neuroethics with a Confucian theory that treats one's self as a relational and contextual construct (Wu & Fukushi, 2012). Morals are deeply embedded in sociocultural contexts, which shape people's mind and behavior (Dewey, 1922). Different sociocultural regions might have their own peculiar processes of constructing and responding to mental impairments and disability. Exploration of these processes is needed to ensure that neuroethics incorporates local culture and morality when addressing disability.

Enhancement of cognition or morality is an important topic in neuroethics. However, some neuroethical discussion of cognitive enhancement may be so far-fetched as to fail the ethics of doing neuroethics; in not acknowledging assumptions explicitly, not validating knowledge through interdisciplinary studies, and not conducting comprehensive reflection (Racine, Rubio, Chandler, Forlini, & Lucke, 2014). Moreover, acceptance of the treatment-enhancement dichotomy in neuroethics may directly conflict with a human variation model of disabilities that embraces neurodiversity. Detailed scholarship on neuro-enhancement might inadvertently sustain the stigmatized views of autism, ADHD, and dyslexia that disabled people try hard to get rid of.

Opportunities for addressing disability in global mental health and neuroethics: A proposal

Opportunities for global mental health

On its official website (http://www.globalmentalhealth.org/), the Movement for Global Mental Health has around 200 institutions and 10,000 members. Also, its leaders and supporters are comprised of a range of different academic disciplines. Although the major themes of global mental health, including a focus on evidence-based practices, task-sharing, equity and human rights, and global concerns and learning, remain unchanged (Patel, 2014b; Patel et al., 2018; Prince et al., 2007), the field has continued to evolve in response to critique. For example, Vikram Patel, one of the major leaders in global mental health, has admitted that mental disorder diagnoses have flaws and has argued we should endeavor to increase their historical, face, predictive and concurrent validities.

Furthermore, given that global mental health requires working at multiple levels (from individual to social), Patel has argued that the dichotomy of biomedical and social determinants of health is flawed. Global mental health has for example emphasized the appropriate use of pharmaceuticals rather than totally rejecting their use. Moreover, the multidisciplinary work of global mental health has included qualitative research that is community based and has adapted its interventions on the basis of inquiry into subjects' experiences (Patel, 2014b). For example, in one of the 2011 Lancet series paper, the authors conducted qualitative research to explore the suffering from stigmatization and human rights violations of subjects with mental and psychosocial disabilities (Drew et al., 2011). In another paper that addresses the credibility gap of global mental health, Patel admitted that the rigid use of formal diagnostic criteria might be counterproductive; outcome of interventions must match the needs of concerned people; care could be offered by community and lay workers in non-professional settings (Patel, 2014a).

Indirectly responding to the issues of the sociocultural penetrating all the way through to mental distress or impairment in disability discourses, Patel is willing to bridge the gap by reviewing the use of mental diagnoses in practice and research without giving up the idea that mental disorders have brain basis and sociocultural determinants. He admitted that the epidemiological figures based on the GBD might be exaggerated when it is about mental disorder rather than mental distress, if people with mental distress (not disorder) are willing to receive help, the help could be tailored with context sensitivity and provided in non-formal settings (Patel, 2014a).

While the United Nations Sustainable Development Goals (UN SDG) includes mental health, worries persist about the risk of adopting interventions to poverty that are reductionist, economistic, individualized and psychologized (Mills, 2018). Around the end of 2018, the Lancet Commission published a report addressing global mental health and sustainable development (Patel et al., 2018). Here is not the space to discuss in details the contents of the report, but it suffices to say that the report is an integrative end product responding to previous debates about global mental health. Recognizing the diversity and complexity of mental health needs, the report emphasized the creation of enabling social and physical environments to promote and protect mental health that is a fundamental human right for all. In addition to its previous major themes such as scaling up, task sharing and investment, it stresses the importance of targeting the barriers and stresses to mental health, social and environmental determinants for mental health in people's different developmental periods, and the collaboration of different disciplines (Patel et al., 2018). Understanding mental health conditions as multilevel interactions between factors of biology and social/physical environment, the report advocates a staging model which aims to offer appropriate care with contextual sensitivity at the concerned stage/pathway of developing mental health conditions through people's life course (Patel et al., 2018). Avoiding psychiatric or cultural imperialism in global mental health does not mean cultural relativism or preservationism (Miller, 2014). An answer for the question of what a culture ought to be should be inquired into with understanding of its historical and dynamic background, because culture is always part and parcel of the people's ideas and artifacts in the making (Yip, Yousuf, Chan, Yung, & Wu, 2015).

The relational individualist construction of legal capacity in Article 12 of the CRPD might contradict the collectivistic construction of selves in different sociocultural regions in protecting other human rights. Contrast to a self that is constituted through the merging of interpersonal networks (Ames, 2011), the CRPD's formulation of relational autonomy in supported decision making still carries the sense of a permanent authentic self that is demarcated from its social networks. Strict respect to the will and preference of persons with psychosocial disabilities, no matter how unreasonable or dangerous they are, might regrettably aggravate the fear toward and stigmatization of these persons (Patel et al., 2018). Therefore, a universal definition of psychosocial disability might not be feasible for global mental health that considers specific sociocultural contexts regarding the recognition of mental impairment and redistribution of resources for intervention, and support for and development of persons with psychosocial disabilities based on capabilities approach (Danermark & Gellerstedt, 2004; Fraser, 1995; Mitra, 2006).

Opportunities for neuroethics

Prior to the development of neuroethics, psychiatric ethics has been an important branch of bioethics. Traditionally, it covers issues of person-level psychiatric care and population-level mental health law and policy. It also has a neuro- part insofar as it addresses treatment of mental disorders with pharmaceuticals and other neurotechnologies (Sadler, Van Staden, & Fulford, 2015). As psychiatry evolves with advances of neuroscience-technology, issues involved with the neuroscience of self and ethics/morality become more challenging, and may consolidate a neuronal/medical model of disability. Scholars in the field of neuroethics are aware of this conceptual trap especially when diagnostic biomarkers for mental disorders, such as those founded on molecular biology and neuroimaging, are yet to be found (Kellmeyer, 2017).

Taking neuroscience as involving multiple levels of observation and intervention, neuroethics must recognize pluralist approaches to understanding human mental conditions (Stein et al., 2015) as well as of the construction of self, morality and culture (Markus & Kitayama, 2010; Wu & Fukushi, 2012). This, for example, means that the construction of self can be construed at different levels (e.g., brain level, cultural level, etc.) simultaneously. Both global mental health and neuroethics are, however, aware of the power of sociocultural context in causing mental distress and improving wellbeing. In dealing with human rights issues in global mental health, neuroethics ought to consider not only the parity, access and distributive justice of neuropsychiatric technologies, but also local sociocultural contexts of morality (Stein & Giordano, 2015). As "morals are social" (Dewey, 1922, p. 321), neuroethics must be reflective in considering the sociocultural contexts of guidelines for principled cosmopolitan neuroethics, including empowerment, non-obsolescence, self-creativity and citizenship (Shook & Giordano, 2014).

It is possible that in different sociocultural contexts, people with psychosocial disabilities may prefer their own approaches to disability. Thus, we have to heed issues in status/identity recognition, resource redistribution, and governance representation (Dahl, Stoltz, & Willig, 2004). Although neuroethics has been criticized for not having a core theme other than the fuzzy question of what brain science can offer (Vidal, 2018), the benefit of such vagueness is that it allows us to examine brain, mind, morality, and sociocultural factors simultaneously. "Neuro" in neuroethics denotes where the scholarship starts, not the boundary of neuroethics. Thus, a pragmatic reconstruction of neuroethics as a field welcomes the inputs of other disciplines (Racine & Sample, 2018).

A proposal for an integrated model of disability through reflective equilibrium

Based on a coherence theory approach, Rawls proposed reflective equilibrium as a methodology for justifying moral judgments (Daniels, 1996). Although considered moral judgment is the starting point of moral belief, as situations change we may have to adjust our moral beliefs or ethical theories to reach a new equilibrium. Combining moral psychology with scientific evidence, Tiberius has argued that it is feasible to extend this method to the justification of moral psychology judgments (Tiberius, 2014). Furthermore, Daniels has advocated for wide reflective equilibrium, "a method that attempts to produce coherence in ordered triple sets of beliefs held by a particular person, namely: (a) a set of considered moral judgments, (b) a set of moral principles, and (c) a set of relevant (scientific and philosophical) background theories" (Daniels, 1996).

As disability per se is a social justice issue, this chapter uses Fig. 1 to represent how a group of people could use wide reflective equilibrium to construct a model of

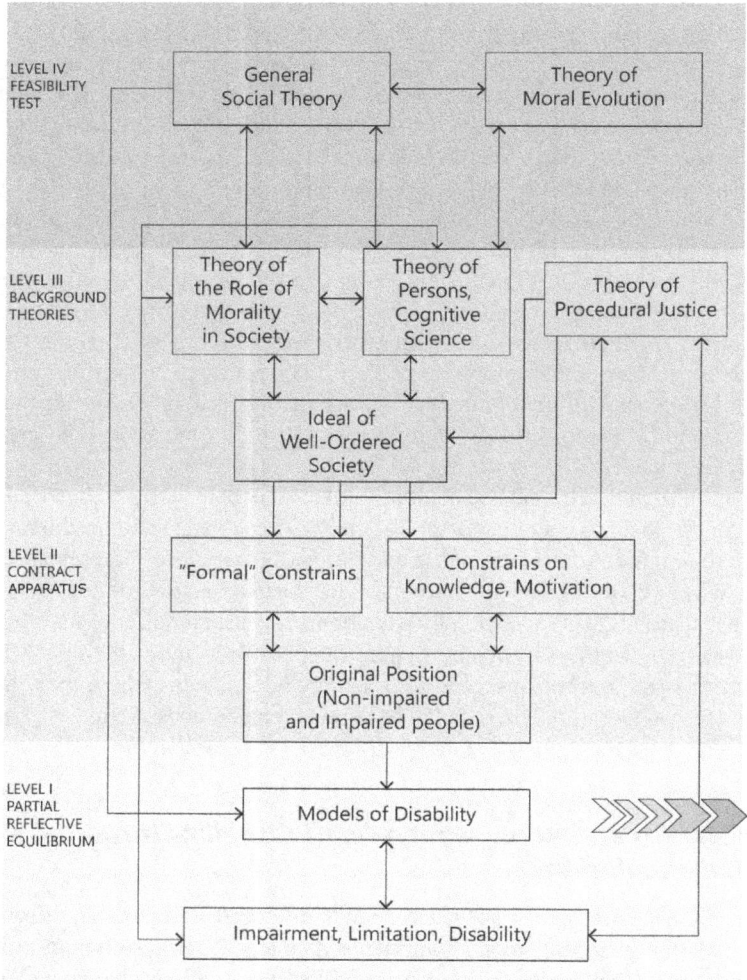

Fig. 1 Constructing a model of disability through wide reflective equilibrium.
Modified from Daniels, N. (1980). Reflective equilibrium and Archimedean points. *Canadian Journal of Philosophy, 10*(1), 88.

disability. At level I, a considered moral judgment about mental impairment, psychosocial disorder and disability has to first reach narrow equilibrium with the disability model. At level II, people with and without impairment could get together behind a thin veil of ignorance to determine a model of disability. This arrangement in Fig. 1 is different from Rawls's thick veil of ignorance for two reasons: (1) people may know whether they have mental impairment; (2) people with mental impairment may not have the "moral power" required by Rawls to reach agreement on the model of disability. During deliberation at the original position, they may be constrained by factors such as public discussion, individual knowledge (behind the thin veil of ignorance) and operations of human psychology like motivations (Daniels, 1996). In advocating for social inclusion and equal recognition of legal capacity with supported decision making, disability scholars have opposed Rawls's downplaying the capability of persons with mental impairment and excluding these persons from deliberations (Nussbaum, 2006; Rawls, 1993; Wong, 2007).

At level III there are the ideals of a well-ordered society, and an emphasis on procedural justice (Daniels, 1996). For us to imagine how we could live together in good enough harmony and wellbeing, these constructs may need to be revised for reaching equilibrium with considered judgments about disability. Especially when it comes to theory of persons, cognitive sciences and neuroethics offer both empirical and normative inputs to check whether considered judgment about models of disability need to be revised. At level IV, general social theories and theory of moral evolution may offer insights through ethnographic studies of sociocultural contexts to check whether level I formulations are feasible (Daniels, 1996).

A wide reflective equilibrium methodology could be extrapolated to populations that are willing to get together to deliberate how they would like to address disability in neuroethics and "glolocal" mental health issues (for the whole movement of global mental health, it is global; for the specified population, it is local). Thus the modified original position depicted in Fig. 1 carries the sense of deliberative democracy to engage science in a way that could offer a variety of formulations of disability for reaching consensus on disability construction and governance (Jasanoff, 2011; Rawls, 1993).

This chapter takes "ethics as a human ecology" (Flanagan, 2008). It emphasizes the close interactions between humans and environment, the prima facie importance of subjective experience, the sociocultural contextuality of human norms, and the necessity of utilizing social and natural sciences to engage and address different conundrums in human lives (Johnson, 2014). "More is different." (Anderson, 1972). Therefore, when addressing phenomena at different levels we must take a pragmatic epistemic approach to disability, recognizing that many phenomena are non-reducible and that it is necessary to use different instruments, explanations and operations for addressing issues at different levels. How we observe and represent things are closely related to how we intervene to address them. This understanding reminds us of the need for humility as we engage local people in utilizing science and technology to engage with human suffering, impairment and disability (Jasanoff, 2005).

Based on the wide reflective equilibrium in Fig. 1, an integrated model of disability is proposed in Fig. 2. Taking a pragmatic multilevel approach to the construction

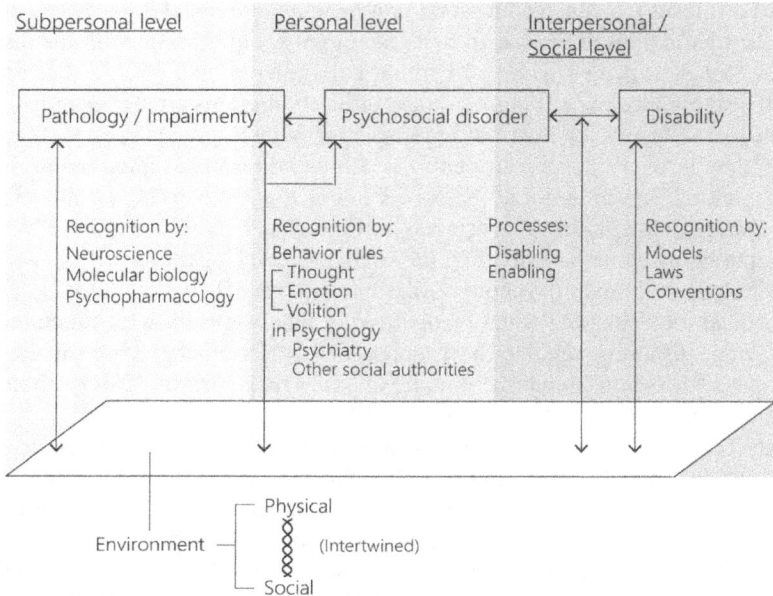

Fig. 2 An integrated model of mental/psychosocial disability.

of disability, this approach is consistent with an interaction model of disability. Importantly, all research and construction of knowledge about pathology and impairment occurs in a specific sociocultural context. Our understanding of the disabling and enabling processes, and the recognition of the disability also goes on in the context. Therefore, we have to be reflective, examining and revising the model of disability dynamically by engaging the public in the relevant context.

Currently, major formal diagnostic systems have incorporated culture or environment in their formulations. The US National Institute of Mental Health advocates adopting Research Domain Criteria (RDoC) for constructing a biology-based assessment system, including consideration of environmental factors. The fifth edition of Diagnostic and Statistical Manual (DSM-5) also has biological and cultural dimensions (Stein et al., 2015). Almost all diagnoses of mental disorders are based on the rules and norms of thought, emotion and volition in a particular society or region (Pilgrim & Tomasini, 2012). The hope that a diagnosis of mental disorder will be based on neuroscientific findings has not come true. Subjective suffering and sociocultural norms actually work together to define mental impairment.

The recognition of mental impairment usually counts on authorities in the psychiatric sciences or other social authorities. In the disability rights movement that demands "nothing about us without us" (Charlton, 1998), people with disabilities should participate and have joint authority in creating discourses of mental pathology and impairment. Thus, the model incorporates voices of people self-identified as users or survivors of mental health services and so are compatible with human variation models of disability. Recognition of pathology, impairment and disability is an important factor in the distribution of epistemic expertise and economic resources. Finally, continuous negotiation is necessary for recognition, representation and resource redistribution of disabilities at both the interpersonal and social levels.

To enhance psychosocial wellbeing for all, a capabilities approach that aims to embed enabling institutions for recovery, resilience, and enhancement (without discriminating against impairment) in society will be useful for appropriate distribution of expertise and resources. With all the caveats mentioned above the Lancet Commission on global mental health and sustainable development is a good demonstration of how a contextually sensitive and multilevel combination of global mental health and neuroscience could form a paradigm to address psychosocial disability and development issues in an ethical way (Patel et al., 2018). Several important issues need to be emphasized in order to strengthen the feasibility of this integrated model of disability that focuses on levels of observations and levels and timings of interventions (Fig. 3).

First, compatible with the Lancet Commission's recommendation, interventions should be implemented at different levels, with efforts to scale up those interventions that are best supported by the evidence. It is also important to examine whether interventions at different levels might conflict with each other. For example, increasing health insurance copayment to control overspending may limit the ability of people in poverty to seek mental health services. Strong marketing of credit cards to boom up economy might render debt-related mental distress in some people (Hodson, Dwyer, & Neilson, 2014; Richardson, Elliott, & Roberts, 2013). As suicide prevention is a very important topic for global mental health and neuroethics, the issue of the right to suicide (including assisted death) needs to be addressed at different levels, in different sectors, and through different stages of life courses (An interview with Tina Minkowitz, 2015; Kim, De Vries, & Peteet, 2016; Shakespeare, 2014; Sisask & Värnik, 2012).

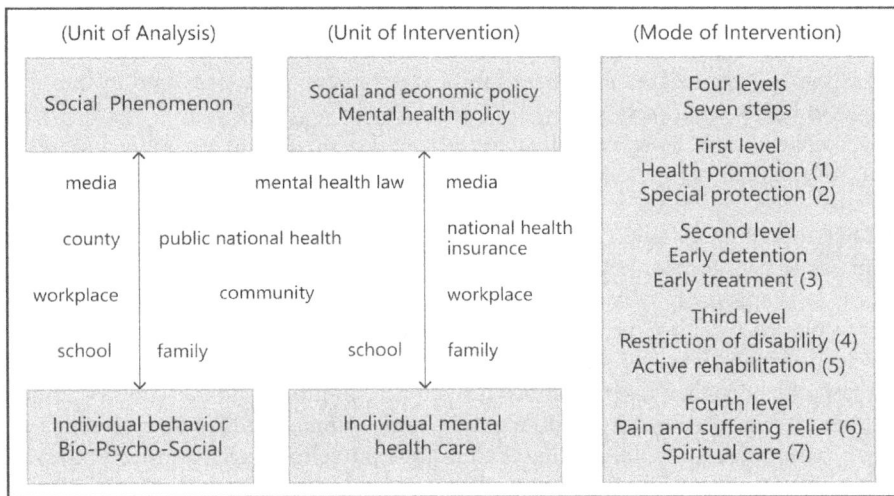

Fig. 3 Multilevel mental health policy.

Second, there is a responsibility for justice in global mental health and neuroethics (Young, 2011). Mutually embedded justice issues in recognition, redistribution and representation run through all the levels. Global mental health and neuroethics have both emphasized the importance of humility and self-reflection. It is important for global mental health and neuroethics to consider how they recognize and represent impairment and disability, and how they propose to redistribute expertise (e.g., among laypersons and professionals) and resources to address mental impairment and psychosocial disability. We live in a changing world, thus we have to adjust our conceptions of disability and distributive justice all the time for sustainable development. What we can achieve pragmatically is to take a comparative justice stance, trying to make our society more just than the past considering all factors (Sen, 2009). It is possible that human rights protection requirements of people with psychosocial disabilities are not all achieved, but continuous exchanges for increasing these people's capabilities and freedom for health and wellbeing must be sustained.

Finally, it is time to examine how models of disability can fit in with different kinds of mental distress or mental disorders in different sociocultural contexts. For example, it is worthwhile to address whether alcohol and substance use problems could be construed as disability in global mental health and neuroethics. Fierce debates have persisted regarding whether alcohol and substance use problems represent moral failure, neuronal or mental disorders, or disabilities (Flacks, 2012; Wasserman, 2004). It is important to take a systemic approach to address alcohol and substance use by adjusting factors concurrently at the subpersonal, individual and social levels (Ahmed, Badiani, Miczek, & Müller, in press). Based on medical, social and interaction models, some alcohol and substance use problems can be construed as disabilities. However, not all countries count and treat alcohol or substance use disorders as such. The United States, but not Canada, excludes these disorders from the coverage of disability social welfare (Flacks, 2012). Moreover, different sectors of same countries might adopt conflicting discourses at the same time. In Taiwan's mental health act, alcohol and substance use disorders are included as official mental diagnoses, but treatment for these disorders are not covered by Taiwan's universal health insurance.

To make things more complicated, advocates for human variation models of disability may argue that alcohol and substance use problems are not impairment, but that people with these problems are disabled by environmental oppressions and barriers. Perhaps good policy making is to accommodate their needs and treat them equally with other people having no "problematic" uses. If a war on drugs is not the best approach, what else could we do by supply side or demand side strategies to reduce disabling processes in society to people with alcohol and substance use "problems"? The considerations demonstrate how complex it is to address alcohol and substance use problems as disability in global mental health and neuroethics. It is necessary for global mental health and neuroethics to explore how to construct models of disability that lead to innovative measures at different levels, in order to increase the capabilities of persons with specific mental impairments and disorders.

Conclusion

Disability is a complicated and challenging issue for global mental health and neuroethics. Analysis of disability models may shed light on how best the intersection of global mental health and neuroscience can address issues surrounding disability. Disability, global mental health, and neuroethics all need transdisciplinary collaboration to make dynamic adjustments to their epistemic frameworks, in order to enhance global mental health by including consideration of local sociocultural contexts as well as the voices of people with mental impairment.

Debates on recognition, representation and resource redistribution in disability studies also reflect key controversies in global mental health and neuroethics. Disability studies can therefore potentially broaden the scope and deepen the discourse at the intersection of global mental health and neuroethics. Whether mental health conditions are best approached as an issue of impairment, morality, normativity, minority, diversity or identity remains contested. Ongoing negotiation is needed to resolve whose perspectives and what sociocultural contexts should be incorporated into debates about impairment and disability. If willing to be flexible and accommodating, global mental health and neuroethics have the opportunity to respond to critiques and to meaningfully address disability.

Corresponding to the argument in Lancet Commission on global mental health and sustainable development, this chapter proposes that global mental health and neuroethics adopt a multilevel integrated model of disability incorporating three major themes:

(1) The construction of models of disability is a dynamic process. Through wide reflective equilibrium, people with mental distress or impairment may join the process to reach overlapping consensus on what disability is. This bottom up process could enrich the contents of neuroethics in achieving the goal of global mental health to enhance sustainable development.

(2) Recognition and representation of impairment and disability must be thoroughly examined in order to ensure that just redistribution policies are epistemically and socioculturally sensitive. Mental impairment is often determined by explicit and implicit behavior rules in specific contexts, and the scientific gaze needs to be supplemented with local understandings. An integrated dimensional approach to mental health problems (from suffering to wellbeing), is needed to address disability.

(3) Disability issues can be observed and addressed at different levels in different stages via different steps. It is important to establish strategies to monitor the conflicts and coherence among interventions. Adopting a comparative justice stance, we could endeavor to adjust our conceptions of disability and justice pragmatically to reach a fair distribution that increase people's capabilities and makes things better. To test whether the integrated model proposed here is a useful instrument, we need to examine its feasibility for addressing specific mental conditions such as addiction and suicide.

The discussion in this chapter demonstrates how difficult it is to address disability in global mental health and neuroethics comprehensively and evenly in limited space. Many ideas touched on in the chapter may be topics for further elaboration. To borrow a Chinese idiom, if the chapter's brick-quality work could attract later related jade-quality scholarship, this would an important achievement.

Acknowledgments

I thank very much Ms. Ching-Ting Liu, LL.B. & B.N., for her collaboration in designing and drawing the figures in the chapter.

References

Ahmed S.H., Badiani A., Miczek K.A., and Müller C.P., Non-pharmacological factors that determine drug use and addiction, *Neuroscience and Biobehavioral Reviews* in press, https://doi.org/10.1016/j.neubiorev.2018.08.015.

Allen, J., Balfour, R., Bell, R., & Marmot, M. (2014). Social determinants of mental health. *International Review of Psychiatry*, 26(4), 392–407.

Altman, B. M. (2001). *Disability definitions, models, classification schemes, and applications*. In *Handbook of disability studies* (pp. 97–122).

Amadio, J., Bi, G.-Q., Boshears, P. F., Carter, A., Devor, A., Doya, K., et al. (2018). Neuroethics questions to guide ethical research in the international brain initiatives. *Neuron*, 100(1), 19–36.

Ames, R. T. (2011). *Confucian role ethics: A vocabulary*. Hong Kong: Chinese University Press.

Amundson, R. (2000). Against normal function. *Studies in History and Philosophy of Science Part C: Studies in History and Philosophy of Biological and Biomedical Sciences*, 31(1), 33–53.

An interview with Tina Minkowitz. (2015). Advancing the rights of users and survivors of psychiatry using the UN convention on the rights of persons with disabilities. In H. Spandler & J. Anderson (Eds.), *Madness, distress and the politics of disablement* (pp. 171–182). Bristol: Policy Press.

Anand, S., & Hanson, K. (1997). Disability-adjusted life years: A critical review. *Journal of Health Economics*, 16(6), 685–702.

Anastasiou, D., & Kauffman, J. M. (2013). The social model of disability: Dichotomy between impairment and disability. *The Journal of Medicine and Philosophy: A Forum for Bioethics and Philosophy of Medicine*, 38(4), 441–459.

Anderson, P. W. (1972). More is different. *Science*, 177(4047), 393–396.

Beaudry, J.-S. (2016). Beyond (models of) disability? *The Journal of Medicine and Philosophy: A Forum for Bioethics and Philosophy of Medicine*, 41(2), 210–228.

Bickenbach, J. E. (1993). *Physical disability and social policy*. Toronto: University of Toronto Press.

Bickenbach, J. E. (2009). Disability, culture and the UN convention. *Disability and Rehabilitation*, 31(14), 1111–1124.

Brief, E., & Illes, J. (2010). Tangles of neurogenetics, neuroethics, and culture. *Neuron*, 68(2), 174–177.

Charlton, J. I. (1998). *Nothing about us without us: Disability oppression and empowerment*. Berkeley: University of California Press.

Cherepanov, E. (2018). *Ethics for global mental health: From good intentions to humanitarian accountability*. Routledge.

Cole, P. (2007). The body politic: Theorising disability and impairment. *Journal of Applied Philosophy*, 24(2), 169–176.

Committee on the Rights of Persons with Disabilities. (2014). *General comment No. 1 (2014). Article 12: Equal recognition before the law* Retrieved from: https://documents-dds-ny.un-.org/doc/UNDOC/GEN/G14/031/20/PDF/G1403120.pdf?OpenElement. February. 2019.

Committee on the Rights of Persons with Disabilities. (2015). *Guidelines on article 14 of the convention on the rights of persons with disabilities* Retrieved from: https://www.ohchr.org/EN/HRBodies/CRPD/Pages/Guidelines.aspx. February 2019.

Conrad, E. C., & De Vries, R. (2011). *Field of dreams: A social history of neuroethics.* In *Sociological reflections on the neurosciences.* Emerald Group Publishing Limited (pp. 299–324).

Curtis, T. R., Dellar, R., Leslie, E., & Watson, B. (2000). *Mad pride: A celebration of mad culture.* London: Spare Change Books.

Dahl, H. M., Stoltz, P., & Willig, R. (2004). Recognition, redistribution and representation in capitalist global society: An interview with Nancy Fraser. *Acta Sociologica, 47*(4), 374–382.

Danermark, B., & Gellerstedt, L. C. (2004). Social justice: Redistribution and recognition—A non-reductionist perspective on disability. *Disability & Society, 19*(4), 339–353.

Daniels, N. (1996). *Justice and justification: Reflective equilibrium in theory and practice.* New York: Cambridge University Press.

Davis, L. J. (2002). *Bending over backwards: Disability, dismodernism & other difficult positions.* New York: New York University Press.

Davis, L. J. (2017). Introduction: Disability, normality, and power. In L. J. Davis (Ed.), *The disability studies reader.* (5th ed., pp. 1–14). New York: Routlefge.

Dewey, J. (1922). *Human nature and conduct: An introduction to social psychology.* New York: Henry Holt.

Drew, N., Funk, M., Tang, S., Lamichhane, J., Chávez, E., Katontoka, S., et al. (2011). Human rights violations of people with mental and psychosocial disabilities: An unresolved global crisis. *The Lancet, 378*(9803), 1664–1675.

Evers, K. (2017). The contribution of neuroethics to international brain research initiatives. *Nature Reviews Neuroscience, 18*(1), 1–2.

Ferrari, A. J., Charlson, F. J., Norman, R. E., Patten, S. B., Freedman, G., Murray, C. J., et al. (2013). Burden of depressive disorders by country, sex, age, and year: Findings from the global burden of disease study 2010. *PLoS Medicine, 10*(11), e1001547.

Flacks, S. (2012). Deviant disabilities: The exclusion of drug and alcohol addiction from the Equality Act 2010. *Social & Legal Studies, 21*(3), 395–412.

Flanagan, O. (2008). *The problem of the soul: Two visions of mind and how to reconcile them.* New York: Basic Books.

Frances, A. (2013). *Saving normal: An insider's look at what caused the epidemic of mental illness and how to cure it.* New York, NY: William Morrow.

Fraser, N. (1995). From redistribution to recognition? Dilemmas of justice in a 'post-socialist'age. *New Left Review,* 68.

Freeman, M. C., Kolappa, K., de Almeida, J. M. C., Kleinman, A., Makhashvili, N., Phakathi, S., et al. (2015). Reversing hard won victories in the name of human rights: A critique of the general comment on article 12 of the UN convention on the rights of persons with disabilities. *The Lancet Psychiatry, 2*(9), 844–850.

Fullagar, S. (2017). Foucauldian theory. In B. M. Z. Cohen (Ed.), *Routledge international handbook of critical mental health* (pp. 39–45). New York: Routledge.

Garland-Thomson, R. (2002). Integrating disability, transforming feminist theory. *NWSA Journal,* 1–32.

Goodley, D. (2017). *Disability studies: An interdisciplinary introduction* (2nd ed.). London: Sage.

Graby, S. (2015). Neurodiversity: Bridging the gap between the disabled people's movement and the mental health system survivors' movement. In H. Spandler, J. Anderson, & B. Sapey (Eds.), *Madness, distress and the politics of disablement* (pp. 231–244). Bristol: Policy Press.

Greene, J., & Cohen, J. (2004). For the law, neuroscience changes nothing and everything. *Philosophical Transactions of the Royal Society, B: Biological Sciences, 359*(1451), 1775.

Grosse, S. D., Lollar, D. J., Campbell, V. A., & Chamie, M. (2009). Disability and disability-adjusted life years: Not the same. *Public Health Reports, 124*(2), 197–202.

Hacking, I. (1983). *Representing and intervening: Introductory topics in the philosophy of natural science.* New York: Cambridge University Press.

Hemmingsson, H., & Jonsson, H. (2005). An occupational perspective on the concept of participation in the International Classification of Functioning, Disability and Health—Some critical remarks. *The American Journal of Occupational Therapy, 59*(5), 569–576.

Hodson, R., Dwyer, R. E., & Neilson, L. A. (2014). Credit card blues: The middle class and the hidden costs of easy credit. *The Sociological Quarterly, 55*(2), 315–340.

Illes, J. (2010). Empowering brain science with neuroethics. *The Lancet, 376*(9749), 1294–1295.

Illes, J. & Hossain, S. (Eds.), (2017). *Neuroethics: Anticipating the future.* New York: Oxford University Press.

Ingleby, D. (2014). How 'evidence-based' is the movement for global mental health? *Disability and the Global South, 1*(2), 203–226.

Jain, S., & Orr, D. M. (2016). Ethnographic perspectives on global mental health. *Transcultural Psychiatry, 53*(6), 685–695.

Jasanoff, S. (2005). *Technologies of humility: Citizen participation in governing science.* In *Wozu experten?* Springer (pp. 370–389).

Jasanoff, S. (2011). *Designs on nature: Science and democracy in Europe and the United States.* Princeton: Princeton University Press.

Johnson, M. (2014). Keeping the pragmatism in neuropragmatism. In T. Solimosi & J. R. Shook (Eds.), *Neuroscience, neurophilosophy, and pragmatism: Brains at work with the world* (pp. 37–56). New York: Palgrave Macmillan.

Jotterand, F., & Ienca, M. (2017). *The biopolitics of neuroethics.* In *Debates about neuroethics* Springer (pp. 247–261).

Kellmeyer, P. (2017). Ethical and legal implications of the methodological crisis in neuroimaging. *Cambridge Quarterly of Healthcare Ethics, 26*(4), 530–554.

Kim, S. Y., De Vries, R. G., & Peteet, J. R. (2016). Euthanasia and assisted suicide of patients with psychiatric disorders in the Netherlands 2011 to 2014. *JAMA Psychiatry, 73*(4), 362–368.

Kirmayer, L. J. (2012). Cultural competence and evidence-based practice in mental health: Epistemic communities and the politics of pluralism. *Social Science & Medicine, 75*(2), 249–256.

Laurie, E. W. (2015). Who lives, who dies, who cares? Valuing life through the disability-adjusted life year measurement. *Transactions of the Institute of British Geographers, 40*(1), 75–87.

Linton, S. (1998). Disability studies/not disability studies. *Disability & Society, 13*(4), 525–539.

Markus, H. R., & Kitayama, S. (2010). Cultures and selves: A cycle of mutual constitution. *Perspectives on Psychological Science, 5*(4), 420–430.

Martiny, K. M. (2015). How to develop a phenomenological model of disability. *Medicine, Health Care and Philosophy, 18*(4), 553–565.

Mathers, C. D., & Loncar, D. (2006). Projections of global mortality and burden of disease from 2002 to 2030. *PLoS Medicine, 3*(11), e442.

Miller, G. (2014). Is the agenda for global mental health a form of cultural imperialism? *Medical Humanities, 40*(2), 131–134.

Mills, C. (2018). From 'Invisible Problem' to global priority: The inclusion of mental health in the sustainable development goals. *Development and Change, 49*(3), 843–866.

Mitra, S. (2006). The capability approach and disability. *Journal of Disability Policy Studies*, *16*(4), 236–247. https://doi.org/10.1177/10442073060160040501.

Mitra, S. (2018). *The human development model of disability, health and wellbeing*. In *Disability, health and human development*. New York: Palgrave Macmillan US (pp. 9–32).

Murray, C. J., & Lopez, A. D. (1994). Quantifying disability: Data, methods and results. *Bulletin of the World Health Organization*, *72*(3), 481.

Murray, C. J., & Lopez, A. D. (1996). Evidence-based health policy—Lessons from the Global Burden of Disease Study. *Science*, *274*(5288), 740–743.

Nussbaum, M. C. (2006). *Frontiers of justice: Disability, nationality, species membership*. Cambridge, MA: Harvard University Press.

Patel, V. (2012). Global mental health: From science to action. *Harvard Review of Psychiatry*, *20*(1), 6–12.

Patel, V. (2014a). Rethinking mental health care: Bridging the credibility gap. *Intervention*, *12*, 15–20.

Patel, V. (2014b). Why mental health matters to global health. *Transcultural Psychiatry*, *51*(6), 777–789.

Patel, V., Saxena, S., Lund, C., Thornicroft, G., Baingana, F., Bolton, P., et al. (2018). The Lancet Commission on global mental health and sustainable development. *The Lancet*, *392*(10157), 1553–1598.

Pilgrim, D., & Tomasini, F. (2012). On being unreasonable in modern society: Are mental health problems special? *Disability & Society*, *27*(5), 631–646.

Prince, M., Patel, V., Saxena, S., Maj, M., Maselko, J., Phillips, M. R., et al. (2007). No health without mental health. *The Lancet*, *370*(9590), 859–877.

Racine, E., Rubio, T. M., Chandler, J., Forlini, C., & Lucke, J. (2014). The value and pitfalls of speculation about science and technology in bioethics: The case of cognitive enhancement. *Medicine, Health Care and Philosophy*, *17*(3), 325–337.

Racine, E., & Sample, M. (2018). Two problematic foundations of neuroethics and pragmatist reconstructions. *Cambridge Quarterly of Healthcare Ethics*, *27*(4), 566–577.

Rawls, J. (1993). *Political liberalism*. New York: Columbia University Press.

Reeve, D. (2012). Psycho-emotional disablism: The missing link? In N. Watson (Ed.), *Routledge handbook of disability studies* (pp. 92–106). New York: Routledge.

Richardson, T., Elliott, P., & Roberts, R. (2013). The relationship between personal unsecured debt and mental and physical health: A systematic review and meta-analysis. *Clinical Psychology Review*, *33*(8), 1148–1162.

Russo, J., & Shulkes, D. (2015). Whtat we talk about when we talk about disability: Making sense of debates in the European user/survivor movement. In H. Spandler & J. Anderson (Eds.), *Madness, distress and the politics of disablement* (pp. 27–42). Bristol: Policy Press.

Sadler, J. Z., Van Staden, W., & Fulford, K. W. M. (Eds.), (2015). *Oxford handbook of psychiatric ethics*. Oxford: Oxford University Press.

Salomon, J. A., Haagsma, J. A., Davis, A., de Noordhout, C. M., Polinder, S., Havelaar, A. H., et al. (2015). Disability weights for the Global Burden of Disease 2013 study. *The Lancet Global Health*, *3*(11), e712–e723.

Sapey, B., Spandler, H., & Anderson, J. (2015). Introduction. In H. Spandler & J. Anderson (Eds.), *Madness, distress and the politics of disablement* (pp. 1–10). Bristol: Policy Press.

Scotch, R. K., & Schriner, K. (1997). Disability as human variation: Implications for policy. *The Annals of the American Academy of Political and Social Science*, *549*(1), 148–159.

Scully, J. L. (2012). Deaf identities in disability studies: With us or without us? In N. Watson (Ed.), *Routledge handbook of disability studies* (pp. 121–133). New York: Routledge.

Sen, A. K. (2009). *The idea of justice*. Harvard University Press.

Series, L. (2015). Relationships, autonomy and legal capacity: Mental capacity and support paradigms. *International Journal of Law and Psychiatry*, *40*, 80–91.

Shakespeare, T. (2014). *Disability rights and wrongs revisited*. New York: Routledge.

Sherry, M. (2006). *If I only had a brain: Deconstructing brain injury*. New York: Routledge.

Shook, J. R., & Giordano, J. (2014). *A principled and cosmopolitan neuroethics: Considerations for international relevance*. BioMed Central.

Sisask, M., & Värnik, A. (2012). Media roles in suicide prevention: A systematic review. *International Journal of Environmental Research and Public Health*, *9*(1), 123–138.

Stein, M. S. (2008). *Distributive justice and disability: Utilitarianism against egalitarianism*. New Haven: Yale University Press.

Stein, D. J., & Giordano, J. (2015). Global mental health and neuroethics. *BMC Medicine*, *13*(1), 44.

Stein, D. J., He, Y., Phillips, A., Sahakian, B. J., Williams, J., & Patel, V. (2015). Global mental health and neuroscience: Potential synergies. *The Lancet Psychiatry*, *2*(2), 178–185.

Summerfield, D.J.T.P. (2012). Afterword: Against "global mental health". *Transcultural Psychiatry*, *49*(3–4), 519–530.

Szasz, T. S. (1960). The myth of mental illness. *American Psychologist*, *15*(2), 113.

Tiberius, V. (2014). *Moral psychology: A contemporary introduction*. Routledge.

Tremain, S. (2001). On the government of disability. *Social Theory and Practice*, *27*(4), 617–636.

United Nations Convention on the Rights of Persons with Disabilities. (2006). Retrieved from: http://www.un.org/disabilities/documents/convention/convention_accessible_pdf.pdf. February 2019.

UPIAS. (1976). *Fundamental principles of disability*. London: Union of the Physically Impaired Against Segregation.

Vehmas, S. (2008). Philosophy and science: The axes of evil in disability studies? *Journal of Medical Ethics*, *34*(1), 21–23.

Vidal, F. (2018). What makes neuroethics possible? *History of the Human Sciences*, https://doi. org/10.1177/0952695118800410.

Wakefield, J. C. (1992). Disorder as harmful dysfunction: A conceptual critique of DSM-III-R's definition of mental disorder. *Psychological Review*, *99*(2), 232–247.

Wallcraft, J., & Hopper, K. (2015). The capabilities approach and the social model of mental health. In H. Spandler & J. Anderson (Eds.), *Madness, distress and the politics of disablement* (pp. 83–97). Bristol: Policy Press.

Wasserman, D. (2004). Addiction and disability: Moral and policy issues. *Substance Use & Misuse*, *39*(3), 461–488.

Wasserman, D. (2018). Can a social model of disability encompass "mental illness"? In C. A. Riddle (Ed.), *From disability to practice: Essays in honor of Jerome E. Bichenbach* (pp. 61–74). Lanham, MD: Lexington Books.

Wasserman, D., Asch, A., Blustein, J., & Putnam, D. (2016). Disability: Definitions, models, experience. In E. N. Zalta (Ed.), *The Stanford encyclopedia of philosophy*. Available from: https://plato.stanford.edu/archives/sum2016/entries/disability/.

White, R. G., Imperiale, M. G., & Perera, E. (2016). The capabilities approach: Fostering contexts for enhancing mental health and wellbeing across the globe. *Globalization and Health*, *12*, 16.

Whitehouse, P. (2011). Empowering whom? Neuroethics at its limits. *The Lancet*, *377*(9764), 468.

Whitley, R. (2015). Global mental health: Concepts, conflicts and controversies. *Epidemiology and Psychiatric Sciences*, *24*(4), 285–291.

Wildeman, S. (2013). Protecting rights and building capacities: Challenges to global mental health policy in light of the convention on the rights of persons with disabilities. *The Journal of Law, Medicine & Ethics, 41*(1), 48–73.

Wong, S. I. (2007). The moral personhood of individuals labeled "mentally retarded": A Rawlsian response to Nussbaum. *Social Theory and Practice, 33*(4), 579–594.

World Health Organization. (2002). *Towards a common language for functioning, disability and health: ICF* Retrieved from: https://www.who.int/classifications/icf/icfbeginnersguide. pdf. February 2019.

World Health Organization. (2011). *World report on disability* Retrieved from: https://www. who.int/disabilities/world_report/2011/en/. February 2019.

Wu, K.C.-C., & Fukushi, T. (2012). Neuroethics in Taiwan: Could there be a confucian solution? *East Asian Science, Technology and Society: An International Journal, 6*(3), 321–334.

Yip, P. S., Yousuf, S., Chan, C. H., Yung, T., & Wu, K.C.-C. (2015). The roles of culture and gender in the relationship between divorce and suicide risk: A meta-analysis. *Social Science & Medicine, 128*, 87–94.

Young, I. M. (2011). *Responsibility for justice*. New York: Oxford University Press.

Zola, I. K. (1989). Aging and disability: Toward a unified agenda. *Journal of Rehabilitation, 55*(4), 6.

Section D

Conclusion

Ethical issues in global mental health

16

Andrea C. Palk, Dan J. Stein
Department of Psychiatry, University of Cape Town, Cape Town, South Africa

Introduction

A consideration of the intersection between global mental health and neuroethics raises broader questions about ethical issues in global mental health itself. The recent emergence of global mental health, as both a distinct field of study, research and practice, and a relatively unified social movement, has been informed by the overarching aims, successes and challenges of the broader field of global health (Koplan et al., 2009; Patel & Prince, 2010). The primary aim of both global health and global mental health has been to address health inequities within and between nations, so as to improve the health and well-being of populations (Benatar, 2011; Patel, 2012; Patel et al., 2018). The implementation of this aim has been informed by attention to the social determinants of health and disease at individual, family, community, national and international levels (Pinto, Birn, & Upshur, 2013a).

The implementation of this aim has also raised a number of ethical issues including the fact that moral and ethical norms, and legal rules, differ across the globe in their stability and applicability. This reality produces tensions regarding the need to balance respect for ethical pluralism with seemingly universally applicable ethical precepts, to avoid charges of ethical imperialism in global health research and practice (Lolas, 2016; Macklin, 2012). In particular, global health endeavors face ethical challenges posed by cultural diversity, including the need to consider and respect explanatory models of disease in particular contexts.

Global mental health and global health also share underlying normative assumptions. Both fields emphasize the moral obligation to redress health inequities and recognize the historical context of colonialism and exploitation in which such inequities arose (Myser, 2015; Pinto, Birn, & Upshur, 2013b). Both are thus strongly informed by a concern for justice and are justified with reference to the recognition that all persons have an equal human right to health. While this overlap provides a rich resource for addressing the ethical issues encountered in the newer field of global mental health, there has been surprisingly little ethical engagement with global mental health as a distinct field. Here we attempt to outline and categorize these ethical issues and challenges.

Despite the considerable overlap between global health and global mental health, the latter intensifies many of the ethical challenges in international research and

Global Mental Health and Neuroethics. https://doi.org/10.1016/B978-0-12-815063-4.00016-2

clinical practice, due to the nature of mental disorders.[a] Ethical issues at the overlap between global mental health and neuroethics are similarly challenging for this reason. Global mental health may also be more ethically complex in comparison with other areas of medicine due to the fact that mental health care is subject to particularly severe resource constraints (Lora et al., 2012; Wittchen & Jacobi, 2005) and often requires longer, ongoing treatment thus necessitating a "care rather than cure" approach (Katz, Lahey, & Campbell, 2014). In addition, because symptoms are manifested behaviorally and variably, mental disorders may be more liable to incorrect or problematic causal ascriptions, and thus, to stigmatizing assumptions (Ngui, Khasakhala, Ndetei, & Roberts, 2010). Mental disorders are also frequently associated with neurocognitive impairments which may pose challenges to securing informed consent from research participants and patients (Katz et al., 2014).

In this concluding chapter we provide an overview of some of the ethical issues raised by the emergence of global mental health as a distinct field as well as supporting calls for a more inclusive bioethics paradigm for considering health on a global scale. In doing this, we draw on ideas put forward by various authors in this volume, as well as on the principles of equity and inclusivity that have been central to the development of global mental health. In particular, we argue that the principle of solidarity is an appropriate guiding principle for global level endeavors. Some of the ethical challenges we discuss are unique to global mental health while others are generic to any global heath endeavor, although where possible, we focus our discussion on the aspects of such ethical concerns that are unique to global mental health. Importantly, health inequities are present not only between low- and middle-income countries (LMICs) and high-income countries (HICs) but also within HICs themselves. Much work addresses the challenges associated with providing equitable access to health care to refugee, migrant and minority populations within such contexts (Robertshaw, Dhesi, & Jones, 2017; Smith & Daynes, 2016; Thornton et al., 2016). However, given that mental health resource scarcities are particularly severe in LMICs, the bulk of the literature engages with these contexts, and our overview will follow suit.

Toward an overview of the major ethical issues in global mental health

Several ethical issues have emerged in relation to global mental health study, research and practice. In considering how best to classify these issues we reviewed previous documents in this area as well as considered some of the ethical challenges

---

[a] A parallel may be drawn with the field of bioethics and neuroethics. While neuroethics may be considered as a subset of bioethics, a strong argument can be made that it warrants consideration as a distinct field in its own right, given the fact that the issues raised are qualitatively unique in comparison with other areas of bioethics (Roskies, 2007). This is due to the fact that because the brain is the organ of thought and consciousness, the possibility of being able to "read," alter or enhance the brain has deeply profound implications for conceptions of personhood, morality, personal identity and free will.

encountered by the broader discipline of global health. Global mental health evokes a range of ethical issues, including questions regarding the normative assumptions that underpin the field, particular challenges related to global mental health research, practice and global collaboration, and cross-cutting concerns related to how to navigate the complex interplay between the nature of mental disorders and the social, political and economic circumstances in particular contexts (see Jotterand et al. and Tomlinson et al. for discussions of this latter theme). Given the considerable overlap in these areas we have organized our discussion in terms of ethical challenges associated with global collaboration in mental health, global mental health research, and global mental health care.

Ethical issues relevant to global collaboration in mental health

Global mental health as cultural and ethical imperialism

Various foundational criticisms of global mental health have been made, particularly from the fields of transcultural psychiatry and anthropology. While some of these criticisms could be applicable to any endeavor with global aspirations, a particular strand is directed at perceived attempts to globalize Western psychiatric nosology, diagnoses, and interventions (Fernando, 2014; Mills, 2014; Mills & Fernando, 2014; Summerfield, 2012). The concern is that a particular conception of mental disorder and health, the biomedical model, is presented as universal with the result that its "exportation" risks sidelining, or ultimately replacing, localized conceptions and responses as well as failing to adequately account for the role played by contextual factors in mental disorders (Campbell & Burgess, 2012; Clark, 2014). Global mental health, the critics claim, is therefore a form of neocolonialism or cultural imperialism (Summerfield, 2013). Furthermore, insofar as it imposes a particular model of health, global mental health contains an implicit value judgment of right and wrong, or better and worse ways of understanding and treating mental disorders, it is thus also a form of ethical imperialism.

Some of these critiques have, however, been described as employing an essentialist or reified conception of culture as immutable and static (Miller, 2014), or, as implying what Appiah describes as a "preservationist ethic," according to which any form of cultural "assimilation" becomes tantamount to "annihilation" (Appiah, 2005). Furthermore, these debates are often framed in polarized terms or "rigid binaries"[*] such as "the biological vs. the social; nature vs. culture; global vs. local; the universal vs. the relative; the biomedical vs. the traditional" (Cooper, 2016). Representing reality in such oversimplified terms is not only an inaccurate reflection of its complexity, but also impedes constructive discussion (Cooper, 2016). In this regard, we have advocated for a more integrated approach to global mental health that avoids the polarities of scientism and skepticism (Stein & Illes, 2015) (see Stein and Palk). Bemme and D'souza also criticize debates that pit the global against the local, arguing that the former is presented in explicitly abstract terms while the universalizing assumptions that inform conceptions of the local are unrecognized and unproblematized (Bemme & D'Souza, 2014). They suggest replacing the global/local polarity with the notion of community, as a means of moving such debates forward. The notion of community is able to encompass varying scales from "global epistemic communities," which are independent of spatial constraints, to the "specificity" that is characteristic of particular, smaller scale communities (Bemme & D'Souza, 2014).

Patel, a pioneer of global mental health, has also responded to criticisms (Patel, 2014). In response to criticisms that the use of the biomedical approach to treating mental disorders pays insufficient attention to the social determinants of mental health, he points out that this sets up a false dichotomy between the biological and the non-biological. While global mental health is founded on the fact that social determinants impact or play a role in nearly all health conditions, it is also the case that these impacts "are ultimately mediated through biological pathways" (Patel, 2014). Patel also contests the claim that global mental health is a front for the extension of the reach of psychiatry and the pharmaceutical industry, pointing out that global mental health practitioners advocate both psychosocial interventions and evidence-based drug interventions, employing generic medications often developed in LMICs (Patel et al., 2003). Furthermore, he draws attention to the fact that global mental health is a multidisciplinary field that is founded in global health rather than psychiatry and is deeply informed by the realization of the importance of including persons with mental disorders in setting its agenda (Patel, 2014).

Power disparities in research collaborations

As is the case with the broader field of global health, global mental health frequently involves collaborations between researchers from HICs and those from LMICs, or between the global north and the global south. Given differential access to funding and other resources between such contexts, there is a risk that power disparities may adversely influence various stages of the research process in such collaborations (Walsh, Brugha, & Byrne, 2016). Walsh et al., suggest that such power disparities are based on differences in economic resources, which have far-reaching effects. Donors generally require the guidance or participation of researchers or institutions based in HICs in such collaborations, implying a lack of trust in the ability of researchers from LMICs, or a lack of institutional legitimacy or prestige (Walsh et al., 2016). While researchers in LMICs have more expertise regarding the context in which research is taking place, referring to what Bourdieu describes as "cultural capital" (Bourdieu, 1977), this is not always given sufficient weight by researchers, institutions or donors from HICs (Walsh et al., 2016).

Recognition of the ethical nature of the challenges associated with such collaborations is not a recent activity. In the late 1980s, for example, the mental health program of the World Health Organization (WHO) presented a list of 10 requirements for equitable and sustainable "cross-cultural collaborative research," highlighting the importance of capacity building, strong ethics oversight and sensitivity to cultural context among other factors (Sartorius, 1988). Similarly, Parker and Kingori have identified eight factors that researchers regard as important for successful collaboration (Parker & Kingori, 2016). Active and meaningful involvement in research, the competence and integrity of leadership and other collaborators, opportunities for capacity building, mutual respect and equality among collaborators, and transparency in discussions are all regarded as crucial. Furthermore, the importance of establishing trust and confidence in collaborators, through ensuring fair and inclusive research practices in all aspects of collaboration, has been highlighted (Parker & Kingori, 2016).

Ethical implications of choosing global mental health as a career

For researchers in both the global north and south, the decision to choose global mental health as a career raises a number of ethical issues. Researchers and practitioners may be faced with ethical dilemmas related to working and delivering care in severely resource-strained settings, and in contexts where worldviews may differ substantially from their own (Loh, Chae, Heckman, & Rhee, 2015). Challenges may also arise due to the need to navigate potential power imbalances with sensitivity so as to avoid unintentional harms or exploitation (Loh et al., 2015). These challenges, coupled with the potentially isolating nature of such work, suggest the possibility of professional and psychological burnout as a risk for global mental health practitioners (Cherepanov, 2017). Varpio and McCarthy have also emphasized the potential for trauma that may be experienced by global health students undertaking electives that involve training at host institutions in LMICs (Varpio & McCarthy, 2018). They found that students had experienced "physical, sexual and emotional trauma," indicating a need for adequate preparation and training as well as safety mechanisms and debriefing procedures (Varpio & McCarthy, 2018).

The training of psychiatrists for global mental health raises other ethical issues. In certain HICs, such as the United States, for example, it has been noted that while there has been a major increase in global health training programs offered at all levels of medical education, this has not been the case for global mental health in psychiatric training (Kerry et al., 2013; Tsai et al., 2014; Van Dyke, Tong, & Mack, 2011). Given the recognition of the global impact of mental disorders, the reality of the treatment gap, and thus, the clear need for more global mental health practitioners, the limited global mental health training on offer in psychiatric curricula is ethically concerning (Tsai et al., 2014). Furthermore, as increased global mental health curricula are introduced in psychiatric training, the selection of content for these curricula will have major implications for the way in which the field will continue to develop. Current training in HICs focuses predominantly on developing the relevant cultural knowledge, sensitivity and flexibility that will equip psychiatrists to navigate different contexts (Griffith et al., 2016). While such "cultural competence" training is a crucial part of global mental health endeavors, it has been criticized (Kirmayer, 2012). In particular, critics argue that it employs oversimplified notions of culture and stereotypes particular ethnic groups, as well as conflating culture and ethnoracial identity (Belkin & Fricchione, 2005; Belkin, Yusim, Anbarasan, & Bernstein, 2011; Kirmayer, 2012). Griffith et al., have provided a number of suggestions for the construction of global mental health curricula (Griffith et al., 2016); importantly, in designing their global mental health curriculum, they consulted with and received critical feedback from mental health colleagues who are members of populations from LMICs (Griffith et al., 2016).

Oversight by RECs in different countries

A feature of multinational research that involves multiple institutions is that it also generally requires ethics approval of protocols from numerous institutional review boards (IRBs) or research ethics committees (RECs). While the need for ethics oversight is indisputable, Ng et al., have drawn attention to the delays and obstacles to research caused by the involvement of multiple RECs in different countries (Ng, Hanlon, Yimer, Henderson, & Fekadu, 2015). Given that different RECs may request competing modifications and frequently only commence with their reviews after protocols have received approval from other RECs, the process of review would benefit from more effective communication and collaboration between participating RECs, or, from an REC located in the context in which the research will take place taking a leading role (Aarons, 2018; Barchi, Kasimatis Singleton, & Merz, 2014; Ng et al., 2015).

One reason for the involvement of multiple RECs has been due to the perception that the quality of ethics oversight in LMICs is inadequate, a perception which is contested by Ng et al., and others given the extensive capacity building and training of RECs in LMICs that has taken place over the last few decades (Klitzman, 2012; Ndebele et al., 2014). Furthermore, a study involving 46 IRBs in the United States indicated low levels of knowledge regarding important contextual factors relevant to research conducted in LMICs (Klitzman, 2012). It is likely that RECs in LMICs may therefore be in a better position to take a leadership role in the collaborative process of review.

Ethical issues related to global mental health research

The ethical challenges posed by global mental health related research largely correspond with those that are encountered by the broader field of global health. The abundant literature that focuses on the latter may therefore serve as a valuable resource in informing an overview of the distinct ethical issues posed by global mental health research (Benatar, 2002; Brisbois & Plamondon, 2018; Hussein & Upshur, 2013; Macklin, 2012; Pang, 2011). Global mental health research encompasses a diverse array of fields with varying aims, levels of risk and potential for benefit. Examples of research relevant to global mental health that have been discussed in the ethics literature include surveillance and epidemiological research (Fairchild et al., 2017; Murray, Kass, Mendelson, & Bass, 2016; World Health Organization, 2017), neuropsychiatric genetics and genomics research (de Vries et al., 2011, 2012; Kong & Singh, 2018) (see de Vries), and its translation into clinical contexts (Kong, Dunn, & Parker, 2017), clinical trials (Carlson, Sweetland, & Wainberg, 2018; Schroeder, Cook, Hirsch, Fenet, & Muthuswamy, 2018), implementation research (D'Souza, Guzder, Hickling, & Groleau, 2018; Gopichandran et al., 2016), health policy and systems research (Pratt, Paul, Hyder, & Ali, 2017) and the implications of "big data" in mental health research (Bereza, 2017; Conway & O'Connor, 2016).

In accordance with the tenets of principlism, all research requires informed consent of participants, based upon a respect for their autonomy, and should avoid or minimize harm as well as ensuring that the burdens and benefits of research participation are justly distributed (Beauchamp, 2013). The way in which these principles are impacted by contextual factors and different worldviews, coupled with the fact that mental health research requires, by definition, the participation of persons with mental disorders, who may be more vulnerable to harm or exploitation, represent the main areas of focus in considering the ethics of research related to global mental health. Ruiz-Casares identifies three areas crucial for ethical global mental health research which we use as a point of departure for our discussion in this section (Ruiz-Casares, 2014).

(i) **Informed consent procedures and disclosure protocols must be "culturally responsible"** (Ruiz-Casares, 2014). This includes making provisions for contextually appropriate forms of decision-making which may be collective rather than individualistic, as is the case in many contexts characterized by communitarian or relational worldviews (Chuwa, 2014; Osuji, 2018; ten Have, 2011). It is also important to ensure that all information related to research participation is appropriately translated and presented to participants in a form that assists understanding and considers local beliefs regarding mental disorders, which may differ from biomedical explanations, as well as taking into consideration any economic or social factors that could impact decisions to participate (Benatar, 2002; Marshall, 2006; Nijhawan et al., 2013; Ruiz-Casares, 2014). While participants in mental health research may have neurocognitive impairments, which could pose challenges to securing their informed consent, studies show extensive variation in the cognitive abilities of persons with mental disorders as well as fluctuating capacity at an individual level (Appelbaum, 2006; Gergel & Owen, 2015). Informed consent procedures should therefore be flexible and responsive to differing levels of decisional capacity as well as tailored to varying levels of education and understanding of mental disorder. Alternatives to text-based or straightforward question and answer forms of informed consent, such as iterative approaches, the use of multimedia, or participatory visual methods, may be more suitable (Black, Davies, Iskander, & Chambers, 2018; Campbell et al., 2017; Jeste et al., 2009; Kongsholm, Lassen, & Sandoe, 2018; Mintz, Sergi, & Wirshing, 2005) (see Rahimzadeh et al.).

In terms of disclosure protocols, the privacy of research participants and confidentiality of any potentially sensitive information regarding particular ethnic groups, if relevant, must be ensured, particularly given the high levels of stigma associated with mental disorders in certain contexts (Lauber & Rössler, 2007; Mascayano, Armijo, & Yang, 2015; Seeman, Tang, Brown, & Ing, 2016). As pointed out by de Vries et al., it is commonly assumed that research which focuses on particular ethnic or minority groups could increase stigmatization toward such groups (de Vries et al., 2012). This concern is particularly salient for genomics research which aims to investigate the genetic variants associated with particular mental disorders in populations that have been underrepresented in such studies (Dalvie et al., 2015; Stevenson et al., 2019). While there has been minimal empirical research of the relationship between such research and stigma in African contexts, de Vries et al., found that such studies may have the potential to exacerbate stigmatizing assumptions, however, this is more likely in the case of certain ethnic groups or disorders that are already subject to high levels of stigmatization (de Vries et al., 2012). This highlights the need for thorough consideration of contextual factors as well as active involvement and consultation with communities before such research commences.

(ii) **Ethical global mental health research requires preliminary risk benefit analyses that pay particular attention to the sociopolitical and economic realities of participants and communities, so as to minimize the potential for harm and ensure equitable distribution of any benefits** (Ruiz-Casares, 2014). This aim will be assisted by ensuring that research is scientifically justifiable and by instilling the importance of the values of integrity and respect as well as providing nuanced cultural and ethical training for researchers that is applicable to the context in which the research will take place (Ruiz-Casares, 2014). A particular concern in multinational research conducted in LMICs is that power disparities may be present not only between researchers from HICs and LMICs, and their respective institutions, as discussed in the previous section, but also between researchers and research participants (Emanuel, Wendler, Killen, & Grady, 2004; Hawkins & Emanuel, 2008; Macklin, 2003). Research in contexts where participants are "lacking in subjectively important social goods" (Kipnis, 2001) risks being exploitative, even if exploitation is unintended and does not result in direct harm. Care must thus be taken to ensure that compensation or perceived benefits, e.g., therapeutic misconceptions, associated with participation, do not serve as undue inducements to research participation (Colom & Rohloff, 2018; Horn, Sleem, & Ndebele, 2014; Kongsholm et al., 2018).

An additional harm-related concern is that global mental health research requires, by definition, the participation of persons with mental disorders. Generally, research that involves the participation of persons with mental disorders requires heightened protective measures to be taken (Council for International Organisations of Medical Sciences (CIOMS) & World Health Organization (WHO), 2016). However, while individuals with mental disorders have traditionally been regarded as vulnerable on account of their being at increased risk of harm or exploitation, due to the perception that their ability to protect their own interests is compromised in some way, there has also been widespread recognition of the harmful, stereotyping and disempowering effects of ascriptions of vulnerability (Kipnis, 2001; Luna, 2009; Mackenzie, Rogers, & Dodds, 2014) (see Dubljević). Most significantly, there has been a realization that vulnerability is a dynamic "situational feature" that arises "from the relationships among participants, investigators, and sociocultural context" (Bracken-Roche, Bell, & Racine, 2016). Global mental health research must therefore anticipate potential harms, with attention to particular contextual features, so as to ensure that research participants with mental disorders are protected, while taking into consideration the potentially harmful effects of overprotective or paternalistic measures.

(iii) In response to the other two areas, **ethical global mental health research requires authentic community engagement and consultation at all stages**, a requirement that has garnered widespread support (Campbell & Burgess, 2012; Holzer, Ellis, & Merritt, 2014; Molyneux et al., 2013; Reynolds & Sariola, 2018; Ruiz-Casares, 2014; Tindana et al., 2015). Consulting with communities prior to and during research has both intrinsic value, as it indicates respect for communities and gains their trust, and instrumental value, insofar as it provides access to the contextual expertise necessary for the success of the research endeavor (Holzer et al., 2014; Molyneux et al., 2013). Pratt and de Vries provide an ethical justification for engagement with all community stakeholders in LMICs that may be affected by research, on the grounds of "shared health governance" in global health research that aims to be "equity oriented" (Pratt & Vries, 2018). They suggest that this engagement should entail: the inclusion of representatives of marginalized groups as well as those who are in a position to "change policy and practice to benefit them", community input in the selection of "research topics and questions" and ensuring that discussions are conducted in such a way that they are not biased by power disparities between stakeholders (Pratt & Vries, 2018). While community engagement is fast become a prerequisite of research in LMICs, the challenges posed by genuine community engagement should also not be underestimated (Aggett, 2018; Parker & Bull, 2009; Reynolds & Sariola, 2018). Particular challenges that have been identified include a lack of "readiness" or "capacity" for engagement of community stakeholders (Lee et al., 2018), difficulties in correctly identifying the "relevant community" and how to ensure that engagement is "fair, inclusive, accountable and appropriate" (Parker & Bull, 2009).

Ethical issues associated with global mental health care

As mentioned above, Katz et al., have argued that global mental health care faces distinct challenges in comparison to other areas of medicine (Katz et al., 2014). In this section, we use their outline of these distinct issues as a frame of reference for our overview of the main ethical issues associated with how the global mental health movement responds to challenges regarding care and practice in LMICs. Our discussion is not exhaustive of the myriad challenges in this area. For example, a systematic review of literature pertaining to the ethical and professional challenges faced by mental health care practitioners in LMICs, conducted by Hanlon et al., revealed various issues ranging from autonomy violations, including involuntary admissions and a lack of adequate informed consent for particular treatments (electro-convulsive therapy in particular), to justice concerns regarding inequities in access to mental health care (Hanlon, Tesfaye, Wondimagegn, & Shibre, 2010). This indicates the sheer diversity of ethical issues encountered in global mental health care.

Ethical issues associated with providing care in severely resource-strained contexts

Devising innovative solutions to the resource scarcities and disparities that constitute the treatment gap in global mental health are, in a sense, the raison d'être of the global mental health movement. One of the major challenges facing global mental health care is the dire shortage of trained psychiatrists in LMICs. A 2007 global study of LMICs reported that nearly 50% of all countries had fewer than "one psychiatrist per 100 000 people, which included all southeast Asian and nearly 90% of African countries" (Jacob et al., 2007). In response to this shortage, as well as to the general resource scarcities in mental health care faced by most LMICs, a particular solution that has been advocated is task sharing, also referred to as task shifting. This entails the training and use of non-specialist health care providers, community health workers, or even lay persons to fulfill duties and roles traditionally performed by specialist practitioners, in order to scale up the provision of mental health care in resource-strained contexts (Patel, 2012).

Task sharing represents an innovative collaborative care approach to a seemingly intractable problem. However, while studies indicate that it has garnered widespread support, several conditions have been identified as necessary for its "acceptability and feasibility" (Mendenhall et al., 2014; Padmanathan & De Silva, 2013; Petersen, Lund, & Stein, 2011). Petersen et al., draw attention to the fact that attempts to increase the provision of mental health services through task sharing must be accompanied by the provision of "mental health literacy" for communities so as to decrease mental illness stigma and ensure uptake of services (Petersen et al., 2011). In addition, the impact that task sharing has on health care providers has ethical implications. In particular, there are concerns that task sharing will place additional burdens on health care workers, who are already overburdened (Mendenhall et al., 2014; Padmanathan & De Silva, 2013).

The use of non-specialists for care provision that is traditionally undertaken by specialists also has deeper ethical implications. Lolas draws attention to the fact that the implicit admission that underpins task sharing is at odds with the discourse of providing the highest standard of care for all, and that the realization that the latter is unattainable, in turn, "reinforces the notion that not all people are equal" (Lolas, 2016). However, if the notion of the highest standard of care is unavoidably relative to context, it may be the case that, as argued by Petersen et al., the non-ideal notion of "good enough care" must be accepted as preferable to no care at all (Petersen et al., 2011).

Ethical implications of stigmatizing causal ascriptions and clashing explanatory models of mental disorder

The lack of biomarkers that can assist in the diagnosis of mental disorders, as well as the fact that they generally produce discernible, sometimes severe, impacts on personality and behavior, has the result that mental disorders are more liable to a wide array of incorrect, and possibly stigmatizing, causal ascriptions (Katz et al., 2014). Ngui et al., observe that in many contexts:

> [l]imited knowledge of the causes, symptoms and treatment of mental illness often leads to common but erroneous beliefs that these conditions are caused by individuals themselves or by supernatural forces, possession by evil spirits, curse or punishment following the individual's family or is part of family lineage
>
> (Ngui et al., 2010).

Moreover, a series of studies that included the views of trainee physicians from various LMICs, located on four different continents, indicated negative and stigmatizing attitudes toward both the field of psychiatry and psychiatric patients (see Roberts, 2010 for an overview of these studies). One study, in particular, found that up to 40% of Nigerian medical students included in the study associated mental disorders with witchcraft, possession or other supernatural explanations (Aghukwa, 2010). These kinds of stigmatizing beliefs severely impact the lives of persons with mental disorders, and mostly importantly, are a major reason for the lack of uptake of mental health care services in many LMICs (Ngui et al., 2010). Furthermore, the negative attitudes toward psychiatry that are revealed by these studies are deeply concerning in terms of their implications for the success of increasing mental health care provision through task sharing in such contexts.

The negative real-world consequences of such causal ascriptions also expose deeper tensions between calls for sensitivity and respect for local explanatory models of illness, and the clear need to address misconceptions regarding mental disorders. This in turn highlights inherent problems with relativist perspectives in general. Global mental health practitioners are thus faced with various dilemmas. While studies indicate that using a biomedical or biogenetic model to explaining the etiology of mental disorders may assist in correcting such beliefs and fostering tolerance, there is also evidence that biogenetic explanations encourage various forms of reductive or deterministic thinking which are at odds with a recognition of the vital role played by social and environmental factors (Kong et al., 2017; Kong & Singh, 2018; Palk, Dalvie, de Vries, Martin, & Stein, 2019). A possible way through this predicament would be to strengthen collaboration between Western medical approaches and indigenous or traditional forms of medicine. The possibility of collaboration with traditional healers and religious spiritual advisors has been explored in sub-Saharan Africa (Sorsdahl et al., 2009) as well as in India and China (Chaturvedi & Patwardhan, 2016).

Toward a more comprehensive paradigm for global mental health ethics

Benatar et al., have emphasized that the moral point of departure for global health is the undeniable fact of "unjust inequalities in the distribution of the conditions necessary for human health and well-being" (Benatar, Daibes, & Tomsons, 2016). They also highlight the fact that these inequalities have arisen within a global history that has resulted in the world being deliberately structured in such a way that it favors certain groups and countries over others (Ndebele et al., 2014). On this interpretation, which is reflective of the broader literature, global health is justified by the principles of rectificatory and distributive justice and grounded in a recognition of human rights. The global mental health literature has also consistently emphasized such insights indicating a similar moral grounding (see Herrera-Ferrá). The other point of departure for global health, mentioned in the introduction, is the reality of a lack of uniformity in moral and ethical norms and legal rules across the globe. In connection with this point, Benatar et al., have questioned the ability of the "dominant bioethical paradigm" to adequately address the challenges faced in global health as well as to provide a common ethical point of reference for all participants in the field of global health, given that the values and principles it espouses are representative of a particular worldview (Benatar et al., 2016) (see McConnell & Savulescu who suggest an alternative welfarist approach in psychiatry). For these reasons they call for the construction of a new paradigm for global health ethics that "increases the capacity for solidarity and shared decision-making" (Benatar et al., 2016).

Given the value that global mental health places on equity, we agree that a more comprehensive and inclusive bioethics paradigm is needed; we therefore support ongoing discussions and contributions to such an endeavor. While the principles of autonomy, justice, beneficence, and non-maleficence should continue to play an important role in global mental health, the answers to questions regarding what constitutes these principles cannot be provided devoid of context (Ruiz-Casares, 2014). Andersen et al., have echoed this sentiment suggesting that more attention be paid to "mutual respect (and benefit), trust, accountability, transparency…[and sustainability]," with the latter justifying various forms of capacity building (Anderson, Johnson, & de Vries, 2017).

Given that a large proportion of global mental health endeavors are directed toward the African continent, we posit that global mental health ethics should pay more attention to the rich resources offered by African moral frameworks (see Fulford & van Staden and Palk & Stein). Various African scholars have argued in support of an African bioethics, or for the importance of including African normative insights in bioethics discussions, as well calling for caution in terms of how this endeavor should proceed (Barugahare, 2018). In particular there have been arguments that more attention should be paid to the value of solidarity (Andoh, 2011; Tosam, Chi, Munung, Oukem-Boyer, & Tangwa, 2018), a respect for "human life invaluableness" (Rakotsoane & van Niekerk, 2017), "eco-bio-communitarianism" (Tangwa, 1996) and other communitarian principles in general, respect for the holistic approach of the "African traditional doctor" (Murove, 2005) and various suggestions based on the southern African conception of relational personhood or ubuntu (Gade, 2012), for example, general harmony (Behrens, 2013), and harmony through respecting the quality of being able to "identify with others and exhibit solidarity with them" (Metz, 2010) (see Coleman, 2017 for a review of the literature on African bioethics).

In keeping with recognition of the communal or relational nature of human existence, and the value of harmonious identification with others as an enabling force, we concur that more attention should be paid to cultivating a sense of solidarity in global mental health endeavors. Furthermore, as an inherently relational concept, solidarity, and the implicit assumptions upon which it rests, could be a fruitful addition to the prevailing Western bioethics paradigm. As pointed out by Benatar et al., the dominant principlist paradigm is unable to provide an adequate justification for the rectificatory obligation that is implicit in global health (Benatar et al., 2016). The obligations implied by global health endeavors are grounded in appeals to distributive justice and an individualist conception of human rights, with the former justified through "weak benevolence-based obligations" and the latter by a social justice matrix which is outside the principlist paradigm (Benatar et al., 2016).

The ethical importance of what is implied by solidarity can be traced back to insights regarding the nature of friendship discussed by Aristotle in his Nicomachean ethics (see 1166a1–33 in Aristotle, 1985). On this interpretation, solidarity entails "one person giving a certain subset of the interests of another person a status in her reasoning that is analogous to the status that she gives to her own interests in her reasoning" (Hussain, 2018). On the one hand, solidarity is linked to the notion of acting in accordance with the common good. This interpretation is present in the argument of Tosam et al., who support solidarity in global health as a means of providing a "united force against global health challenges" (Tosam et al., 2018). Their argument is based on the fact that the effects of global health disparities and diseases prevalent in poor countries are not localized to these contexts due to globalization; a point that is evidenced by the way in which communicable diseases are able to spread rapidly throughout the world. On this account, global solidarity is a pragmatic and protective mechanism that responds to the reality that all persons are equally vulnerable. On the other hand, solidarity may also be regarded as valuable as an end in itself. This interpretation associates it with "interdependence within a group, nation, class, etc., or a feeling of affinity with and willingness to support and assist other people" (Mautner, 2005). This account of solidarity is able to more effectively ground the rectificatory obligations implicit in global health.

There are various implications for global mental health of including solidarity as a guiding principle in the prevailing bioethics paradigm. Solidarity in global mental health collaborations acknowledges the historical context that has produced power disparities between countries. Solidarity also justifies an obligation to respectfully build the capacity of researchers and institutions in such contexts so as to rectify previous injustices. In global mental health research, solidarity as interdependence implies reciprocity so as to acknowledge the consequences of the fact that the development of HICs was afforded through the extraction of human and material resources from the developing world. Reciprocity requires that research is relevant to the needs of communities and includes their genuine participation in all aspects of the research endeavor. Finally, solidarity in global mental health care justifies increasing global mental health training in HICs, and choosing to specialize in this area, on the basis of the instrumental value of addressing the negative global impact of mental disorders, the obligation to redress past injustices, and the intrinsic goodness of identifying with the suffering of others. While the above observations require further substantive discussion, our suggestions serve to indicate that the inclusion of solidarity as a guiding principle is able to provide a more effective and appropriate normative foundation for global mental health than the dominant principlist account alone.

Conclusion

In this chapter we have attempted to present a broad overview of the various ethical issues encountered in global mental health. In doing this, we utilized the abundance of literature that has engaged with the broader field of global health in order to identify similarities and differences between the two areas, as well as the growing literature and critical engagement with specific areas of global mental health itself. First, we discussed ethical issues associated with global collaboration in mental health. This included looking at some of the criticisms of the normative assumptions that allegedly underpin global mental health, challenges posed by power disparities in research collaborations, the ethical implications of choosing global mental health as a career and challenges posed by the oversight of multiple RECs based in different countries in international collaborations. Second, we discussed cross-cutting issues related to global mental health research using a contextualized account of principlism as a framework. The discussion was further organized in terms of areas crucial for ethical global mental health research and included the necessity of culturally responsible informed consent procedures and disclosure protocols, contextually informed risk benefit analyses and ensuring authentic community engagement at all stages of the research process. Third, we discussed ethical issues associated with global mental health care by using the distinct challenges that face global mental health in comparison to global health care as a point of departure. This included looking at ethical issues associated with providing care in severely resource-strained contexts and the ethical implications of the tendency of mental disorders to be particularly liable to stigmatizing causal ascriptions.

In the second part of the chapter we discussed calls for a more appropriate and comprehensive bioethics paradigm for global health endeavors by considering the principles of equity, inclusivity and rectification that have been central to the development of the field. In particular, we argued that global mental health ethics should pay more attention to the rich resources offered by African moral frameworks and to the relational notion of solidarity which has both instrumental and intrinsic value.

We concluded by arguing for the inclusion of solidarity as a guiding principle that is able to provide a more effective and appropriate normative foundation for global mental health than the dominant principlist account alone. We note that our overview and discussion of a more comprehensive paradigm for global mental health is not exhaustive and that there are numerous ways in which the issues we have engaged with may be categorized as well as other principles that may be relevant. However, we hope that this overview will contribute to ongoing discussion and the construction of a distinct global mental health ethics.

References

Aarons, D. (2018). Research in epidemic and emergency situations: A model for collaboration and expediting ethics review in two Caribbean countries. *Developing World Bioethics*, *18*(4), 375–384. https://doi.org/10.1111/dewb.12157.

Aggett, S. (2018). Turning the gaze: Challenges of involving biomedical researchers in community engagement with research in Patan, Nepal. *Critical Public Health*, *28*(3), 306–317. https://doi.org/10.1080/09581596.2018.1443203.

Aghukwa, C. N. (2010). Medical students' beliefs and attitudes toward mental illness: Effects of a psychiatric education. *Academic Psychiatry*, *34*(1), 67–69. https://doi.org/10.1176/appi.ap.34.1.67.

Anderson, F. W. J., Johnson, T. R. B., & de Vries, R. (2017). Global health ethics: The case of maternal and neonatal survival. *Best Practice & Research. Clinical Obstetrics & Gynaecology*, *43*, 125–135. https://doi.org/10.1016/j.bpobgyn.2017.02.003.

Andoh, C. T. (2011). Bioethics and the challenges to its growth in Africa. *Open Journal of Philosophy*, *01*(02), 67–75. https://doi.org/10.4236/ojpp.2011.12012.

Appelbaum, P. S. (2006). Decisional capacity of patients with schizophrenia to consent to research: Taking stock. *Schizophrenia Bulletin*, *32*(1), 22–25. https://doi.org/10.1093/schbul/sbi063.

Appiah, A. (2005). *The ethics of identity*. Princeton, NJ: Princeton University Press.

Aristotle. (1985). *Nicomachean ethics. Hackett classics*. Indianapolis: Hackett.

Barchi, F., Kasimatis Singleton, M., & Merz, J. F. (2014). Fostering IRB collaboration for review of international research. *The American Journal of Bioethics*, *14*(5), 3–8. https://doi.org/10.1080/15265161.2014.892168.

Barugahare, J. (2018). African bioethics: Methodological doubts and insights. *BMC Medical Ethics*, *19*(1), 98. https://doi.org/10.1186/s12910-018-0338-6.

Beauchamp, T. L. (2013). *Principles of biomedical ethics* (7th ed.). New York: Oxford University Press.

Behrens, K. G. (2013). Towards an indigenous African bioethics. *South African Journal of Bioethics and Law*, *6*(1). https://doi.org/10.7196/sajbl.255.

Belkin, G. S., & Fricchione, G. L. (2005). Internationalism and the future of academic psychiatry. *Academic Psychiatry: The Journal of the American Association of Directors of Psychiatric Residency Training and the Association for Academic Psychiatry*, *29*(3), 240–243. https://doi.org/10.1176/appi.ap.29.3.240.

Belkin, G., Yusim, A., Anbarasan, D., & Bernstein, C. (2011). Teaching "global mental health:" psychiatry residency directors' attitudes and practices regarding international opportunities for psychiatry residents. *Academic Psychiatry*, *35*(6), 400–403. https://doi.org/10.1176/appi.ap.35.6.400.

Bemme, D., & D'Souza, N. A. (2014). Global mental health and its discontents: An inquiry into the making of global and local scale. *Transcultural Psychiatry*, *51*(6), 850–874. https://doi.org/10.1177/1363461514539830.

Benatar, S. R. (2002). Reflections and recommendations on research ethics in developing countries. *Social Science and Medicine*, *54*(7), 1131–1141. https://doi.org/10.1016/s0277-9536(01)00327-6.

Benatar, S. R. (2011). Global health ethics. In K. Moodley (Ed.), *Medical ethics, law and human rights: A South African perspective pretoria* (pp. 339–349). Van Schaik Publishers.

Benatar, S., Daibes, I., & Tomsons, S. (2016). Inter-philosophies dialogue: Creating a paradigm for global health ethics. *Kennedy Institute of Ethics Journal*, *26*(3), 323–346. https://doi.org/10.1353/ken.2016.0027.

Bereza, E. (2017). The use of clinical databases in disease outcomes research: Is the ethics of IRB review keeping up? *Multiple Sclerosis*, *23*(10), 1325–1327. https://doi.org/10.1177/1352458517707264.

Black, G. F., Davies, A., Iskander, D., & Chambers, M. (2018). Reflections on the ethics of participatory visual methods to engage communities in global health research. *Global Bioethics*, *29*(1), 22–38. https://doi.org/10.1080/11287462.2017.1415722.

Bourdieu, P. (1977). Outline of a theory of practice. *Cambridge studies in social anthropology*: *Vol. 16*. Cambridge: Cambridge University Press.

Bracken-Roche, D., Bell, E., & Racine, E. (2016). The "vulnerability" of psychiatric research participants: Why this research ethics concept needs to be revisited. *Canadian Journal of Psychiatry*, *61*(6), 335–339. https://doi.org/10.1177/0706743716633422.

Brisbois, B., & Plamondon, K. (2018). The possible worlds of global health research: An ethics-focused discourse analysis. *Social Science and Medicine*, *196*, 142–149. https://doi.org/10.1016/j.socscimed.2017.11.034.

Campbell, C., & Burgess, R. (2012). The role of communities in advancing the goals of the movement for global mental health. *Transcultural Psychiatry*, *49*(3–4), 379–395. https://doi.org/10.1177/1363461512454643.

Campbell, M. M., Susser, E., Mall, S., Mqulwana, S. G., Mndini, M. M., Ntola, O. A., et al. (2017). Using iterative learning to improve understanding during the informed consent process in a South African psychiatric genomics study. *PLoS ONE*, *12*(11), e0188466. https://doi.org/10.1371/journal.pone.0188466.

Carlson, C., Sweetland, A., & Wainberg, M. (2018). Ethical challenges in global mental health clinical trials. *The Lancet Psychiatry*, *5*(11), 866–867. https://doi.org/10.1016/S2215-0366(18)30300-6.

Chaturvedi, S., & Patwardhan, B. (2016). Building bridges for integrative medicine. *The Lancet Psychiatry*, *3*(8), 705–706. https://doi.org/10.1016/s2215-0366(16)30145-6.

Cherepanov, E. (2017). Ethics for global mental health specialists. *Intervention*, *15*(1), 17–33. https://doi.org/10.1097/WTF.0000000000000142.

Chuwa, L. (2014). *African indigenous ethics in global bioethics. Interpreting Ubuntu. Advancing global bioethics 1*. Dordrecht: Springer Dordrecht.

Clark, J. (2014). Medicalization of global health 2: The medicalization of global mental health. *Global Health Action*, *7*, 24000. https://doi.org/10.3402/gha.v7.24000.

Coleman, A. M. E. (2017). What is "African bioethics" as used by Sub-Saharan African authors: An argumentative literature review of articles on African bioethics. *Open Journal of Philosophy*, *07*(01), 31–47. https://doi.org/10.4236/ojpp.2017.71003.

Colom, M., & Rohloff, P. (2018). Cultural considerations for informed consent in paediatric research in low/middle-income countries: A scoping review. *BMJ Paediatrics Open*, *2*(1), e000298. https://doi.org/10.1136/bmjpo-2018-000298.

Conway, M., & O'Connor, D. (2016). Social media, big data, and mental health: Current advances and ethical implications. *Current Opinion in Psychology*, *9*, 77–82. https://doi.org/10.1016/j.copsyc.2016.01.004.

Cooper, S. (2016). Global mental health and its critics: Moving beyond the impasse. *Critical Public Health*, *26*(4), 355–358. https://doi.org/10.1080/09581596.2016.1161730.

Council for International Organisations of Medical Sciences (CIOMS), World Health Organization (WHO). (2016). *International ethical guidelines for health-related research involving humans*. Geneva: CIOMS.

Dalvie, S., Koen, N., Duncan, L., Abbo, C., Akena, D., Atwoli, L., et al. (2015). Large scale genetic research on neuropsychiatric disorders in African populations is needed. *eBioMedicine*, *2*(10), 1259–1261. https://doi.org/10.1016/j.ebiom.2015.10.002.

de Vries, J., Bull, S. J., Doumbo, O., Ibrahim, M., Mercereau-Puijalon, O., Kwiatkowski, D., et al. (2011). Ethical issues in human genomics research in developing countries. *BMC Medical Ethics*, *12*, 5. https://doi.org/10.1186/1472-6939-12-5.

de Vries, J., Jallow, M., Williams, T. N., Kwiatkowski, D., Parker, M., & Fitzpatrick, R. (2012). Investigating the potential for ethnic group harm in collaborative genomics research in Africa: Is ethnic stigmatisation likely? *Social Science and Medicine*, *75*(8), 1400–1407. https://doi.org/10.1016/j.socscimed.2012.05.020.

D'Souza, N. A., Guzder, J., Hickling, F., & Groleau, D. (2018). The ethics of relationality in implementation and evaluation research in global health: Reflections from the Dream-A-World program in Kingston, Jamaica. *BMC Medical Ethics*, *19*(Suppl 1), 50. https://doi.org/10.1186/s12910-018-0282-5.

Emanuel, E. J., Wendler, D., Killen, J., & Grady, C. (2004). What makes clinical research in developing countries ethical? The benchmarks of ethical research [Perspective]. *Journal of Infectious Diseases*, *189*(5), 930. https://doi.org/10.1086/381709.

Fairchild, A. L., Haghdoost, A. A., Bayer, R., Selgelid, M. J., Dawson, A., Saxena, A., et al. (2017). Ethics of public health surveillance: New guidelines. *The Lancet Public Health*, *2*(8), e348–e349. https://doi.org/10.1016/s2468-2667(17)30136-6.

Fernando, S. (2014). Globalization of psychiatry—A barrier to mental health development. *International Review of Psychiatry*, *26*(5), 551–557. https://doi.org/10.3109/09540261.2014.920305.

Gade, C. B. N. (2012). What is Ubuntu? Different interpretations among South Africans of African descent. *South African Journal of Philosophy*, *31*(3), 484–503. https://doi.org/10.1080/02580136.2012.10751789.

Gergel, T., & Owen, G. S. (2015). Fluctuating capacity and advance decision-making in bipolar affective disorder—Self-binding directives and self-determination. *International Journal of Law and Psychiatry*, *40*, 92–101. https://doi.org/10.1016/j.ijlp.2015.04.004.

Gopichandran, V., Luyckx, V. A., Biller-Andorno, N., Fairchild, A., Singh, J., Tran, N., et al. (2016). Developing the ethics of implementation research in health. *Implementation Science*, *11*(1), 161. https://doi.org/10.1186/s13012-016-0527-y.

Griffith, J. L., Kohrt, B., Dyer, A., Polatin, P., Morse, M., Jabr, S., et al. (2016). Training psychiatrists for global mental health: Cultural psychiatry, collaborative inquiry, and ethics of alterity. *Academic Psychiatry*, *40*(4), 701–706. https://doi.org/10.1007/s40596-016-0541-z.

Hanlon, C., Tesfaye, M., Wondimagegn, D., & Shibre, T. (2010). Ethical and professional challenges in mental health care in low- and middle-income countries. *International Review of Psychiatry*, *22*(3), 245–251. https://doi.org/10.3109/09540261.2010.482557.

Hawkins, J. S. & Emanuel, E. J. (Eds.), (2008). *Exploitation and developing countries: The ethics of clinical research*. Princeton, NJ: Princeton University Press.

Holzer, J. K., Ellis, L., & Merritt, M. W. (2014). Why we need community engagement in medical research. *Journal of Investigative Medicine*, *62*(6), 851–855. https://doi.org/10.1097/JIM.0000000000000097.

Horn, L., Sleem, H., & Ndebele, P. (2014). *Research vulnerability*. In M. Kruger, P. Ndebele, & M. Horn (Eds.), *Research ethics in Africa Stellenbosch: African SUN MeDIA* (pp. 81–90).

Hussain, W. (2018). The common good. In *The Stanford encyclopedia of philosophy*. https://plato.stanford.edu/archives/spr2018/entries/common-good/ (Accessed March 18, 2019).

Hussein, G., & Upshur, R. (2013). Ethical challenges in global health research. In A. Pinto & R. Upshur (Eds.), *An introduction to global health ethics* (pp. 103–116). Oxford: Routledge.

Jacob, K. S., Sharan, P., Mirza, I., Garrido-Cumbrera, M., Seedat, S., Mari, J., et al. (2007). Mental health systems in countries: Where are we now? *The Lancet*, *370*(9592), 1061–1077. https://doi.org/10.1016/S0140-6736(07)61241-0.

Jeste, D. V., Palmer, B. W., Golshan, S., Eyler, L. T., Dunn, L. B., Meeks, T., et al. (2009). Multimedia consent for research in people with schizophrenia and normal subjects: A randomized controlled trial. *Schizophrenia Bulletin*, *35*(4), 719. https://doi.org/10.1093/schbul/sbm148.

Katz, C. L., Lahey, T. P., & Campbell, H. T. (2014). An ethical framework for global psychiatry. *Annals of Global Health*, *80*(2), 146–151. https://doi.org/10.1016/j.aogh.2014.04.002.

Kerry, V. B., Walensky, R. P., Tsai, A. C., Bergmark, R. W., Bergmark, B. A., Rouse, C., et al. (2013). US medical specialty global health training and the global burden of disease. *Journal of Global Health*, *3*(2), https://doi.org/10.7189/jogh.03.020406.

Kipnis, K. (2001). *Vulnerability in research subjects: A bioethical taxonomy*. In *Ethical and policy issues in research involving human participants* (pp. G1–G13). Bethesda, MD: National Bioethics Advisory Commission.

Kirmayer, L. J. (2012). Cultural competence and evidence-based practice in mental health: Epistemic communities and the politics of pluralism. *Social Science and Medicine*, *75*(2), 249–256. https://doi.org/10.1016/j.socscimed.2012.03.018.

Klitzman, R. L. (2012). US IRBS confronting research in the developing world. *Developing World Bioethics*, *12*(2), 63–73. https://doi.org/10.1111/j.1471-8847.2012.00324.x.

Kong, C., Dunn, M., & Parker, M. (2017). Psychiatric genomics and mental health treatment: Setting the ethical agenda. *The American Journal of Bioethics*, *17*(4), 3–12. https://doi.org/10.1080/15265161.2017.1284915.

Kong, C., & Singh, I. (2018). The ethics of global psychiatric genomics: Multilayered challenges to integrating genomics in global mental health and disability—A position paper of the Oxford Global Initiative in Neuropsychiatric GenEthics (NeuroGenE). *American Journal of Medical Genetics. Part B, Neuropsychiatric Genetics*, https://doi.org/10.1002/ajmg.b.32697.

Kongsholm, N. C. H., Lassen, J., & Sandoe, P. (2018). "I didn't have anything to decide, I wanted to help my kids"—An interview-based study of consent procedures for sampling human biological material for genetic research in rural Pakistan. *AJOB Empirical Bioethics*, *9*(3), 113–127. https://doi.org/10.1080/23294515.2018.1472148.

Koplan, J. P., Bond, T. C., Merson, M. H., Reddy, K. S., Rodriguez, M. H., Sewankambo, N. K., et al. (2009). Towards a common definition of global health. *The Lancet*, *373*(9679), 1993–1995. https://doi.org/10.1016/S0140-6736(09)60332-9.

Lauber, C., & Rössler, W. (2007). Stigma towards people with mental illness in developing countries in Asia. *International Review of Psychiatry*, *19*(2), 157–178. https://doi.org/10.1080/09540260701278903.

Lee, C., Mellor, T., Dilworth-Anderson, P., Young, T., Brayne, C., & Lafortune, L. (2018). Opportunities and challenges in public and community engagement: The connected for cognitive health in later life (CHILL) project. *Research Involvement and Engagement*, *4*, 42https://doi.org/10.1186/s40900-018-0127-x.

Loh, L., Chae, S., Heckman, J., & Rhee, D. (2015). Ethical considerations of physician career involvement in global health work: A framework. *Journal of Bioethical Inquiry*, *12*(1), 129–136. https://doi.org/10.1007/s11673-014-9591-7.

Lolas, F. (2016). Global mental health: Challenges for a global ethics. *Acta Bioethica*, *22*(1), 9–14. https://doi.org/10.4067/S1726-569X2016000100002.

Lora, A., Kohn, R., Levav, I., McBain, R., Morris, J., & Saxena, S. (2012). Service availability and utilization and treatment gap for schizophrenic disorders: A survey in 50 low- and middle-income countries. *Bulletin of the World Health Organization*, *90*(1), 47. https://doi.org/10.1590/S0042-96862012000100012.

Luna, F. (2009). Elucidating the concept of vulnerability: Layers not labels. *International Journal of Feminist Approaches to Bioethics*, *2*(1), 121–139. https://doi.org/10.3138/ijfab.2.1.121.

Mackenzie, C., Rogers, W., & Dodds, S. (Eds.), (2014). *Vulnerability: New essays in ethics and feminist philosophy*. New York: Oxford University Press.

Macklin, R. (2003). Bioethics, vulnerability, and protection. *Bioethics*, *17*(5–6), 472–486. https://doi.org/10.1111/1467-8519.00362.

Macklin, R. (2012). *Ethics in global health: Research, policy, and practice*. New York: Oxford University Press.

Marshall, P. A. (2006). Informed consent in international health research. *Journal of Empirical Research on Human Research Ethics*, *1*(1), 25–42. https://doi.org/10.1525/jer.2006.1.1.25.

Mascayano, F., Armijo, J. E., & Yang, L. H. (2015). Addressing stigma relating to mental illness in low- and middle-income countries. *Frontiers in Psychiatry*, *6*, 38. https://doi.org/10.3389/fpsyt.2015.00038.

Mautner, T., Solidarism. (2005). *The penguin dictionary of philosophy* (2nd ed.). London: Penguin.

Mendenhall, E., De Silva, M., Hanlon, C., Petersen, I., Shidhaye, R., Jordans, M., et al. (2014). Acceptability and feasibility of using non-specialist health workers to deliver mental health care: Stakeholder perceptions from the PRIME district sites in Ethiopia, India, Nepal, South Africa, and Uganda. *Social Science & Medicine (1982)*, *118*(C), 33–42. https://doi.org/10.1016/j.socscimed.2014.07.057.

Metz, T. (2010). African and Western moral theories in a bioethical context. *Developing World Bioethics*, *10*(1), 49–58. https://doi.org/10.1111/j.1471-8847.2009.00273.x.

Miller, G. (2014). Is the agenda for global mental health a form of cultural imperialism? *Medical Humanities*, *40*(2), 131. https://doi.org/10.1136/medhum-2013-010471.

Mills, C. (2014). *Decolonizing global mental health: The psychiatrization of the majority world*. Routledge, ISBN: 978-1-84872-160-9.

Mills, C., & Fernando, S. (2014). Globalising mental health or pathologising the global south? Mapping the ethics, theory and practice of global mental health. *Disability and the Global South*, *1*(2), 188–202.

Mintz, J., Sergi, M., & Wirshing, D. (2005). A videotape intervention to enhance the informed consent process for medical and psychiatric treatment research. *American Journal of Psychiatry*, *162*(1), 186–188. https://doi.org/10.1176/appi.ajp.162.1.186.

Molyneux, S., Bull, S. J., & Organizing Committee for the Community Engagement and Consent Workshop. (2013). Consent and community engagement in diverse research contexts. Reviewing and developing research and practice. *Journal of Empirical Research on Human Research Ethics*, *8*(4), 1–18. https://doi.org/10.1525/jer.2013.8.4.1.

Murove, M. F. (2005). African bioethics: An explanatory discourse. *Journal for the Study of Religion, 18*(1), 16–36.

Murray, S. M., Kass, N., Mendelson, T., & Bass, J. (2016). The ethics of mental health survey research in low- and middle- income countries. *Global Mental Health (Cambridge, England), 3*, e12. https://doi.org/10.1017/gmh.2016.6.

Myser, C. (2015). Defining "global health ethics": Offering a research agenda for more bioethics and multidisciplinary contributions-from the global south and beyond the health sciences-to enrich global health and global health ethics initiatives. *Journal of Bioethical Inquiry, 12*(1), 5–10. https://doi.org/10.1007/s11673-015-9626-8.

Ndebele, P., Wassenaar, D., Benatar, S., Fleischer, T., Kruger, M., Adebamowo, C., et al. (2014). Research ethics capacity building in Sub-Saharan Africa: A review of NIH Fogarty-funded programs 2000–2012. *Journal of Empirical Research on Human Research Ethics, 9*(2), 24–40. https://doi.org/10.1525/jer.2014.9.2.24.

Ng, L. C., Hanlon, C., Yimer, G., Henderson, D. C., & Fekadu, A. (2015). Ethics in global health research: The need for balance. *The Lancet Global Health, 3*(9), e516–e517. https://doi.org/10.1016/S2214-109X(15)00095-9.

Ngui, E. M., Khasakhala, L., Ndetei, D., & Roberts, L. W. (2010). Mental disorders, health inequalities and ethics: A global perspective. *International Review of Psychiatry, 22*(3), 235–244. https://doi.org/10.3109/09540261.2010.485273.

Nijhawan, L. P., Janodia, M. D., Muddukrishna, B. S., Bhat, K. M., Bairy, K. L., Udupa, N., et al. (2013). Informed consent: Issues and challenges. *Journal of Advanced Pharmaceutical Technology & Research, 4*(3), 134–140. https://doi.org/10.4103/2231-4040.116779.

Osuji, P. I. (2018). Relational autonomy in informed consent (RAIC) as an ethics of care approach to the concept of informed consent. *Medicine, Health Care, and Philosophy, 21*(1), 101–111. https://doi.org/10.1007/s11019-017-9789-7.

Padmanathan, P., & De Silva, M. J. (2013). The acceptability and feasibility of task-sharing for mental healthcare in low and middle income countries: A systematic review. *Social Science and Medicine, 97*, 82–86. https://doi.org/10.1016/j.socscimed.2013.08.004.

Palk, A. C., Dalvie, S., de Vries, J., Martin, A. R., & Stein, D. J. (2019). Potential use of clinical polygenic risk scores in psychiatry—Ethical implications and communicating high polygenic risk. *Philosophy, Ethics, and Humanities in Medicine, 14*(1), 4. https://doi.org/10.1186/s13010-019-0073-8.

Pang, T. (2011). Global health research: Changing the agenda. In S. Benatar & G. Brock (Eds.), *Global health and global health ethics* (pp. 285–292). Cambridge: Cambridge University Press.

Parker, M., & Bull, S. (2009). Ethics in collaborative global health research networks. *Clinical Ethics, 4*(4), 165–168. https://doi.org/10.1258/ce.2009.009025.

Parker, M., & Kingori, P. (2016). Good and bad research collaborations: Researchers' views on science and ethics in global health research. *PLoS ONE, 11*(10), e0163579. https://doi.org/10.1371/journal.pone.0163579.

Patel, V. (2012). Global mental health: From science to action. *Harvard Review of Psychiatry, 20*(1), 6–12. https://doi.org/10.3109/10673229.2012.649108.

Patel, V. (2014). Why mental health matters to global health. *Transcultural Psychiatry, 51*(6), 777–789. https://doi.org/10.1177/1363461514524473.

Patel, V., Chisholm, D., Rabe-Hesketh, S., Dias-Saxena, F., Andrew, G., & Mann, A. (2003). Efficacy and cost-effectiveness of drug and psychological treatments for common mental disorders in general health care in Goa, India: A randomised, controlled trial. *The Lancet, 361*(9351), 33–39. https://doi.org/10.1016/S0140-6736(03)12119-8.

Patel, V., & Prince, M. (2010). Global mental health: A new global health field comes of age. *Journal of the American Medical Association, 303*(19), 1976–1977. https://doi.org/10.1001/jama.2010.616.

Patel, V., Saxena, S., Lund, C., Thornicroft, G., Baingana, F., Bolton, P., et al. (2018). The Lancet Commission on global mental health and sustainable development. *The Lancet*, https://doi.org/10.1016/s0140-6736(18)31612-x.

Petersen, J. I., Lund, J. C., & Stein, J. D. (2011). Optimizing mental health services in low-income and middle-income countries. *Current Opinion in Psychiatry, 24*(4), 318–323. https://doi.org/10.1097/YCO.0b013e3283477afb.

Pinto, A., Birn, A. E., & Upshur, R. (2013a). An introduction to global health ethics. In A. D. Pinto & R. Upshur (Eds.), *An introduction to global health ethics* (pp. 3–15). Abingdon, Oxon: Routledge.

Pinto, A. D., Birn, A.-E., & Upshur, R. E. G. (2013b). The context of global health ethics. In A. D. Pinto & R. E. G. Upshur (Eds.), *An introduction to global health ethics* (pp. 3–15). New York: Routledge.

Pratt, B., Paul, A., Hyder, A. A., & Ali, J. (2017). Ethics of health policy and systems research: A scoping review of the literature. *Health Policy and Planning, 32*(6), 890–910. https://doi.org/10.1093/heapol/czx003.

Pratt, B., & Vries, J. (2018). Community engagement in global health research that advances health equity. *Bioethics, 32*(7), 454–463. https://doi.org/10.1111/bioe.12465.

Rakotsoane, F. C. L., & van Niekerk, A. A. (2017). Human life invaluableness: An emerging African bioethical principle. *South African Journal of Philosophy, 36*(2), 252–262. https://doi.org/10.1080/02580136.2016.1223983.

Reynolds, L., & Sariola, S. (2018). The ethics and politics of community engagement in global health research. *Critical Public Health, 28*(3), 257–268. https://doi.org/10.1080/09581596.2018.1449598.

Roberts, L. (2010). Stigma, hope, and challenge in psychiatry: Trainee perspectives from five countries on four continents. *Academic Psychiatry, 34*(1), 1–4. https://doi.org/10.1176/appi.ap.34.1.1.

Robertshaw, L., Dhesi, S., & Jones, L. L. (2017). Challenges and facilitators for health professionals providing primary healthcare for refugees and asylum seekers in high-income countries: A systematic review and thematic synthesis of qualitative research. *BMJ Open, 7*(8), e015981. https://doi.org/10.1136/bmjopen-2017-015981.

Roskies, A. L. (2007). Neuroethics beyond genethics. Despite the overlap between the ethics of neuroscience and genetics, there are important areas where the two diverge. *EMBO Reports, 8*(S52–6). https://doi.org/10.1038/sj.embor.7401009.

Ruiz-Casares, M. (2014). Research ethics in global mental health: Advancing culturally responsive mental health research. *Transcultural Psychiatry, 51*(6), 790–805. https://doi.org/10.1177/1363461514527491.

Sartorius, N. (1988). Experience from the mental health programme of the World Health Organization. *Acta Psychiatrica Scandinavica, 78*(S344), 71–74. https://doi.org/10.1111/j.1600-0447.1988.tb09004.x.

Schroeder, D., Cook, J., Hirsch, F., Fenet, S., & Muthuswamy, V. (2018). Ethics dumping: Introduction. In D. Schroeder, J. Cook, F. Hirsch, S. Fenet, & V. Muthuswamy (Eds.), *Ethics dumping case studies from north-south research collaborations*. Cham: Springer International Publishing.

Seeman, N., Tang, S., Brown, A. D., & Ing, A. (2016). World survey of mental illness stigma. *Journal of Affective Disorders, 190*, 115–121. https://doi.org/10.1016/j.jad.2015.10.011.

Smith, J., & Daynes, L. (2016). Borders and migration: An issue of global health importance. *The Lancet Global Health*, *4*(2), e85–e86. https://doi.org/10.1016/s2214-109x(15)00243-0.

Sorsdahl, K., Stein, D. J., Grimsrud, A., Seedat, S., Flisher, A. J., Williams, D. R., et al. (2009). Traditional healers in the treatment of common mental disorders in South Africa. *The Journal of Nervous and Mental Disease*, *197*(6), 434–441. https://doi.org/10.1097/ NMD.0b013e3181a61dbc.

Stein, D. J., & Illes, J. (2015). Beyond scientism and skepticism: An integrative approach to global mental health. *Frontiers in Psychiatry*, *6*, 166. https://doi.org/10.3389/fpsyt.2015.00166.

Stevenson, A., Akena, D., Stroud, R. E., Atwoli, L., Campbell, M. M., Chibnik, L. B., et al. (2019). Neuropsychiatric Genetics of African Populations-Psychosis (NeuroGAP-Psychosis): A case-control study protocol and GWAS in Ethiopia, Kenya, South Africa and Uganda. *BMJ Open*, *9*(2), e025469. https://doi.org/10.1136/bmjopen-2018-025469.

Summerfield, D. (2012). Afterword: Against "global mental health". *Transcultural Psychiatry*, *49*(3–4), 519–530. https://doi.org/10.1177/1363461512454701.

Summerfield, D. (2013). "Global mental health" is an oxymoron and medical imperialism. *BMJ [British Medical Journal]*, *346*(2), https://doi.org/10.1136/bmj.f3509.

Tangwa, G. B. (1996). Bioethics: An African perspective. *Bioethics*, *10*(3), 183–200. https://doi. org/10.1111/j.1467-8519.1996.tb00118.x.

ten Have, H. A. (2011). Global bioethics and communitarianism. *Theoretical Medicine and Bioethics*, *32*(5), 315–326. https://doi.org/10.1007/s11017-011-9190-0.

Thornton, R. L., Glover, C. M., Cene, C. W., Glik, D. C., Henderson, J. A., & Williams, D. R. (2016). Evaluating strategies for reducing health disparities by addressing the social determinants of health. *Health Affairs*, *35*(8), 1416–1423. https://doi.org/10.1377/ hlthaff.2015.1357.

Tindana, P., de Vries, J., Campbell, M., Littler, K., Seeley, J., Marshall, P., et al. (2015). *Community engagement strategies for genomic studies in Africa: A review of the literature*. University of Cape Town.

Tosam, M. J., Chi, P. C., Munung, N. S., Oukem-Boyer, O. O. M., & Tangwa, G. B. (2018). Global health inequalities and the need for solidarity: A view from the global south. *Developing World Bioethics*, *18*(3), 241–249. https://doi.org/10.1111/dewb.12182.

Tsai, A. C., Fricchione, G. L., Walensky, R. P., Ng, C., Bangsberg, D. R., & Kerry, V. B. (2014). Global health training in US graduate psychiatric education. *Academic Psychiatry*, *38*(4), 426–432. https://doi.org/10.1007/s40596-014-0092-0.

Van Dyke, C., Tong, L., & Mack, K. (2011). Global mental health training for United States psychiatric residents. *Academic Psychiatry*, *35*(6), 354–359. https://doi.org/10.1176/appi. ap.35.6.354.

Varpio, L., & McCarthy, A. (2018). How a needs assessment study taught us a lesson about the ethics of educational research. *Perspectives on Medical Education*, *7*(Suppl 1), 34–36. https://doi.org/10.1007/s40037-017-0356-y.

Walsh, A., Brugha, R., & Byrne, E. (2016). "The way the country has been carved up by researchers": Ethics and power in north-south public health research. *International Journal for Equity in Health*, *15*(1), 204. https://doi.org/10.1186/s12939-016-0488-4.

Wittchen, H.-U., & Jacobi, F. (2005). Size and burden of mental disorders in Europe—A critical review and appraisal of 27 studies. *European Neuropsychopharmacology*, *15*(4), 357–376. https://doi.org/10.1016/j.euroneuro.2005.04.012.

World Health Organization. (2017). *WHO guidelines on ethical issues in public health surveillance*. Geneva: World Health Organization.

Index

Note: Page numbers followed by f indicate figures, t indicate tables, and b indicate boxes.